Chronic Illness in Children and Adults

A *Psychosocial Approach*

Chronic Illness in Children and Adults

A *Psychosocial Approach*

Debra P. Hymovich, RN, PhD, FAAN
Professor, University of South Florida
College of Nursing
Tampa, Florida

Gloria A. Hagopian, RN, EdD
Associate Professor of Oncological Nursing
University of Pennsylvania
School of Nursing
Philadelphia, Pennsylvania

W. B. SAUNDERS COMPANY

Harcourt Brace Jovanovich, Inc.

PHILADELPHIA   LONDON   TORONTO   MONTREAL   SYDNEY   TOKYO

W. B. SAUNDERS COMPANY

Harcourt Brace Jovanovich, Inc.

The Curtis Center
Independence Square West
Philadelphia, PA 19106

Library of Congress Cataloging-in-Publication Data

Hymovich, Debra P.
    Chronic illness in children and adults: a psychosocial approach /
Debra P. Hymovich, Gloria A. Hagopian.
        p. cm.
    Includes bibliographical references.
    ISBN 0-7216-2355-7
    1. Chronic diseases—Nursing. I. Hagopian, Gloria Ann.
II. Title.
    [DNLM: 1. Adaptation, Psychological. 2. Chronic Disease—
psychology. 3. Long Term Care. 4. Models, Theoretical. 5. Social
Adjustment. 6. Social Environment. WT 30 H996c]
    RC108.H96 1992
    155.9'16—dc20
    DNLM/DLC   91-25280
    for Library of Congress   CIP

CHRONIC ILLNESS IN CHILDREN AND ADULTS—
A Psychosocial Approach...ISBN   0-7216-2355-7

Last digit is the print number: 9   8   7   6   5   4   3   2   1

Contributors

MARGARET GREY, DrPh, FAAN

Associate Professor, University of Pennsylvania
School of Nursing, Philadelphia

Chapter 7 Suprasystems and Chronic Conditions

TERRI LIPMAN, PhD, RN

Lecturer, University of Pennsylvania
School of Nursing, Philadelphia

Clinical Nurse Specialist
St. Christopher's Hospital for Children
Philadelphia, Pennsylvania

*Chapter 15A Hymovich's Contingency Model of Long-Term Care
   Clinical Assessment Guide*

CHRIS CONN, RN, MS

Visiting Instructor, University of South Florida
College of Nursing,
Tampa, Florida

Clinical Nurse Specialist
Tampa General Rehabilitation Center
Tampa, Florida

Preface

THE PURPOSE OF THIS BOOK is to provide a model to analyze the impact of chronic conditions on the many people who are affected by them, and to suggest a systematic approach for psychosocial assessment and intervention. The emphasis is on promoting psychosocial adjustment to chronic conditions for those who are chronically ill and for their families. Although the model and approaches suggested are not ends in themselves, it is hoped the reader will see them as an initial step to meeting the need for comprehensive, adequate, and equitable services in our society.

This book is a blend of concepts, theories, and clinical applications. It is our hope that the book will provide readers with a selection of the evidence that is available on the care of patients with chronic conditions and their families.

A book like this requires choices about the amount to cover, the amount of detail, and the level of complexity. We had several goals in mind when we wrote this book. First, we wanted to provide an overview of important concepts, with an extensive bibliography so that readers could search in depth for the topics of interest to them. We chose to cite classic references as well as recent sources that would be readily obtainable by most readers. Some of the references cited, although secondary, contain extensive bibliographies and literature reviews. Readers who want more background or depth in any of these areas are encouraged to explore these references.

Research evidence related to some of these topics is incomplete and does not provide definitive guidelines for clinical practice. A review of the literature reveals many publications that describe general clinical impressions or several case studies rather than systematic research. As far as possible, we used original data sources to document what is and is not known. Next, we wanted to provide meaningful and practical information that could be applied to practice, so we included theoretical concepts that have implications for clinical practice. Thus, this book is a blend of concepts, theories, and clinical applications. We hope that it will provide readers with a selection of the available evidence on care of patients with chronic illness and their families. We also hope that it will encourage constant questioning of interventions and stimulate research to fill in the gaps of our knowledge.

There may be advantages to having separate books related to chronic conditions in children and chronic conditions in adults, but there are also advantages to a book that covers the life span. There is literature from both child and adult chronic illness that is relevant to both groups, and family literature cuts across all ages. Many concepts know no age barrier. Although nurses and other health care professionals may be caring for only one family member, they need to understand the influence of other family members, including their health status, on the identified client. For example, pediatric nurses may be caring for well children whose parents are chronically ill, or adult clinicians may be caring for parents whose child has a chronic illness. In either case, the impact of the illness permeates family life and daily activities.

We have raised many questions and had frequent and long discussions about the relationships of the components of the Contingency Model of Long-Term Care. For example, does time pervade everything, or is it a mediating variable? Based on research findings in the literature and our own research and practice, we made some decisions, changed them, made some more, and so on. We concluded that the categories are not mutually exclusive, and one cannot always arrange things in neat categories. We also decided that lack of sufficient data precluded describing the relationships of many of the model's concepts. Since many of the variables are contingent upon each other, the name of Contingency Model of Long-Term Care seemed descriptive of current conceptualizations. We are sure that as time passes and more data becomes available, our thinking will change.

This book is written for those who care for and about children and adults with chronic conditions and their families. The book should be useful in both graduate and undergraduate programs. It can be used as a supplement to undergraduate textbooks as well as a course textbook in either graduate or undergraduate programs. We also believe it is appropriate for the practicing nurse in a variety of settings—inpatient, outpatient, community, and long-term care. Other disciplines may also find the book helpful. Although the book focuses on chronic illness and disability, many of the concepts, assessments, and interventions are likely to be appropriate for any patient at any stage in the continuum.

DEBRA P. HYMOVICH, R.N., PH.D., F.A.A.N.
GLORIA A. HAGOPIAN, R.N., ED.D.

Contents

SECTION IV

Contingency Variables: Stressors and Coping Strategies

10
STRESSORS AND POTENTIAL STRESSORS ——————— 137

11
COPING STRATEGIES ——————————— 170

14
LEVEL OF FUNCTIONING ———————————————————— 248

15
CASE EXAMPLES USING THE CONTINGENCY MODEL
OF LONG-TERM CARE ———————————————————— 263

SECTION I
Introduction

Section I provides the reader with an overview of Hymovich's Contingency Model of Long-Term Care, concepts related to chronic illness, the magnitude of chronic conditions in the United States, and an overview of the nursing component of the model.

Chapter 1 includes an overview of the development, assumptions, and components of the Contingency Model of Long-Term Care. The model is based on assumptions regarding individual perceptions, system characteristics, needs of people with chronic conditions and their families, the health care team, and internal motivation. Each component of the Contingency Model is described: systems (individual, family, community, society); identifying characteristics; time; contingency variables (orientation to life [values, attitudes, and beliefs], stressors, coping strategies, strengths, needs); level of functioning; and nursing care. The model is presented as a guide for clinical practice and research with chronically ill individuals and their families.

Chapter 2 provides an overview of chronic illness as a leading cause of morbidity and mortality in the United States. Included in the chapter are an overview of the magnitude of the problem, trends and issues influencing care, and implications for nursing. Terms used throughout the book, such as *disease, illness, disability, impairment, handicap,* and *chronic illness* are defined. Also included in the second chapter are selected trends influencing the care persons with chronic conditions receive, and will receive in the future. Implications of these trends and issues for nursing practice, education, and research are mentioned.

Chapter 3 is an overview of the nursing care component of the Contingency Model of Long-Term Care. Included in this chapter are the areas requiring periodic reassessment and an overview of the assessment process.

1 Overview of the Contingency Model of Long-Term Care

Living with a chronic condition can be challenging and threatening both for those who are affected with the condition and for their families. Because chronic conditions affect every aspect of being (physical, emotional, social, financial, spiritual), they pose a threat to everything vital to the person. At the same time, chronic conditions present a challenge to overcome—to incorporate living with an illness into one's life-style. Since these conditions extend over time, they require "continued adjustments and readjustments, appraisals and reappraisals" (Turk & Speers, 1983, p. 211).

The conceptual framework of this book, Hymovich's Contingency Model of Long-Term Care, organizes knowledge about chronic illness and disability from diverse sources for nurses to use. The authors found the model served in arranging and categorizing a vast array of information for nursing assessment and intervention. The model was developed to facilitate understanding relationships within and among the numerous systems concerned with chronic conditions. Each part of the model can be analyzed separately or as a unit related to other parts within the model. The model has been used clinically with families of children with chronic conditions and, more recently, with chronically ill and disabled adults. Nurses who have reviewed the model at various stages of development believe it is appropriate for persons of any age throughout the life span. While the authors believe the Contingency Model of Long-Term Care can be used to guide observations and interpretations when any family member has a chronic condition, continued testing is needed and recommended.

According to the model, nursing care for those with chronic health problems varies with the circumstances. No single viewpoint provides an adequate umbrella for the multiple and varied situations, issues, and stressors likely to occur. The model emphasizes assessment of system contingency variables, level of functioning, and perceptions in planning and implementing interventions. The nurse who uses the model is guided in thinking analytically, perceiving each situation from many perspectives (individual, family, community, and society), and recognizing a variety of ways to manage a given situation. The model allows for fluidity, flexibility, and modifications as situations change.

This chapter provides the background of the Contingency Model of Long-Term Care and an overview of the entire model. The overview describes its concepts and the relationships among the components. Each component is discussed in greater detail in remaining chapters.

Background

A number of proposed models and guidelines using assessment and adaptation to chronic conditions have appeared in the literature. Some models were developed by nurses (Craig & Edwards, 1983; Crate, 1965; Lawrence & Lawrence, 1979; MacVicar & Archibald, 1976), and some by other professionals (Lefton & Lefton, 1979; McCubbin & Patterson, 1982; Rolland, 1988). While the usefulness of these models in clinical practice is occasionally documented, many have had little consistent use in research or practice. It is beyond the scope of this book to review these models, but concepts from them relevant to the Contingency Model of Long-Term Care are discussed in appropriate chapters.

Notable work in chronicity was initiated by Quint (1969). Although she did not present a conceptual model, she was one of the first nurses to work with the concept of chronicity. Quint began identifying a theory of chronicity based on the collection and analysis of empirical data of women with breast cancer and children with juvenile diabetes mellitus. She recognized the social context of chronic illness as a critical element in developing a meaning of chronicity. This social context is a vital component of the Contingency Model of Long-Term Care. Quint assumed that people with chronic conditions had a negatively valued social status and that there was some hierarchy of undesirable statuses due to chronic illnesses. For example, currently, a person with diabetes or congenital heart disease is likely to have a more desirable status than a person with cancer or AIDS.

Awareness context is another important concept in Quint's theory. Awareness determines one's actions, regardless of whether or not these actions are perceived to be appropriate or inappropriate by the health care provider. Quint also described time, another important component of the Contingency Model, as a central dimension in any theory of chronicity.

Development of the Contingency Model of Long-Term Care

The Contingency Model of Long-Term Care was developed to synthesize a variety of approaches for understanding, assessing, and intervening with chronically ill persons at various system levels. As currently conceived, the model draws on concepts from a variety of sources, including psychology, sociology, nursing, and management. It is based on Hymovich's research (1979, 1984) to develop a systematic approach for assessing and intervening with families of chronically ill children and on the evolving model's use in clinical practice (Lipman, 1989; Sciarillo, 1980). It is a complex model because the needs of those with chronic conditions and their significant others are complex and contingent upon multiple factors. The model was created to help nurses develop organized and thoughtful assessment and intervention programs. Care plans related to specific needs of family members can be readily transmitted to all team members, avoiding gaps or overlaps of information or imparting too much or contradictory information to clients.

The authors propose this model to provide direction for understanding, conducting research, and working clinically with adults and children who have chronic conditions, and with others involved in their care. The model is believed to be sufficiently comprehensive, so it can be used to plan and provide optimum care for individuals with a wide variety of chronic conditions of varying severity and stage. It can be used to organize research and theoretical concepts related to health, nursing care, and chronic conditions. It aims to include families at any developmental level in a variety of settings.

Figure 1–1 presents a simplified conceptual model to illustrate relationships among its major components. The model's development and use in

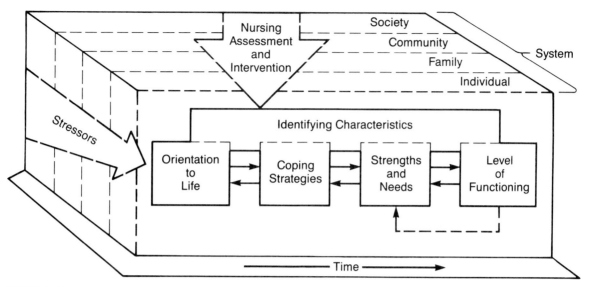

FIGURE 1–1 Hymovich's Contingency Model of Long-Term Care

research and practice have been discussed in detail elsewhere (Hymovich, 1976a, 1976b, 1979, 1981, 1984, 1986, 1987; Lipman, 1989; Sciarillo, 1980). The following section provides a brief overview of its development.

Background of the Model

The earliest form of the model was developed in 1976 and expanded in 1979. These early formulations were based primarily on reviews of the theoretical literature and clinical nursing practice. In time, the need to develop the model in a systematic manner became apparent, along with the recognized need to develop instruments to assess the outcome of nursing interventions with families of chronically ill children. As the model grew, its use became clear for adults with chronic conditions as well as for children. Research is currently under way to expand and refine the framework for use with adults (Baines, 1989; Hymovich, unpublished).

The initial approach to the model's development was inductive, using guidelines for developing grounded theory described by Glaser and Strauss (1967). Grounded theory is a form of field methodology to generate theoretical constructs that explain action in the social context under study. Theory is generated from data by a constant comparative method of collecting, analyzing, and conceptualizing the data. That is, as data are collected, they are ana-

lyzed and conceptualized. These analyses and conceptualizations direct further data collection, until all elements of the theory have been identified and described.

An eclectic framework, derived from the literature, guided early decisions regarding data collection. The framework contained three major dimensions: developmental tasks, impact variables (perceptions, resources, coping), and nursing care needed by the family (Hymovich, 1979). Open-ended interviews with parents of chronically ill children were conducted to determine parent perceptions of the impact of their child's condition on the family, family stressors, and ways in which family members coped with the condition. Additional data were collected from nurses and social workers (Schadt, 1980) and chronically ill children. After the initial components of the model were developed, an extensive review of the chronic illness literature, related to both children and adults, was undertaken. Over the years, with continued research and refinement, the current model evolved. The expanded model, described here, draws heavily from the earlier work and the theoretical literature related to systems, families, human development, and stress and coping. The concepts of these various theories have been adapted to make them consistent with this model. The model is still evolving and will continue to evolve as new data are added to the knowledge base.

Assumptions of the Model and Their Implications

Listed below are assumptions upon which the model is based, and the implications of these assumptions for clinical practice. While it is recognized that not everyone will agree with these assumptions, we believe it is important for the reader to understand the authors' beliefs.

Assumption 1. People behave according to the facts as they perceive them, not as the facts are perceived by others.

Perceptions are unique to each individual; therefore a person's subjective views determine what is considered a stressor or a satisfaction. This assumption suggests that family members, health professionals, and others providing services to families are likely to have differing views of what the condition means and how to deal with it. The subjective nature of experiences often makes it difficult for health care professionals to understand their clients' experiences (Mechanic, 1986). To provide meaningful and relevant care, health professionals need to assess their clients' perceptions **and,** at the same time, be aware of their own perceptions.

Assumption 2. All systems have both unique and common responses and characteristics.

There are general experiences affecting most persons with chronic conditions; however, these experiences are interpreted subjectively. While clients tend to think of their experiences as unique, they are often surprised and relieved to find that others have similar responses.

While commonalities exist among systems, each system also has unique characteristics. Assumptions and generalizations about individual, family, community, and social systems are an insufficient base for long-term care. Although generalizations can serve as guidelines for the appropriate areas to assess, they need to be supplemented by individual system assessments. Consequently, it is important to plan and implement care based on information obtained from a thorough assessment of unique characteristics, in turn based on sound knowledge of theory and research related to commonalities.

Assumption 3. All family members should have the opportunity to be active participants in health care.

Nursing care cannot be limited to the person with the chronic condition. Health providers need to identify ways of including significant others who are part of the patient's support system. Since people affect and are affected by the family system in which they live, the family system should have the opportunity to be the unit of nursing care.

Assumption 4. The needs of people with chronic conditions, and their families, are complex and require a team approach.

No single person can meet all needs required by clients who are chronically ill. Therefore, no one individual can provide all necessary care. An understanding of the complex nature of the physical condition, as well as its developmental, psychological, social, economic, and spiritual impact, facilitates the determination of appropriate team members. Team communication and coordination are integral components of nursing care.

Assumption 5. The patient and family are integral parts of the health care team.

Nursing care plans should not be developed in isolation; they are best prepared in collaboration with patients and their families. All team members, including the family, must be informed of, and in agreement with, the plan of care. Realistic goals are in harmony with the values, attitudes, hopes, and beliefs of the patient and family. Mutually set goals are more likely to be achieved than those developed by health care professionals in isolation.

Assumption 6. It is possible to influence a person's internal motivation.

Client behavior is determined by external and internal values, attitudes, and beliefs. Although many of these motivations come from within the person, the authors believe it is possible for health care providers to identify appropriate techniques for changing behavior as needed to improve health status. By being aware of the principles of teaching and learning and by applying them, health care professionals can influence and capitalize on readiness for learning, thus contributing to the person's motivation for self-care.

Components of the Contingency Model of Long-Term Care

The primary focus of the Contingency Model of Long-Term Care is on family functioning when a family member has a chronic condition. The level of functioning changes as a family system copes with various daily stressors, and is contingent upon the resources and coping of other systems. The model has five major dimensions: Systems and their Identifying Characteristics, Time, Contingency Variables (Orientation to Life, Stressors, Coping Strategies, Strengths, Needs), and Level of Functioning (Performance of Developmental and Situational Tasks), and Nursing Care (see Figure 1–1). This model implies that nothing is mutually exclusive. Therefore each variable is contingent on all other variables. Concepts, while important, do not stand alone, but rather are interdependent. The relationships among the various components of the model are currently being studied.

Systems

A **system** is a complex of elements or components that interact with each other in a more or less stable way within any particular period of time (Buckley, 1967; von Bertalanffy, 1968). Systems can be arranged in a hierarchy so that the point of reference can be divided into subsystems and suprasystems. A **subsystem** is a system in the hierarchy beneath the point of reference, whereas a **suprasystem** is above the point of reference.

Systems can be either open or closed. **Open systems** have permeable boundaries and interact (exchange matter and energy) with the outside environment, while **closed systems** have tight boundaries, are self-contained, and do not interact with the environment but exchange information only within themselves (Hymovich & Chamberlin, 1980; Pasquali et al, 1985; von Bertalannfy, 1968). **Entropy** refers to energy available within a system. In a closed system, no energy is able to enter, and the system deteriorates. As the degree of entropy increases, the system's structure and ability to do work diminish. Total disorganization is called maximum entropy. On the other hand, an open system receives energy from the outside, thus ensuring its continuing existence. The utilization of energy is called negative entropy or **negentropy.** As negentropy increases, the system's structural and functional integrity also increases, making the system stronger. Systems are regulated through a feedback mechanism that occurs within the system (internal feedback) and passes outside its boundary to the environment (external feedback).

A major component of the model is the **family system,** its subsystems and the suprasystems that influence family adjustment when one of its members has a chronic condition. These systems were identified by family members interviewed early in the model's development and appear frequently in the literature. The family is a system of interdependent interacting individuals who are related to one another by marriage, birth, adoption, or mutual consent. The family system is composed of individual members (**individual systems**) and subsystems of paired positions, such as husband-wife, parent-child, and sibling (child-child) (See Figure 1–2). The individual system is composed of the person's biological, emotional, social, cognitive, and spiritual subsystems.

The community and societal suprasystems have an impact on family functioning and are important aspects of family life when someone is chronically ill. The **community system** is composed of the family's neighborhood, health, recreational, educational, vocational, social, and political institutions that affect its functioning. **Society** is the large political, economic, and social system under which each of the other systems (individual, family, community) function. The elements of each system are discussed in greater detail in Chapters 4 through 7.

Identifying characteristics Each system has **identifying characteristics,** a complex set of variables that help define and describe it. These characteristics are important in determining how the system responds to a chronic condition and affects its level of functioning. These identifying characteristics and other variables influence what people know, believe, and think about their condition, its effect on them, symptoms they regard as serious, and what they should do about the symptoms. Among the characteristics of the family unit to consider when planning nursing care are family structure, developmental level, race, roles, and relationships. Characteristics of individual members relevant to clinical practice include age, sex, personality, cognitive abilities, and educational level (See Figure 1–3). Identifying characteristics of the individual system and family systems, and guidelines for assessing these characteristics, are discussed in detail in Chapters 4 (Individual System) and 5 (Family System).

Time Systems evolve over time, and each has a past, present, and future. **Time** is "an indefinite, unlimited duration in which things are considered as

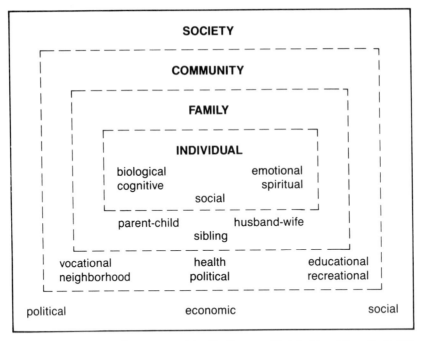

FIGURE 1–2 Systems Component of the Contingency Model of Long-Term Care. The broken lines denote the openness of the systems to one another; the unbroken line delimits the boundaries of the systems component of the model.

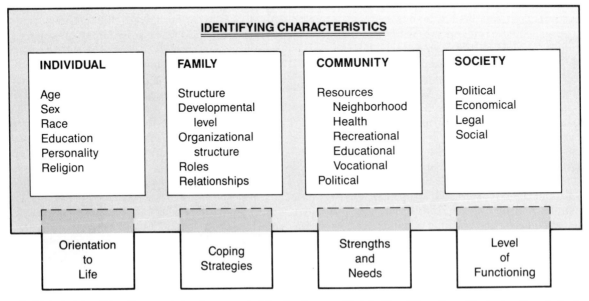

FIGURE 1–3 Identifying Characteristics Component of the Contingency Model of Long-Term Care. The broken lines indicate that Orientation to Life, Coping Strategies, Strengths, Needs, and Level of Functioning overlap with the Identifying Characteristics and may, at times, be used to identify a system.

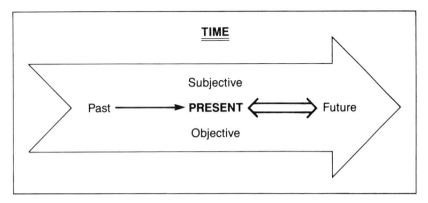

FIGURE 1–4 Time Component of the Contingency Model of Long-Term Care. The wide arrow depicts Time as moving forward; the smaller unidirectional arrow indicates past influences on the present, which is the point of reference for interaction; the double arrow indicates that what happens in the present, or happened in the past, influences the system's future, and that system goals for the future are determined by decisions made in the past and present.

happening in the past, present, or future" (Guralnik, 1984, p. 1489). Although health care providers interact with a system in the present, psychosocial needs can be met only if one understands the system's past and has some idea of its future (See Figure 1–4). In addition, all client and health care provider activities require time and are influenced by the amount of time available to accomplish them. Amount of time varies with the event that may take place over minutes, hours, days, months, or even years. Chronic conditions can last for months, years, or a lifetime, but selected aspects of the care, such as hospitalization, may last a shorter time.

Although time is a somewhat elusive concept, it can be defined and measured objectively with clocks and calendars, or subjectively, according to one's personal perception of time passage. The components of time and their clinical implications are discussed in Chapter 8.

Contingency Variables

Contingency variables are mediators influencing the impact a chronic condition has on system functioning; they affect or may be affected by it. These variables are the system's orientation to life, stressors, coping strategies, strengths, and needs.

Orientation to life The first contingency variable relates to how the system views the world. This **orientation to life** includes values, attitudes, and beliefs of system members regarding pertinent issues

such as life, death, health, illness, hospitalization, and health care personnel (See Figure 1–5). The presence of a chronic condition in a family member may challenge deeply held values, thus threatening the family's functioning, integrity, and autonomy. In place of old values, chronically ill persons and their families may struggle to substitute new ones that help them make sense out of their experiences. "If one accepts the premise that behavior is determined, rather subjectively, by an individual's own values and beliefs, then such intervening variables exert tremendous influence on decision-making or choice of action" (Rosser, 1971, p. 387).

Attitudes, values, and beliefs of members of society, such as overprotectiveness, stigmatization, or social exclusion, can contribute to difficulties when patients try to resume their ordinary social roles. For example, employers may exclude workers with chronic conditions who are physically capable of doing the work. These values, attitudes, and beliefs and their clinical applications are discussed in Chapter 9. As noted in Figure 1–5, there is an overlapping of Values, Attitudes, and Beliefs with the Spiritual component of one's being as the central core.

Stressors **Stressors** are contingency variables that represent a source of concern or difficulty for the system (See Figure 1–6). They are any stimuli (or the absence of stimuli in the environment or internal to the system) that can tax or exceed the system's resources for adapting and for accomplishing tasks and that elicit a response from the system. Stressors

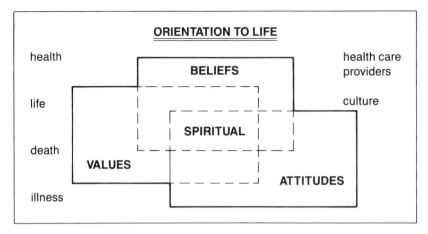

FIGURE 1–5 Orientation to Life Component of the Contingency Model of Long-Term Care. The broken lines depict the overlapping nature of Values, Attitudes, and Beliefs; the Spiritual component of one's being is within the central core. Examples of the components of Orientation to Life are in lower case type.

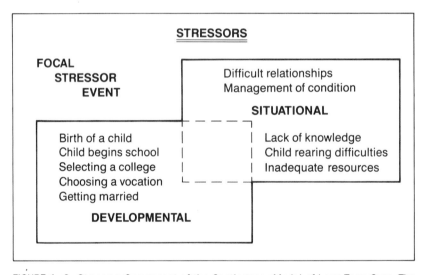

FIGURE 1–6 Stressors Component of the Contingency Model of Long-Term Care. The broken lines depict the overlapping nature of the developmental and situational stressors. Examples of stressors are in lower case type.

may be either developmental or situational, actual (focal) or potential. **Potential stressors** are events or conditions that, for some individuals under certain circumstances, have a probability of becoming stressors.

Developmental stressors are stressful events that occur during the normal course of growth and development and can strain or surpass the system's ability to cope. Sending a child to school, deciding a

vocation, selecting a college, and getting married have the potential to be developmental stressors.

Situational stressors are stressful events that arise as the result of a stressful event and can strain or surpass the system's ability to cope. They are superimposed on developmental stressors and tasks. Physical disorders, especially chronic ones, are stressful to the patient and to those who provide support and care. Stressors for chronically ill persons and their families might include: lack of knowledge and information, child-rearing difficulties, inadequate resources, difficult family relationships, and management of the condition.

For clinical assessment purposes, situational stressors are circumstances or events that family members indicate are problematic or potentially problematic for themselves or other family members. These perceptions determine whether a particular event is a stressor for the system because events construed as stressors for one system may be sources of satisfaction for others. A situation that is a stressor at one time may not be one at some later date. For example, one family may have an adequate support system while another may not. Therefore, support systems could be either stressors or strengths, depending upon the situation for any given family. Or a community that has inadequate recreational facilities for the handicapped at one time may develop them at a later time, thereby creating a resource rather than a stressor.

A specific kind of stressor is the **focal stressor or focal stressor event.** Focal stressors are circumstances or events that cause the individual or family system to evaluate its situation and determine the presence of a need. Focal stressors can be any actual or potential developmental or situational stressors that strain or surpass the system's ability to cope and precipitate a need for assistance. Numerous stressors could be focal for a family system requiring health care services at various times throughout the course of the condition. Focal stressors include concerns about diagnosis, symptoms, management of the condition, or hospitalization. They also include such things as running out of a medication or equipment that requires a prescription or going to a health agency for replenishment of supplies. Selected individual and family stressors are discussed in detail in Chapter 10 and in their implications for clinical practice in Chapter 12.

Coping strategies   **Coping** is a cognitive, affective, and behavioral process to manage perceived stressors or potential stressors in the environment or internal to the system that tax or exceed the system's current resources for responding (See Figure 1–7). Clinically, **coping strategies** may be defined as system members' cognitive, affective, or behavioral means of minimizing or relieving their perceived stressors. The strategies may be either emotion focused or problem focused. Coping strategies are not static, but change according to situational demands on a person and the person's perception of the situation. Knowledge of system coping strategies can aid nursing recommendations to help clients decide how best to utilize the knowledge and information they have. It may also be possible to teach alternative coping strategies for reducing stressors. Selected

FIGURE 1–7 Coping Strategies Component of the Contingency Model of Long-Term Care. The broken lines depict the overlapping nature of the emotion-focused and problem-focused coping strategies. Examples of coping strategies are in lower case type.

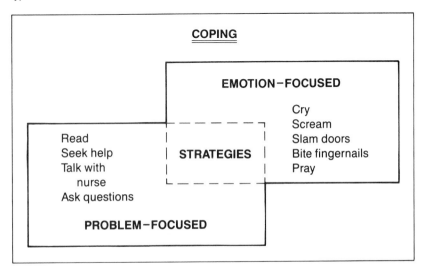

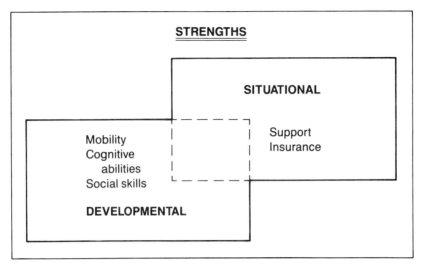

FIGURE 1–8 Strengths Component of the Contingency Model of Long-Term Care. The broken lines depict the overlapping nature of the developmental and situational strengths. Examples of strengths are in lower case type.

coping strategies used by family members are discussed in Chapter 11 and in their clinical applications in Chapter 12.

Strengths   **Strengths** are system assets, capabilities, and resources (See Figure 1–8). They may be identified subjectively by the individual or objectively by others (e.g., family member, friend, health care professional). Strengths form the foundation for system growth and can be reinforced or built on to help various system members cope with stressors that tax or exceed their current abilities. In the past, research focused on system limitations and weaknesses. Consequently the literature contains more information about these areas than about strengths. Only recently has there been increasing recognition of strengths and abilities. Documenting strengths, as well as needs, is necessary when the focus of care is on strengthening abilities. It can be hypothesized that, as strengths increase, needs will decrease. These strengths and implications for assessment and intervention are discussed in Chapter 13.

Needs   Another contingency variable, closely related to strengths, is needs. **Needs** are motivating forces that initiate behavior with the purpose of maintaining internal consistency and harmony with the external environment. They are identified by the system and health team members as conditions requiring resources or relief (See Figure 1–9). Needs

are felt as tensions that can be reduced by specific sources of satisfaction. As needs increase, so does the system's tension. A system's level of functioning depends upon the extent to which it is able to satisfy its needs.

Needs particularly relevant to the Contingency Model of Long-Term Care are generally based on limitations that individuals perceive they have in coping with their developmental and situational stressors. Needs can also be objectively identified by health care providers. Human needs arise within the individual and are based on cultural background, personality, social class, and events external to the individual, such as crises (Williamson, 1978). Illness events alter perception of needs by shifting system priorities (Maslow, 1968). For example, relieving one's pain during illness may become more important than socializing with a friend. In this situation, pain would be the focal stressor, and the need would be to relieve pain.

Identifying and meeting needs is an important challenge for nurses working with chronically ill patients and their families, especially as needs change over time. The more specific and well defined the needs, the easier it will be to plan appropriate nursing care. Like stressors, needs may be either developmental (related to normal aspects of growth and development) or situational (related to chronic condition stressors and tasks) and are related to the focal stressor and other contingency variables. Identified

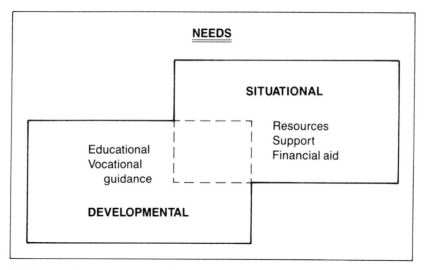

FIGURE 1—9 Needs Component of the Contingency Model of Long-Term Care. The broken lines depict the overlapping nature of the developmental and situational needs. Examples of needs are in lower case type.

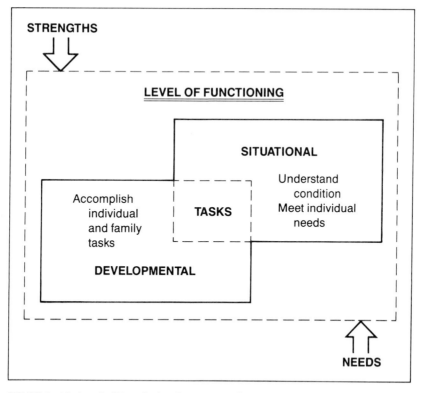

FIGURE 1—10 Level of Functioning Component of the Contingency Model of Long-Term Care. The broken lines depict the overlapping nature of the developmental and situational tasks. Strengths and needs impinge upon the level of functioning, as depicted by the arrows. Examples of tasks are in lower case type.

needs can be used as the basis for planning and providing nursing care that is relevant to the perspective of the client. Specific needs and their clinical implications are discussed in Chapter 13.

Level of Functioning

Level of functioning refers to the system's current performance and is determined by the extent to which it is accomplishing its developmental and situational tasks. The boundaries of task accomplishment are contingent upon the system's strengths and needs (See Figure 1–10). The system's level of functioning may change over time as the individual and family develop, the chronic condition progresses, or new focal stressors occur. Individual and family level of functioning are discussed more fully in Chapter 14.

Tasks   Tasks are certain duties a given system is expected to accomplish to continue its growth and functioning. All systems are required to accomplish two kinds of tasks, developmental and situational.

    Developmental tasks of individual and family systems are growth responsibilities arising at a particular stage in the life cycle. If the tasks are achieved successfully, the individual or family will feel satisfied, achieve appropriate approval from society, and be successful in accomplishing later tasks. If the system fails to accomplish these tasks, unhappiness, disapproval by society, and difficulty with later tasks are likely to occur (Duvall, 1977).

    Hymovich and Chamberlin (1980) identified five individual and five family developmental tasks they believe span all developmental levels. More specific tasks for each developmental level have been identified by various theorists, such as Aldous (1978), Duvall (1977), Erikson (1968), Piaget (1971), and Havighurst (1953). These general and specific tasks form the basis for nursing assessments and interventions related to other components of the model. These tasks, listed in Table 1–1, are explained more fully in subsequent chapters.

    Situational tasks are functional requirements that arise as a result of stressors, such as illness, hospitalization, disaster, or death in the family, and are superimposed on developmental tasks. Examples of situational tasks to be accomplished by chronically ill persons and family members include learning to understand and manage the disease, mastering feel-

Table 1–1   Individual and Family Developmental Tasks

INDIVIDUAL DEVELOPMENTAL TASKS

1. Develop and maintain healthy growth and nutrition patterns
2. Learn to manage one's body satisfactorily
3. Learn to understand and relate to the physical world
4. Develop self-awareness and a satisfying sense of self
5. Learn to relate to others

FAMILY DEVELOPMENTAL TASKS

1. Meet the basic physical needs of the family (e.g., food, health care, shelter, and money)
2. Assist all family members develop their own potential
3. Meet the emotional needs of all family members
4. Maintain and adapt family organization and management to meet family needs
5. Function in the community

Source: Adapted from Hymovich & Chamberlin, 1980.

ings associated with the condition, and incorporating the condition into one's lifestyle.

    There are also developmental and situational tasks to be carried out by communities and societies. A task of the community would be to assure adequate resources to meet basic needs of the chronically ill, whereas a task of society is to establish policies related to the chronically ill and handicapped.

Nursing Care

Nursing care, the final major component of the model, involves both process and content (see Figure 1–11). Nursing care refers to deliberate activities of a nurse to help the individual and family systems meet their needs. The process includes assessment over time of individual and family identifying characteristics, contingency variables, and level of functioning. Plans for nursing interventions are contingent on the ongoing assessment and reassessment (evaluation) process. An overview of this nursing process as it relates to the care of the chronically ill and disabled and their families is presented in Chapter 3.

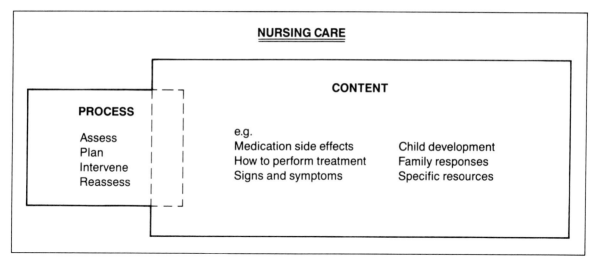

FIGURE 1–11 Nursing Care Component of the Contingency Model of Long-Term Care. The broken lines depict the overlapping nature of the nursing process and content. Examples of nursing process and content are in lower case type.

Use of the Contingency Model of Long-Term Care

The current state of knowledge about chronic conditions, contingency variables, level of functioning, and nursing care leaves us with many unknowns. However, it is still necessary to provide care to clients with chronic conditions, and knowledge presently available forms the basis for suggestions and guidelines for nursing interventions. Wherever possible, research findings formed the basis for suggestions offered in this book. Although some information will likely be modified or disputed in the future, it is the best available at present. We encourage readers to critically evaluate the recommendations for their own practice. We also urge the reader to keep up to date with recent research findings and to contribute to the developing body of knowledge. Keeping good data records about clients and establishing and participating in ongoing research will help evolve more-definitive answers.

By use of the Contingency Model of Long-Term Care, we believe, nurses can systematically assess and provide intervention unique to the needs of each family. The model should not be seen as an end in itself, but as a guide or map to help organize information about client needs, recognize areas to cover during assessment, and formulate interdisciplinary care plans for persons with chronic conditions and their families. It can also be used to assess the needs of communities and society.

Summary

This chapter provides an introduction to the Contingency Model of Long-Term Care and an overview of its assumptions and components. The model is based on the following assumptions: (1) People behave according to the facts as they perceive them, not as the facts are perceived by others; (2) all systems have both unique and common characteristics; (3) all family members should have the opportunity to be active participants in health care; (4) the needs of people with chronic conditions are complex and require a team approach; (5) the patient and family are integral parts of the health care team; and (6) it is possible to influence a person's internal motivation.

There are five major components of the model. The first component is the System and its Identifying Characteristics. Four systems are relevant to nursing care: the individual system, family system, community system, and societal system. The focus of the model is on the family system and its individual members. Time is the second major component of the model and refers to the system's past, present, and future. Five contingency variables influence family functioning when a chronic condition is present: orientation to life (values, attitudes, and beliefs), stressors, coping strategies, strengths, and needs. Level of functioning, the fourth component, refers to the system's adaptation to the chronic condition throughout its course. Nursing care is the final component of the model. Nursing care refers to the deliberate assessment and intervention activities of the nurse to assist the individual and family systems meet needs.

The model is presented as a guideline for clinical practice and for research with chronically ill individuals and their families.

References

Aldous, J. (1978). *Family careers: Developmental change in families.* New York: Wiley.

Baines, B. (1989). Personal correspondence.

Buckley, W. (1967). *Sociology and modern systems theory.* Englewood Cliffs, NJ: Prentice-Hall.

Craig, H.M., & Edwards, J.E. (1983). Adaptation in chronic illness: An eclectic model for nurses. *J Adv Nurs, 8,* 397–404.

Crate, M.A. (1965). Nursing functions in adaptation to chronic illness. *Am J Nurs, 65*(10), 72–75.

Duvall, E.M. (1977). *Marriage and family development.* Philadelphia: Lippincott.

Erikson, E. (1968). *Identity: Youth and crisis.* New York: Norton.

Glaser, B.G., & Strauss, A.L. (1967). *The discovery of grounded theory: Strategies for quality of life.* Chicago: Aldine.

Guralnik, D.B. (Ed.). (1984). *Webster's new world dictionary of the American language* (2nd ed). New York: Simon & Schuster.

Havighurst, R.J. (1953). *Human development and education.* New York: Longmans, Green.

Hymovich, D.P. (1976a). A framework for measuring outcomes of intervention with the chronically ill child and his family. In G.D. Grave & I.B. Pless (Eds.), *Chronic childhood illness: Assessment of outcomes* (pp. 91–93). (DHEW Publication No. (NIH)-76-876). Washington, D.C.: Fogarty International Center Series on Teaching of Preventive Medicine.

Hymovich, D.P. (1976b). Parents of sick children: Their needs and tasks. *Pediatr Nurs, 2,* 9–13.

Hymovich, D.P. (1979). Assessment of the chronically ill child and family. In D.P. Hymovich & M.U. Barnard (Eds.). *Family health care: General perspectives* (Vol. 1). (2nd ed.). New York: McGraw-Hill.

Hymovich, D.P. (1981). Assessing the impact of chronic childhood illness on the family and parent coping. *Image, XIII,* 71–74.

Hymovich, D.P. (1984). Development of the chronicity impact and coping instrument: Parent questionnaire. *Nurs Res, 33,* 218–222.

Hymovich, D.P. (1986). Child and family teaching: Special needs and approaches. *Hospice J, 2*(1), 103–120.

Hymovich, D.P. (1987). Assessing families of children with cystic fibrosis. In M. Leahey & L.M. Wright (Eds.). *Family nursing series: Vol. I. Families and chronic illness.* Springhouse, PA: Springhouse.

Hymovich, D.P. (Unpublished work in progress). *Parents with Cancer: Their Stressors, Strengths, and Needs.*

Hymovich, D.P., & Chamberlin, R.W. (1980). *Child and family development: Implications for care.* New York: McGraw-Hill.

Lawrence, S.A., & Lawrence, R.M. (1979). A model of adaptation to the stress of chronic illness. *Nurs Forum, 18*(1), 33–43.

Lefton, E., & Lefton, M. (1979). Health care and treatment for the chronically ill: Toward a conceptual framework. *J Chronic Dis, 32,* 334–339.

Lipman, T.H. (1989). Assessing family strengths to guide plan of care using Hymovich's framework. *J Pediatr Nurs, 4*(3), 186–196.

McCubbin, H.I., & Patterson, J.M. (1982). Family adaptation to crisis. In H.I. McCubbin, A.E. Cauble, & J.M. Patterson (Eds.), *Family stress, coping, and social support* (pp. 26–47). Springfield, IL: Charles C Thomas.

MacVicar, M.G., & Archibald, P. (1976). A framework for family assessment in chronic illness. *Nurs Forum, 15*(2), 180–194.

Maslow, A.H. (1968). *Toward a psychology of being* (2nd. ed.). New York: Van Nostrand Reinhold.

Mechanic, D. (1986). *From advocacy to allocation: The evolving American health care system.* New York: Macmillan.

Pasquali, E.A., Arnold, H.M., DeBasio, N., & Alasi, E.G. (1985). *Mental health nursing: A holistic approach.* St. Louis: Mosby.

Piaget, J. (1971). *The child's conception of time.* New York: Ballentine Books.

Quint, J.C. (1969). Some thoughts on a theory of chronicity. *Proceedings of the first nursing theory conference* (pp. 67). University of Kansas Medical Center Department of Nursing Education, March 20–29.

Rolland, J.S. (1988). A conceptual model of chronic and life-threatening illness and its impact on families. In C.S. Chilman, E.W. Nunnally, & F.M. Cox (Eds), *Chronic illness and disability* (pp. 17–68). Newbury Park, CA: Sage.

Rosser, J.M. (1971). Values and health. *J Sch Health, 41,* 386–390.

Schadt, A.B. (1980). Nursing and social work interventions with families of chronically ill children. Unpublished master's thesis. University of Colorado.

Sciarillo, W.C. (1980). Using Hymovich's framework in the family-oriented approach to nursing care. *MCN, 5,* 242–248.

Turk, D.C., & Speers, M.A. (1983). Diabetes mellitus: A cognitive-functional analysis of stress. In T.G. Burish & L.A. Bradley (Eds.). *Coping with chronic disease* (pp. 191–217). New York: Academic Press.

von Bertalanffy, L. (1968). *General systems theory.* New York: Braziller.

Williamson, Y.M. (1978). Methodological dilemmas in tapping the concept of patient needs. *Nurs Res, 27*(3), 172–177.

2 Impact of Chronic Conditions on the Systems

The presence of chronic illness and disability has a tremendous impact on American society. Today, people are living with formerly fatal illnesses and experiencing longer periods of limited or curtailed activities. When a chronic condition is present, everyone is affected by it, including the children and adults with the condition, their families, health care personnel, community service personnel, community citizens, and elected political representatives. Psychosocial challenges faced by people with chronic conditions are complex and demanding, as are the challenges they place on the health care system and society. Communities and societies are faced with an urgent need to develop approaches to provide adequate and equitable services to all, not only to meet the medical demands of the conditions but the emotional, social, and spiritual needs as well. The increasing number of people requiring long-term care, along with the changing age profile and prevalence patterns of disease in the United States, creates many challenges. Health professionals are responsible for helping persons maintain as much function as possible within the context of their conditions, as well as for seeking cures for the illnesses (Mechanic, 1986). The rising costs of long-term care and the ineffectiveness of current approaches to care necessitate action to change the current status of the services provided for the chronically ill (Reif &

Estes, 1982). Nurses play an important role in ensuring that the individual and diverse needs of those affected by these long-term conditions are met.

This chapter presents an introduction to terminology associated with long-term or chronic conditions, a broad overview of the magnitude of chronic illness and disability, and current trends related to these conditions. This information is followed by a brief overview of nursing implications that is expanded upon in later chapters.

Definition of Terms

Many terms used throughout this book are subject to a variety of definitions and conceptualizations. To eliminate redundancy and wordiness, the terms **person, patient, client,** and **individual** are used interchangeably to identify the person (adult or child) with the chronic condition who is receiving or needs assistance from health care providers. **Family** is used to designate a system of interdependent interacting individuals who are related to one another by marriage, birth, adoption, or mutual consent.

There are various conceptualizations of the terms *health* and *illness* and, consequently, various definitions. Among the issues in conceptualizing these terms is whether health and illness are dichotomous (separate, discrete) variables or whether they occur on a continuum, with health on one end and illness on the other.

Health is defined by the World Health Organization as a "state of complete physical, mental, and social well-being (WHO, 1980). This somewhat utopian definition would allow few people to qualify and provides little direction for measurement. However, it is consistent with Twaddle and Hessler's (1977) view that health is an ideal toward which people are oriented, but which they are not expected to attain. We are defining health as the ability to function physically, psychologically, and socially in a manner that is deemed satisfying to the individual. In other words, we are defining it as a subjective state of being. This is consistent with the Dimond and Jones (1983) belief that evaluations of health depend upon the perceptions, value orientations, and situations of the persons involved.

Illness can be defined as the "psychosocial experiences and meaning of perceived disease" (Kleinman, Eisenberg, & Good, 1978). Illness refers to secondary personal and social responses to a disease. It involves a person's subjective perceptions and

feelings. According to Watson (1988), "Illness is not necessarily disease. Illness is subjective turmoil or disharmony within a person's inner self or soul at some level or disharmony within the spheres of the person, for example, in the mind, body, and soul, either consciously or unconsciously" (p. 48).

Chronic illness (long-term illness, chronic condition, chronic health problem) refers to any long-term or permanent disability that interferes with the person's ordinary physical, psychological, or social functioning. It is a condition that has one or more of the following characteristics: It is permanent; leaves residual disability; is caused by a nonpathological alteration; requires special training for rehabilitation; is expected to require a long period of supervision, observation, or care (National Commission on Chronic Illness, 1956). In 1972, Mattsson defined chronic illness as "a disorder with a protracted course which can be progressive and fatal, or associated with a relatively normal life span despite impaired physical or mental functioning" (p. 801). Pless and Pinkerton (1975) operationally defined it as "a physical, usually non-fatal condition which lasted for longer than three months in a given year or necessitated a period of continuous hospitalization of more than one month" (pp. 90–91). Within the context of the Contingency Model of Long-term Care, chronic illness is defined as a chronic condition or long-term health problem leading to actual or potential interference with a system's level of functioning. Chronic conditions vary in severity and progression and necessitate continuing adjustment of the individual and group systems they affect. This book focuses on psychosocial aspects of chronic care rather than on the physiological components of care.

In 1980, the World Health Organization attempted to classify terminology related to long-term illnesses. The goal was to make it possible to assess patient status at more than one time in order to detect changes in response to intervention over time, thus providing an outcome measure. The original model of the International Classification of Diseases (ICD) was a sequence of

$$Etiology \rightarrow Pathology \rightarrow Manifestation$$

However, this sequence failed to account for the morbidity associated with many illnesses, such as diabetes mellitus or arthritis, that can be controlled but not prevented or cured. The ninth revision of the classification identified the following sequence to represent the experience of people with long-term and progressive or irreversible disorders:

$$\text{Disease} \rightarrow \text{Impairment} \rightarrow \text{Disability} \rightarrow \text{Handicap}$$

Although these terms are often used interchangeably, there are important conceptual and semantic differences that should be recognized (Pless & Pinkerton, 1975).

Disease is a term with various synonyms, such as *defect, disorder,* and *condition.* These terms describe the pathological process representing the basic underlying disturbance at the cellular level. Disease may be defined as anatomic and physiologic dysfunction of organ systems.

Impairment is "any loss or abnormality of psychological, or anatomical structure or function" (WHO, 1980, p. 46). It is a more inclusive term than *disease* or *disorder* because it is not contingent on etiology. It includes abnormalities of body structure and appearance, or the functioning of organs, such as an absent limb, cough, shortness of breath, pain, or swelling, which can be caused by a variety of diseases.

Disability reflects the consequences of the impairment of the person's functional performance and activities. It is "any restriction or lack resulting from an impairment of ability to perform an activity in the manner or within the range considered normal for a human being" (WHO, 1980, p. 143). Disabilities represent disturbances as they directly affect the person involved. Disability is as much a social definition as it is a physical status (Mechanic, 1986). For example, a disability associated with arthritis would be difficulty in walking, but a disability associated with chronic obstructive lung disease or cystic fibrosis would be difficulty in breathing.

The definition of **developmental disability** stems from federal legislation of the 1960s and 1970s and encompasses a wide range of conditions. The scope of developmental disabilities varies with the criteria for definition and may or may not include intellectual impairment (Schilling, Paul, & Kirkham, 1988). According to the Developmental Disabilities Assistance and Bill of Rights Act of 1978, a developmental disability is "a substantial chronic disability" likely to continue indefinitely that results from a physical and/or a mental impairment manifested in a person before 22 years of age. The developmentally disabled person has substantial limitations in at least three of the following life activities: self-care, mobility, learning, capacity for self-direction, capacity for independent living, receptive and expressive language, and economic self-sufficiency.

Handicap refers to the social disadvantages a person experiences as a result of an impairment or disability. A handicap reflects interaction with, and adaptation to, the person's surroundings. It is defined by the World Health Organization (1980) as "a disadvantage for a given individual resulting from an impairment or a disability, that limits or prevents the fulfillment of a role that is normal (depending on age, sex, and social and cultural factors) for that individual" (p. 183). Handicaps are classified according to the key social roles of individuals: orientation, physical independence, mobility, occupation, social integration, and economic self-sufficiency. For example, a person who is unable to see would be handicapped in driving an automobile, but a child who cannot walk would be handicapped in running a race. Unfortunately, people who are handicapped in one or two ways may be considered handicapped in all aspects of their lives by others.

Long-term care generally refers to "a range of services that address the health, social, and personal care needs of persons who are unable to care for themselves because of a physical or mental impairment caused by a chronic condition" (Reif & Estes, 1982, p. 151).

To summarize, disease embodies and interferes with the functioning of the body, whereas illness is a personal experience with the disease that may or may not involve disability and handicap. Although illness is observable to the individual (perceived illness) and to others (observed illness), the presence of disease can only be inferred from its manifestations (Magi & Allander, 1981). Generally, the focus of medical care is the disease and its treatment (observed illness), while to the individual with the condition, disability and handicap may be of great consequence in daily functioning (perceived illness). Nurses play a significant role in helping clients and families achieve a balance, within the health care system, of their medically defined disease needs and their self-defined illness needs.

Magnitude of the Problem

Chronic illness is the number one health problem in the United States today, with nearly 50% of the population having one or more chronic conditions (Forsyth, Delancy, & Gresham, 1984). Esti-

Table 2–1 Persons with Selected Chronic Conditions*

Condition	Number of conditions	Total	Under 18 years	18–44 years	45–64 years	65–74 years	75+ years
Heart disease	18,458	78.1	21.7	39.3	123.2	250.0	319.4
Hypertension	28,969	122.6	1.9	67.2	250.6	385.2	409.2
Varicose veins	6,856	29.0	—	22.6	56.3	76.2	71.9
Hemorrhoids	9,909	41.9	.9	46.7	73.2	70.2	64.1
Bronchitis	11,379	48.1	63.2	36.5	45.8	62.9	55.4
Asthma	9,690	41.0	51.1	36.4	36.3	46.4	36.3
Sinusitis	34,386	145.5	65.8	170.4	187.0	168.6	170.7
Dermatitis	9,547	40.4	42.0	44.3	35.4	33.6	25.2
Arthritis	30,911	130.8	2.0	47.9	284.6	443.3	540.1
Diabetes	6,585	27.9	2.4	8.7	63.7	91.9	106.5
Migraine	8,516	36.0	14.6	49.4	45.5	21.3	20.1
Urinary disease	7,736	32.7	6.8	32.8	45.4	58.3	92.3
Visual impairment	8,352	35.3	12.2	28.7	46.3	69.3	136.3
Cataract	5,031	21.3	.6	1.5	21.1	84.3	233.2
Hearing impairment	20,732	87.7	20.1	51.8	136.2	244.2	378.4
Tinnitus	6,315	26.7	3.6	15.3	49.2	83.2	88.3
Orthopedic problems	27,381	115.9	32.5	132.2	161.6	158.4	195.7

*In the United States in 1986 per 1,000 persons
Source: National Center for Health Statistics, 1987.

mates of incidence and prevalence of chronic illness vary widely because the statistics depend on the definitions used, populations studied, and methods used for data collection. An estimated 36 million persons, or 17% of the population, in this country have a chronic health problem resulting in some limitation of activity. There are 7.66 million persons, or 3.6% of the population, who have a functional deficit serious enough to prevent them from carrying out their major activity (e.g., school, occupation) (Reif & Estes, 1982).

Many chronic diseases begin in youth or middle age with varying degrees of impairment, persist throughout life, and are often not fatal. Table 2–1 lists a number of chronic conditions of this nature.

Some chronic conditions are more serious than others. Arteriosclerotic heart disease and cancer, for example, each occur in 1 of every 4 adults and are the first and second leading causes of death in the United States. Arthritis, which affects 1 in every 10 persons, is the leading cause of immobility (Hanson, 1987). The human immunodeficiency virus (HIV) has created a catastrophic public health threat, with more than one million people believed to be infected. According to the Centers for Disease Control (1988), 66.1% of the reported cases are gay or bisexual men, 16.4% are intravenous drug users,

2.1% are heterosexual partners, and 2.1% are blood recipients. The total number of new cases reported in 1988 was 35,238, with 400 cases reported in children. A rising rate of AIDS-related tuberculosis is expected to increase (Cote et al, 1990).

Chronic conditions are a leading cause of death as well as morbidity. The Centers for Disease Control report that 52% of the United States population die from nine chronic diseases: stroke, heart disease, pulmonary disease, lung cancer, female breast cancer, cervical cancer, colorectal cancer, and cirrhosis of the liver. Table 2–2 reports the estimated death rates for the leading causes of death by age group in 1988.

Disabled individuals are the poorest, least educated, but largest, majority in America (Bush & Dukakis, 1988; Oda, 1989). They are more than twice as likely to drop out of school, be unemployed, and live in poverty. In 1984, 50% of all disabled adults had household incomes of $15,000 or less, compared with 25% for the nondisabled; 40% had not finished high school, 25% worked full-time, and 10% worked part-time. In 1980 2.9 million noninstitutionalized disabled workers and 1.9 million of their dependents were receiving disability benefits from the Social Security Administration, a 60% increase since 1972 (Dittmar, 1989).

Table 2–2   Estimated Age Specific Death Rates for Leading Causes of Death*

Cause	Age not stated	Under 1 year	1–14 years	15–24 years	25–34 years	35–44 years	45–54 years	55–64 years	65–74 years	75–84 years	85+ years
All causes	883.0	1,001.9	33.5	104.8	133.6	217.6	486.4	1,246.3	2,731.2	6,324.4	15,577.7
Heart disease	312.2	23.6	1.4	2.8	7.3	33.0	131.4	405.6	985.6	2,554.4	7,119.1
Cancer	196.6	1.3	3.5	5.0	10.8	44.3	157.2	456.5	845.4	1,324.8	1,664.5
Cerebral vascular disease	61.1	1.0	0.1	0.9	2.1	7.1	20.4	51.9	155.7	544.4	1,710.3
Accidents	39.7	23.8	14.0	51.3	37.3	32.1	31.2	34.4	50.8	110.8	273.7
Chronic lung disease	33.3	0.5	0.3	0.4	0.6	1.8	8.8	50.2	151.6	301.3	399.9
Pneumonia and influenza	31.5	14.5	0.6	0.5	2.1	3.6	7.3	19.3	60.7	263.5	1,090.2
Diabetes	16.1	—	0.1	0.4	1.7	3.7	9.3	26.4	62.3	127.8	203.9
Suicide	12.3	—	0.6	12.8	15.5	14.3	14.8	15.7	16.8	28.9	19.7
Chronic liver disease	10.6	0.3	0.0	0.2	2.4	10.3	20.0	30.1	35.7	31.0	18.3
Atherosclerosis	9.6	—	—	—	0.0	0.1	0.9	3.8	16.2	74.1	428.8
Homicide	9.0	7.3	1.6	15.1	16.3	10.9	7.5	5.3	4.4	4.3	6.1
Renal Disease	8.9	5.2	0.1	0.2	0.8	1.1	2.7	9.0	25.1	79.5	207.3
Septicemia	8.1	6.5	0.3	0.3	0.3	1.3	3.4	9.9	28.2	80.4	230.9
Perinatal problems	7.5	474.0	0.4	0.1	—	—	—	—	—	—	—
AIDS	6.6	{0.7}		1.8	13.1	17.3	9.4	{2.1}			

*In the United States in 1988 per 100,000 population in specified age group
Source: Adapted from National Center for Health Statistics. (1989). *Monthly vital statistics report*. U.S. Department of Health and Human Services, 37(13), July 26, 1989, pp. 20–21.

Individual System

Children   The overall estimate of rates for **any** chronic disorder for children under 18 years of age is 10% to 22%. This rate includes sensory impairments; mental retardation; and speech, learning, and behavior disorders. Between 500,000 and 1,000,000 youngsters under 16 years of age have a severe chronic illness, representing a prevalence rate of 1% to 1.5% (Pless & Perrin, 1985). About 1% of the total childhood population (10% of the chronically ill) have disabilities severe enough to interfere with the ability to carry out ordinary tasks appropriate for their age. An estimated 7.7% of children under 17 years of age are limited in activity because of chronic illness (National Center for Health Statistics, 1982). The frequency of genetic disease is approximately 5.6 per 1,000 births, and the frequency of major congenital anomalies is about 3% among newborn infants (Swint, 1982). The incidence of birth defects among liveborn infants not amenable to prenatal diagnosis in the general population is 2% to 4% (Paucker, 1982). Anello (1981) predicts there

will be a major reduction in hereditary and congenital defects through gene splicing in the future.

Three large surveys of chronically ill children (Haggerty, Roghmann, & Pless, 1975; Pless & Douglas, 1971; Rutter, Graham, & Yule, 1970) indicated the prevalence of chronic illness in children under the age of 16 years to range from 5% to 20%, depending upon the sampling methods used. The most common disorders involve the respiratory system and allergies, followed by sensory and motor disorders. Rates of psychiatric and behavioral disorders were somewhat higher (12% to 16%) for chronically ill children than for the general population (7%). Early studies of children with chronic disorders indicated higher rates of psychiatric difficulties than found in the general population, and the presence of brain injury or epilepsy increased the risk of developing a psychiatric disorder (Rubenstein, 1984; Rutter et al, 1970). Identified psychosocial risk factors for psychiatric disorders were gender (males at higher risk than females), chronic marital discord, social disadvantages (e.g., overcrowding, parental unemployment), paternal criminality, maternal psychiatric illness, repeated admissions for institutional care, and lack of opportunities for social stimulation (Rubenstein, 1984). Studies of children with cerebral palsy, head injuries, and cancer suggest a relationship between brain damage, lower intelligence quotients (IQ), and reading difficulties. When a pattern of school failure and lack of accomplishment develops, the child's self-esteem is likely to suffer, and behavior problems may begin as a way of coping with the frustration. The other possibility is that children who have brain disorders and cognitive difficulties have disturbed behavior because they do not understand the nuances of their behavior and socialization. The disturbed behavior is then reinforced by the environment's response to it.

Adults The epidemiology of adult chronic illness differs from that of childhood chronic illness (Pless & Perrin, 1985). Adult chronic illness is characterized by a relatively large number of common disorders (e.g., arthritis, hypertension, diabetes) and a few rare diseases. On the other hand, childhood chronic illnesses consist of only a few common disorders (e.g., asthma, seizures) and many that are rare (e.g., sickle cell anemia, spina bifida). Nurses and other health professionals are likely to see adults with common chronic illnesses and children with a variety of uncommon disorders.

Middle-aged Adults

Generally, adults are diagnosed with chronic illness during their most productive years. However, their chronic conditions are likely to result in loss of productivity. For example, approximately 37 million of the 227 million people in the United States have some type of arthritis (Metropolitan, 1986), which often interferes with their daily living and work-related activities. Other common chronic disorders are respiratory diseases and diabetes mellitus (Parker, 1985). Diabetes mellitus affects more than 5.2 million people in the United States, and another 5 million may have diabetes but do not know it. Diabetes represents the third most common chronic disease requiring the management of the family physician and the ninth most common reason for patient visits to doctors' offices (Galazka & Eckert, 1984).

Older Adults

In 1985, 23 million Americans, 11% of the population, were over 65, and it is estimated that there will be 55 million (18%) by 2030 (Ellison, 1985). Of those over 65, 86% (nearly 20 million) have at least one chronic health problem (Butler & Lewis, 1982). Almost 85% of the 25.5 million elderly people in the United States suffer from at least one chronic disease (Dychtwald, 1986). Some 6% of Americans between 65 and 74 years, and 13% of those over 75 years of age, are incontinent (Harris, 1986).

The 10 most common chronic conditions of persons over 65 are arthritis, hypertensive disease, hearing impairments, heart conditions, chronic sinusitis, visual impairments, arteriosclerosis, diabetes mellitus, and varicose veins (Soldo & Manton, 1985). An estimated 2 million elderly need help with one or more activities of daily living, and 5 million people are involved in caring for elderly family members (Brody, 1985). The elderly are also likely to suffer from more than one chronic disorder. Among the multiple disorders are multiple sensory losses (vision, hearing), arteriosclerotic valvular disease, and diabetes (Ellison, 1985).

Societal Trends Influencing Long-Term Care

Some of the most significant trends facing society have been identified by John Naisbitt (1982) in his book, *Megatrends.* Four trends are particularly relevant to the psychosocial aspects of persons with chronic conditions and their families: the shifts from an industrial to an information society, from institutional help to self-help, from a forced technology to a "high-tech, high-touch" technology, and from a representative democracy to a participative democracy. These trends, as well as trends toward an aging population and theory- and research-based nursing practice, are discussed below.

Informational Society

American society is changing from an industrial to an informational society. With innovations in communication systems (telephones, beepers, televisions) and computer technology, increased accessibility and availability to clients and health providers in remote areas can be anticipated. This means there will be new and innovative ways to monitor patients at home, and consumers and health care providers will have increased access to information. With these changes will come increased opportunities for education and advances in the processes of teaching and communicating.

In step with this change, society is becoming increasingly research oriented. New knowledge, new drugs, and new medical equipment for diagnosis and treatment of chronic illness are appearing. As the acquisition of fundamental knowledge about the nature of diseases and cures for them grows, it is reasonable to anticipate some changes in the types and severity of illness that will be seen in the future. Medical care needs "a better balance between prevention and treatment, promotion of function and cure, and educational as compared to technical approaches to care" (Mechanic, 1986, p. 23). Nursing care needs to include a balance between psychosocial care and technical care to meet the needs of patients and their families.

Self-help

A second trend in society is the shift from institutional help to self-help. More people with chronic illnesses are taking care of themselves in their homes rather than in institutions. Patients treated at home and in institutions are sicker than they were in the past. The burden of care is shifting from institutional personnel to the chronically ill person or family member or, in some cases, community members to provide care.

It is estimated that family members care for 60% to 80% of the chronically ill persons who receive care at home, with this percentage increasing with the severity of the functional impairment of the person receiving care (Reif & Estes, 1982). However, population projections indicate that the number of available caretakers will decrease, leaving fewer people to provide care in the home.

An estimated 500,000 mutual aid groups are available to develop and share self-care skills with peers who have similar problems. Increased interest in self-care is emerging from consumer activism and from professional commitment to increasing consumer involvement (Parcel et al, 1986). The trend toward education for self-care has been attributed to increased acceptance by health professionals of patient education programs and increasing awareness on the part of consumers that they are capable of carrying out complex procedures, such as the care of a person dependent on a ventilator or home dialysis (Green et al, 1977). Other contributing factors are the new applications of behavior modification techniques emphasizing self-management or self-regulation, the growth of self-help groups, and the change in nursing's emphasis toward encouraging self-care.

Two trends in national health policy are likely to continue this trend toward self-directed care. They are the shift in health care financing from a fee-based, retrospective approach to a prospective or capitation system; and an increased priority and support for health promotion and disease prevention programs and services (Parcel et al, 1986).

Adults have always participated in activities to maintain life, health, and well-being. In today's society, adults are expected to be responsible and self-reliant, to care for themselves as well as their dependents. Self-care activities are learned relative to the beliefs, habits, and practices that identify the cultural way of life of the group to which the individual belongs. Nutrition, grooming, and exercise at the individual level and sanitation, sewage disposal and water purification at the community level are all health-related self-care measures. As consumers became more oriented toward health and prevention of illness, demanded more input into health care, and wanted to be partners in health care, the notion of self-care has gained in popularity. As nursing has become increasingly based in research and theory, Orem's self-care theory (1991) evolved to put nursing in the unique position of assisting patients in meeting their self-care needs.

"**Self-care** is the practice of activities that individuals initiate and perform on their own behalf in maintaining life, health and well-being " (Orem, 1991, p. 117). Adults normally take care of their own health needs, and self-care contributes to one's own health. When people become ill, self-care demands may exceed their ability to meet the demands, and nursing may be needed to help them regain a steady state.

Over 70 million Americans, nearly half of the adult population, already perform at least some self-care (Andreoli & Musser, 1985). To foster self-care, health care professionals need to listen to family members and respect their differing perspectives. There is increasing need to educate people so that they can care for themselves to the greatest extent possible. As this self-care trend continues, increased family involvement in decision making will place a burden on providers to assure that the families have adequate information to make these decisions. Clients will need to know how to work within the system and to manipulate it to obtain needed services. Programs in homes, community agencies, work sites, and schools will be needed to promote health and prevent chronic diseases. These important services are not currently reimbursed by health insurers unless they are ordered by a physician. Nurses need to take an active role advocating for changes in reimbursement and in finding alternative ways to finance these services.

High Touch and High Technology

A third trend is the movement from a forced technology to a "High/Tech, High/Touch" technology. Recent technological innovations include robots to deliver home and hospital services, communication devices for those unable to speak, and innovative assistive devices for ambulation. As technology increases, the need for human touch also increases; thus, high touch (care) becomes an essential component of nursing in order to provide balance in a highly technological society. For each new technological advance, a high-touch intervention is needed.

High touch refers to seeing the person as a human being, separate from the machines and pathology. High touch requires increased understanding, concern, caring, and psychosocial support for persons with chronic conditions and their families. As Naisbitt (1982) stated, society must "learn to balance the material wonders of technology with the spiritual demands of . . . human nature" (p. 36). For example, Larkin (1987) reports that following a myocardial infarction, persons felt nurses and physicians were interested only in their heart muscles and not in them as people.

Technology advanced more rapidly in the past 50 years than in the previous 5,000 years (Anello, 1981). Six categories of emerging technological changes have been identified (McCormick, 1983): (1) drugs, such as vaccines for influenza, arthritis, hepatitis, and cancer, and endorphins for mental health, sleep, and pain management; (2) devices, such as ambulatory cardiac monitoring, communication devices for nonspeaking patients, robots delivering services, and rehabilitation devices; (3) medical procedures with diagnostic and therapeutic implications such as high-frequency ventilators, electrical stimulation, and nuclear magnetic resonance (NMR); (4) surgical procedures, principally transplants, implants, and genetic microsurgery for genetic engineering; (5) organizational systems, including hospital information systems and microcomputers; and (6) supportive systems such as supply regulators for delivery of products to hospitals, cities, and communities. An example of the rapid increase is the number of patients receiving dialysis. In the mid-1960s approximately 1,000 patients received dialysis, compared with about 63,000 in 1983 (Mechanic, 1986). These changes are already forcing us to think about choices in expenditures of our limited resources and the ethical issues involved.

Advances in medical technology have increased the life span of persons with diseases such as cancer, cystic fibrosis (CF), end-stage renal disease (ESR), diabetes, spina bifida, and hypertension. Infants with respiratory distress syndrome (RDS), adults following cardiac arrest, and those of all ages requiring transplants of hearts, kidneys, and livers are examples of people of various ages benefitting from technology. People are living longer with chronic illness; consequently patients and their families must face challenges that were not previously anticipated (Drotar, 1981). Diseases such as cystic fibrosis are no longer strictly childhood disorders. Approximately 75% to 80% of the youngsters with this disorder survive into late adolescence or early adulthood, with 50% now living beyond the age of 18 years, and some having lived into their 50s (Philips et al, 1985; Pinkerton et al, 1985; Strauss & Wellish, 1981). Therefore, a future-oriented approach is needed with this population to prepare youngsters and their families for their continuing development. Nurses working with adults will be caring for more of these individuals as they make the transition from pediatric to adult care. However, one should keep in mind that the poor cannot even afford primary care, much less take advantage of biomedical progress.

Participative Democracy

The fourth trend discussed by Naisbitt (1982) is the move from a representative democracy to a participatory democracy, in which people participate in arriving at decisions that affect their lives. This change means consumers will have a growing voice in planning and evaluating services for themselves and their family members. The use of referenda and initiatives have had unprecedented growth, allowing people direct access to political decision making. Already many consumer groups, including those with chronic conditions and their families, are becoming increasingly vocal and politically active about their needs. Health care providers need to become assertive and strengthen their voice and role regarding clients' needs as they relate to various systems. The growth of social movements has led to modification of social definitions and social policies that enable persons with disabilities to pursue conventional activities (e.g., school, occupation) successfully (Mechanic, 1986).

Changing Age Distribution

The increasing elderly population has been identified by Andreoli and Musser (1985) as an important factor influencing nursing practice and the care of the chronically ill. As noted above, 11.3% of the American population in 1980 was 65 years or older. By the year 2030, 20% of Americans will be 65 years or older, and by 2040, the "old-old" (75 years and over) will be the majority elderly population (U.S. Dept of Commerce, 1982). Compared with other age groups, the elderly have more chronic diseases and use more health care services. As the population of elderly increases, their utilization of services can be expected to increase, as will the number of days they remain hospitalized. Hospital admissions will be for acute and complicated illnesses requiring care by nurses skilled in critical care.

It is also estimated that the number of elderly in nursing homes will quadruple by the year 2050 (Shields & Kick, 1982). By 2040, a fivefold increase in the number of persons over 85 who are in nursing homes or functionally dependent in the community is anticipated (Soldo & Manton, 1985). These nursing home residents will require more rehabilitative, psychosocial, and custodial nursing care than medical care, indicating growing need for nurses skilled in these areas.

Demand will grow for nontraditional nurses in ambulatory care settings. As the trend toward deinstitutionalizing the elderly increases, nurses will be needed in homes, adult day care centers, hospices, day hospitals, and community-based mental health centers.

Increased Demand for Long-Term Care Services

With the implementation of the prospective payment system (PPS) for hospitals, patients are being discharged earlier and sicker than in the past (Harrington, 1988). These early discharges, the complexity of home care required by patients, and the increasing high technology moving into the home are placing a tremendous burden on the rapidly proliferating home health services. Care that was previously being delivered by visiting nurses is now being provided by families, proprietary, chain, and hospital-based organizations. Costs of such care are also increasing rapidly. It was estimated that costs would rise from $9 billion in 1985 to $16 billion in 1990 (Harrington, 1988).

High quality home health care means "meeting the individual's physical, medical, psychosocial, and rehabilitative needs and effectively encouraging maximal functional independence" (Harrington, 1988, p. 165). Yet, many problems have been identified with these services, including inadequate availability and access. Harrington (1988) summarized the findings of a report by the American Bar Association listing problems with the quality of home health services. Among the identified problems are: tardiness, failure to report for work, inadequate or improper care, insensitivity, disrespect, abusiveness, intimidation, theft, and financial exploitation.

Impact on the Nursing System

Clinical Practice Based on Theory and Research

Nurses have striven to attain the status and ideals of a profession. Basic to any profession is the development of a body of knowledge that can be applied to its practice. Nursing has grown as a field of scientific inquiry since the early 1970s. With the preparation of nurses at the doctoral level and the development of doctoral programs in nursing, the profession has imposed rigorous standards upon itself. Today, nursing has established itself as a scientific discipline and is demanding nursing theory development and research-based clinical practice. There now exists a body of nursing knowledge comprised of concepts and theories that support nursing practice. As this trend continues, nurses will question current practice in chronic care and provide new answers. It is expected that quality of care will be enhanced with cost-effective programs derived from research. With sound documentation of efficient and effective nursing practice, nurses can increase their influence in the political arena and lobby for changes within the health care system.

Implications for Nursing

The changing age profile and the prevalence patterns of disease in the United States challenge health professionals (1) to help patients maintain as much function as possible within the context of their illnesses and (2) to seek cures for the illnesses. Changes in nursing practice, education, and research are needed and can be anticipated in the future. Consequently, a fluid model, such as the Contingency Model for Long-Term Care, allows for creativity in planning and implementing care based on these changes. The following section introduces selected nursing practice, education, and research developments.

Nursing Practice

Nursing roles and relationships have been changing in response to nursing, interdisciplinary, and consumer needs. Nursing specialties are developing according to age groups, medical problems, and clinical settings (Hymovich, 1985). The trend toward home care is having a major impact on nursing practice within the hospital and the community. As growing numbers of children and adults are living with chronic illnesses and even cures (e.g., childhood cancer), emphasis is shifting from helping families cope with death to helping them cope with a person with a chronic illness (Wallace et al, 1984). In addition, the increasing technology and related complexity of nursing tasks are requiring shifts in nursing roles and responsibilities.

Holistic nursing care, with a focus on the patient and family (respect, dignity, humanity, privacy) is an ever-increasing need. The caring, supporting, and comforting aspects of the nursing profession are essential in today's society. Increased involvement of all professions in coordinating and integrating the health care team to prevent fragmentation of care to families is required. Also needed is increased collaboration, cooperation, and communication among all health care professionals. A delicate balance between technology (high/tech) and caring (high/touch) is critical. The situations related to many patients will call into question nurses' moral and ethical values.

In long-term care, the current emphasis is on treating the manifestations of illness once it occurs. There has been limited attention to the psychosocial and economic factors leading to increased risk for chronic illnesses. Nurses can play an important role in reducing the risks for chronic illness and by working intensively with those at risk because of low income, poor nutrition and housing, and limited social support.

Nursing Education

According to McCormick (1983), nursing education should include four broad categories: science; remedial and healing arts; focus or direction of knowledge (from cell to society); and professional conditions and controls (code of ethnics, attributes of education, regulation and licensure). Nurses need to understand society in its local, national, and international context. Nurses need to speak the language of politicians, business people, and artists in order to communicate effectively with patients as well as play a role in changing public policy (Anello, 1981).

Nurses need to be competent in using technology, including computers. Clinical specialists who know technical equipment should be available to advise and teach nurses who use such equipment infrequently. The specialists should also encourage the staff to spend time attending to the psychosocial needs of patients and families (Campbell & Leatt, 1982). High-tech nursing must also include the high-touch aspect of nursing. Nurses need to convey genuine care and concern for clients and their families.

Nurses also need to become skilled in working with a team of specialists including physicians, sociologists, psychologists, and computer analysts, as well as planning committees. Knowledge of human relations, organizational management, administrative behavior, control, planning, and coordination is imperative (Anello, 1981).

Political savvy and effectiveness are other skills nurses must learn (Andreoli & Musser, 1985). Nurses need to inform politicians about the state of our health care system and its needs, and become vocal advocates of necessary legislation. Nurses need to ensure that one of the nation's most vulnerable group of citizens, those with chronic conditions, have access to health care where and when it is needed. Davis (1988) suggests that nurses present a united front by resolving nursing's internal issues (e.g., entry into practice, licensure), serving as advocates for the underprivileged, demonstrating that nursing services are cost effective, and developing innovative and humanistic nursing approaches that are responsive to a competitive health system.

Content pertinent to care of the chronically ill and their families should be provided at all levels of nursing education programs, in-service education, and continuing-education programs (Hymovich, 1985). Such content includes updated information about chronic conditions; their impact on families, community, and society; and intervention strategies to minimize stressors and enhance coping and level of functioning. In addition, approaches to help nurses cope with their own stressors in working with the chronically ill need to be included in education programs at all levels.

Nursing Research

As mentioned earlier, the profession of nursing has established itself as a scientific discipline and demands practice based on sound research. This book attempts to bring together selected research from nursing and other disciplines that can be used to provide nursing care. However, research in nursing care for the chronically ill is still in its infancy. Nurses must continue to question their practice and document cost-effective ways to deliver high-quality health care to the chronically ill. While nurses are beginning collaborative research projects with one another as well as with other members of the health care team, increased effort in this area is needed.

Summary

Chronic conditions are a leading cause of morbidity and mortality in the United States. This chapter presented an overview of the magnitude of the problem, terminology, trends and issues influencing care, and implications for nursing. **Disease** (defect, disorder, condition) was described as a term that embodies and interferes with the functioning of the body, whereas **illness** was defined as a personal experience with the disease that may or may not involve disability and handicap. **Chronic illness** (long-term illness, chronic condition, chronic health problem) refers to any long-term or permanent disability that interferes with the person's ordinary physical, psychological, or social functioning. **Impairment** involves "loss or abnormality of psychological, or anatomical structure or function" (WHO, 1980, p. 46). **Disability** reflects the consequences of the impairment in terms of the person's functional performance and activities, while **handicap** refers to the social disadvantages a person experiences as a result of an impairment or disability.

Trends influencing the care people with chronic conditions receive, and will receive in the future, are the shifts from (1) an industrial to an information society, (2) institutional help to self-help, (3) forced technology to high/tech, high/touch technology, and (4) representative democracy to participative democracy. In addition, the country's changing age distribution and the trend toward theory- and research-based clinical nursing practice are influencing patient and family care. Implications of these trends for nursing practice, education, and research are mentioned.

References

Andreoli, K.G., & Musser, L.A. (1985). Trends that may affect nursing's future. *Nurs Health Care, 6*(1), 47–51.

Anello, M. (1981). Nursing and the changing scene. *Nurs Leadership, 4*(3), 19–24.

Brody, E.M. (1985). Patient care as a normative stress. *Gerontologist, 26*, 19–29.

Bush and Dukakis on disability issues. (1988). *J Rehabil, 54*(3), 10–12.

Butler, R.N., & Lewis, M. (1982). *Aging and mental health.* St. Louis: Mosby.

Campbell, S., & Leatt, P. (1982). The role of complex equipment in nurses work: Toward the development of a measure. *Nurs Papers, 14*(3), 36–45.

Centers for Disease Control, Center for Infectious Diseases. (1988). *Acquired Immunodeficiency Syndrome Weekly Surveillance Report-United States AIDS Program.*

Cote, T.R., Nelson, M.R., Anderson, S.P., & Martin, R.J. (1990). The present and the future of AIDS and tuberculosis in Illinois. *Am J Public Health, 80*(8), 950–953.

Davis, G.C. (1988). Nursing values and health care policy. *Nurs Outlook, 36*(6), 289–292.

Developmental Disabilities Assistance and Bill of Rights Act. (1978). Washington, DC: United States Department of Health, Education, and Welfare.

Dimond M., & Jones M. (1983). *Chronic illness across the life span.* Norwalk, CT: Appleton-Century-Crofts.

Dittmar, S.S. (1989). Scope of rehabilitation. In S.S. Dittmar (Ed.) *Rehabilitation Nursing: Process and application* (pp. 2–15). St. Louis: Mosby.

Drotar, D. (1981). Psychological perspectives in chronic childhood illness. *J Pediatr Psychol, 6*, 211–228.

Dychtwald, K. (1986). *Wellness and health promotion for the elderly.* Rockville, MD: Aspen Publishers.

Ellison, S.A. (1985). Geriatric oncology: A developmental approach. *Cancer Nurs. Suppl 1*, 28–32.

Forsyth, G.L., DeLancy, K.D., & Gresham, M.L. (1984). Vying for a winning position: Management style of the chronically ill. *J Nurs Health, 7*, 181–188.

Galazka, S.S., & Eckert, J.K. (1984). Diabetes mellitus from the inside out: Ecological perspectives on a chronic disease. *Fam Syst Med, 2*(1), 28–36.

Green, L.W., Werlin, S.H., Schauffler, H.H., & Avery, C.H. (1977). Research and demonstration issues in self-care: Measuring the decline of mediocentrism. *Health Educ Q, 5,* 161–188.

Haggerty, R.J., Roghmann, K.J., & Pless, I.B. (1975). *Child health and the community.* New York: Wiley.

Hanson, S.M.H. (1987). Family nursing and chronic illness. In L.M. Wright & M. Leahy (Eds.), *Families and chronic illness* (pp. 2–32). Springhouse, PA: Springhouse.

Harrington, C. (1988). Quality, access, and costs: Public policy and home health care. *Nurs Outlook, 36*(4), 164–166.

Harris, T. (1986). Aging in the eighties, prevalence and impact of urinary problems in individuals age 65 years and over. *Advancedata,* No. 121, August 27, 1986. USDHHS.

Hymovich, D.P. (1985). Nursing care. In N. Hobbs & J.M. Perrin (Eds.), *Issues in the care of children with chronic illness* (pp. 478–497). San Francisco: Jossey-Bass.

Kleinman, A.M., Eisenberg, L., & Good, B. (1978). Culture, illness and care. *Ann Intern Med, 88,* 251–258.

Larkin, J. (1987). Factors identifying one's ability to adapt to chronic illness. *Nurs Clin North Am, 22*(3), 535–542.

McCormick, K.A. (1983). Preparing nurses for the technological future. *Nurs Health Care, 4*(7), 379–382.

Magi, M., & Allander, E. (1981). Towards a theory of perceived and medically defined need. *Sociol Health Illness, 3*(1), 49–71.

Mattsson, A. (1972). Long term illness in childhood: A challenge to psychosocial adaptation. *Pediatrics, 50,* 801–805.

Mechanic, D. (1986). *From advocacy to allocation: The evolving American health care system.* New York: Macmillan.

Metropolitan Washington Chapter of the Arthritis Foundation. (1986). *Fact sheet on arthritis.* Arlington, VA.

Naisbitt, J. (1982). *Megatrends—Ten new directions for transforming lives.* New York: Warner Books.

National Center for Health Statistics. (1982). *Current estimates from the health interview survey* (Series 10, Number 141). DHEW.

National Center for Health Statistics. (1987). DHEW.

National Center for Health Statistics. (1989). *Monthly vital statistics report. 37*(13) pp. 20–21. DHEW.

National Commission on Chronic Illness. (1956). *Chronic illness in the United States: Care of the long-term patient. Vol. II.* Cambridge: Harvard University Press.

Oda, D.S. (1989). The imperative of a national health strategy for children: Is there a political will? *Nurs Outlook, 37,*(5), 206–208.

Orem, D.E. (1991). *Nursing: Concepts of practice* (4th ed.). St. Louis: Mosby-Year Book.

Parcel, G.S., Bartlett, E.E., & Bruhn, J.G. (1986). The role of health education in self-management. In K.A. Holroyd & T.L. Creer (Eds.), *Self-management of chronic disease* (pp. 3–27). Orlando: Academic Press.

Parker, S.R. (1985). Future directions in behavioral research related to lung diseases. *Ann Behav Med, 7,* 21–25.

Paucker, S.P. (1982). Prenatal genetics diagnosis by amniocentesis: The human problem. In B.J. McNeil & E.B. Cravalho (Eds.), *Critical issues in medical technology* (pp. 317–324). Boston: Auburn House.

Phillips, S., Bohannon, W.E., Gayton, W.F., et al. (1985). Parent interview findings regarding the impact of cystic fibrosis on families. *J Dev Behav Pediatr, 6,* 122–127.

Pinkerton, P., Trauer, T., Duncan, F. et al. (1985). Cystic fibrosis in adult life: A study of coping patterns. *Lancet, 2,* 761–763.

Pless, I.B., & Douglas, J.W.B. (1971). Chronic illness in childhood: I Epidemiological and clinical characteristics. *Pediatrics, 47,* 405–414.

Pless, I.B., & Perrin, J.M. (1985). Issues common to a variety of illnesses. In N. Hobbs & J.M. Perrin (Eds.), *Issues in the care of children with chronic illness* (pp. 41–60). San Francisco: Jossey-Bass.

Pless, I.B., & Pinkerton, P. (1975). *Chronic childhood disorder—Promoting patterns of adjustment.* London: Henry Kimpton Publishers.

Reif, L., & Estes, C.L. (1982). Long-term care: New opportunities for professional nursing. In L.H. Aiken (Ed.), *Nursing in the 1980s: Crises, opportunities, challenges* (pp. 147–181). Philadelphia: Lippincott.

Rubenstein, B. (1984). When a child has a serious illness: Psychiatric aspects of chronic handicaps. In E. Aronowitz & E.M. Bromberg (Eds.), *Mental health and long-term illness* (pp. 45–65). Canton, MA: Prodist.

Rutter, M., Graham, P., & Yule, W. (Eds.). (1970). *A neuropsychiatric study in childhood.* London: Spastic International Medical Publications.

Schilling, R.F., Paul, S.P., & Kirkham, M.A. (1988). The impact of developmental disabilities and other learning deficits on families. In C.S. Chilman, E.W., Nunnally, & F.M. Cox (Eds.), *Chronic illness and disability* (pp. 156–170). Newbury Park, CA: Sage.

Shields, E.M., & Kick, E. (1982). Nursing care in nursing homes. In L.H. Aiken (Ed.), *Nursing in the 1980s: Crises, opportunities, challenges* (pp. 195–209). Philadelphia: Lippincott.

Soldo, B.J., & Manton, K.G. (1985). Health status and service needs of the oldest old: Current patterns and future trends. *Memor Fund Q/Health Soc, 63*(2), 286–319.

Strauss, G.D., & Wellish, D.K. (1981). Psychosocial adaptation in older cystic fibrosis patients. *J Chronic Dis, 34,* 141–146.

Swint, J.M. (1982). Antenatal diagnosis of genetic disease: Economic considerations. In B.J. McNeil & E.B. Cravalho (Eds.), *Critical issues in medical technology* (pp. 325–342). Boston: Auburn House.

Twaddle, A.C., & Hessler, R.M. (1977). *Sociology of health*. St. Louis: Mosby.

U.S. Department of Commerce Bureau of the Census. (1982). *1980 Census supplemental reports: Age, sex, race, and Spanish origin of the population by regions, divisions, and states*. PC 80-S1-1, Washington, DC: Bureau of the Census.

Wallace, M.H., Bakke, K., Hubbard, A., & Pendergrass, T.W. (1984). Coping with childhood cancer: An educational program for parents of children with cancer. *Oncol Nurs Forum, 11*(4), 30–35.

Watson, J. (1988). *Nursing: Human science and human care*. Publication 15-2236. New York: National League for Nursing.

World Health Organization. (1980). *International classification of impairments, disabilities, and handicaps*. Geneva: World Health Organization.

3 Overview of Nursing Care

Nursing care, a major component of the Contingency Model of Long-Term Care, contains two main elements, process and content. These elements and their principal categories are illustrated in Figure 3–1. The process categories are nursing process and nursing strategies. The **nursing process** consists of assessment, planning, intervention, and reassessment or evaluation. The primary **nursing strategy** categories are (1) establishing and maintaining trust, (2) providing support and guidance, (3) providing information, (4) providing anticipatory guidance, (5) facilitating stress reduction, (6) fostering independence through self-care, (7) facilitating access to resources, (8) modifying attitudes, (9) assisting all system members, (10) providing direct care, and (11) collaborating with others. The **content** component of nursing care contains details of the process, such as specific information to be imparted about side effects of medications. The broken lines between these elements in Figure 3–1 illustrate their overlapping relationships. For example, nursing intervention may involve facilitating access to resources, which includes providing accurate information about community resources, whom to contact, and how to contact the appropriate personnel.

Several questions need to be addressed periodically to ensure comprehensive care for clients with chronic conditions. Summarized in Box 3–1, these questions, modified from Pless and Pinkerton (1975) are:

(a) **Who** are the recipients of the care? It is important to determine whether the nursing care is for the patient with the chronic condition, another family member (sibling, parent, spouse, child), or the entire family unit, including extended-family members. Other recipients might be friends, neighbors, school children or personnel, and members of various community groups.

(b) **Who** should provide the care? Who are the appropriate health professionals to be working with the patients and their families? The Commission on Chronic Illness recognizes the need for a team approach in caring for the complex needs of the chronically ill. The makeup of the team may vary for different clients and at different times, depending upon the identified needs of the clients, with families remaining as the central members. Team coordination is essential. Although nurses may or may not be the coordinator for any given family, they can take responsibility to see that someone serves that function.

(c) **What** are the **goals** of the nursing care? What are the short-term and long-term **objectives** for the individual patient and family? Appropriate goals depend upon the mediators and contingency variables identified by clients and health professionals. Nurses need to consider both short-term and long-term goals. A long-term plan that can be modified when necessary should be developed. Goals involve both high technology and high touch. They are aimed at minimizing the impact of the condition on all family members and enhancing their coping abilities by (1) treating the disease itself, (2) meeting the psychosocial needs of individual and family, and (3) preventing the disease process, treatments, and

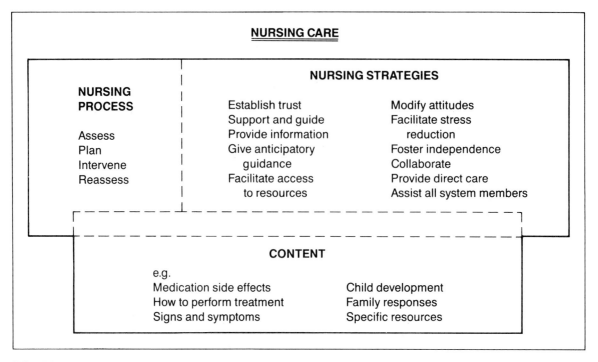

FIGURE 3–1 Nursing Care Component of the Contingency Model of Long-Term Care. The broken lines depict the overlapping nature of nursing process and content.

various people involved in the program from interfering with individual development and disrupting the family unit (Pless & Pinkerton, 1975).

(d) **How** should the nursing care take place? That is, what has to be done to meet the goals? Nursing processes may include mutual goal setting, counseling, supporting, teaching, listening, collaborating, and referring, as well as providing direct care. The processes should be culturally relevant and planned to capitalize on individual and family strengths and decrease needs.

Actual techniques for accomplishing goals vary with the individual and family and are contingent on their orientation to life, coping strategies, strengths, needs, and level of functioning. However, there are certain commonalities based on needs that are appropriate for all clients. These nursing activities are to (1) establish and maintain trust; (2) provide information; (3) provide support and guidance, including anticipatory guidance; (4) assure access to adequate resources, and (5) assist system members to acquire necessary skills.

(e) **When** is the appropriate time for nursing care to occur? Not all people with stressors related to chronic conditions need or want formal psychoso-

cial nursing interventions. When intervention is indicated, appropriate timing is a major consideration. People in crisis may be more amenable to certain interventions, but others may be too numb to benefit at these times. Appropriate timing should be based on assessment of the family members' readiness and motivation. Timing is especially crucial with early hospital discharge, because the shock of diagnosis often inhibits learning. If patients and their families are taught about the necessary care within this early period, they are likely to hear little of it. Although they may have been taught, it does not necessarily follow that they have learned. Alternative strategies for teaching under these circumstances are needed.

(f) **Where** should the nursing care take place? That is, what is the most appropriate location? It may be the home, hospital, clinic, community (school, community agency), regional center, or elsewhere.

(g) **What** is the outcome of the nursing care and **how** will it be measured? Outcome should be measured by objectives. According to Mechanic (1986), a person's illness behavior and coping capacities may be more powerful determinants of medical outcomes than many of the biological indicators of disease. A nursing care plan should include information on how the effectiveness of the outcome will be measured, and when the outcome is anticipated. Because care plans should be developed with the clients, it is necessary to determine whether the clients were able to accomplish their goals, and what modifications needed to be made.

Long-term nursing outcome will be more a function of the social environment than of the underlying pathology or prescriptions of health care workers. Mechanic (1986) suggests that outcome depends more on how others react to the situation than to the psychological state of the patients.

Goals of Nursing Care

The overall goal of nursing care is to assist persons with chronic conditions and their families adapt to the condition and its effects on their daily lives so that they may accomplish their developmental and situational tasks to the extent possible within the limits of the condition. This objective may be realized by enhancing coping abilities and alleviating or minimizing the impact of stressors on each system. Specific goals for the individual and family are (1) to minimize their stressors; (2) increase their ability to cope with stressors; (3) maximize their strengths; and (4) accomplish, within the limits of the chronic condition, their developmental and situational tasks.

Rehabilitation and Habilitation

Rehabilitation and habilitation are often important components of care for those with chronic condi-

tions. **Rehabilitation** "is an approach, a philosophy, an attitude, and a process" to facilitate a person's movement toward health (Dittmar, 1989, p. 2). The family's collaborative role is crucial in any rehabilitation program (Versluys, 1980). Goals of rehabilitation treatment are to (1) strengthen family relationships by developing an arena for mutual sharing of activities, (2) solve problems related to practical and emotional aspects of rehabilitation, (3) encourage expression of everyone's feelings, and (4) identify and practice new living skills through task assignments within the hospital or community (Versluys, 1980).

The **habilitation** process involves establishing fundamental capabilities, knowledge, experiences, and attitudes needed for as near normal living as possible (Whitehouse, 1953). People needing habilitation are those who have never achieved a status equal to the development of their peers (Whitehouse, 1976). The habilitation approach stresses development of assets and the indoctrination of mature behavior and attitudes. The difference between habilitation and rehabilitation is mainly the difference between education and reeducation.

Assessment

Assessment involves appraising the situation and making some judgment (diagnosis) about that appraisal. Assessment of the patient's and family's frame of reference, as well as the perceptions of health team members, can facilitate planning effective and acceptable nursing interventions.

Comprehensive assessment includes obtaining objective and subjective information, over time, about each variable in the model: System Identifying Characteristics, Contingency Variables (Orientation to Life, Stressors, Coping Strategies, Strengths, Needs), and Level of Functioning. Since all members do not necessarily have similar perceptions of the situation, subjective information is gathered from family members as well as from the patient. When this is not possible, patient or care-giver perceptions may provide the only source of subjective information.

According to Strauss et al (1984), persons have three biographies, and health care personnel usually know only a small portion of these biographies. However, these biographies affect the person's interaction with all members of the health care system, so information about each biography is important.

Table 3–1 Components of a Comprehensive
Client Assessment

- Previous life experiences, especially those related to health, illness, crises, health care personnel and facilities, and death
- Time orientation, including past medical history, present illness, and anticipated future outcomes
- Orientation to life (values, attitudes, and beliefs)
- Focal stressors
    Include chronological events related to the illness.
- Previous and current coping strategies
- Perceived resources and strengths
- Perceived needs
- Level of functioning in accomplishing individual and family developmental and situational tasks, including past and present functioning
    (a) Encounters with family, friends, and others
    (b) Satisfaction with functioning
- Goals (short-term, long-term)

The biographies are (1) chronological events related to the illness; (2) experiences with health care personnel and facilities; and (3) a social biography of encounters with family, friends, and others. This information is incorporated in an assessment using the Contingency Model of Long-Term Care. Focus of assessment involves patient and family stressors, coping strategies, strengths, and needs in relation to each of their developmental and situational tasks. Specific areas to be assessed are listed in Table 3–1.

Assessment of satisfactions related to each developmental and situational task provides some measure regarding the importance of possible suggestions for intervention. For example, a person who indicates little involvement in community activities and is satisfied with that situation has needs different from those of the person who is involved in activities but is dissatisfied, or the person who is not involved but would like to be. After reviewing nearly 200 articles related to families and health care, Schwenck and Hughs (1983) concluded that knowing the family's definition of the situation was key to knowing how the family would respond to a member's illness. Many families are capable of caring for those with chronic conditions at home by using current support networks, with little outside intervention other than health care intervention. However, positive feedback from health care providers is also important. As one woman said, "It's nice to hear the

doctor tell us we're doing a good job, even though we know it ourselves. Our lives are so tied up in the medical system that it's important to hear it from them."

Clients may require help in identifying strengths as well as needs. Assessing and reinforcing strengths and coping abilities is an important nursing role "despite the fact that, in this era of cost containment, improved life quality may be an outcome that is overlooked, ignored, and undervalued" (Shekleton, 1987, p. 579). In fact, self-assessment of one's strengths is in itself strengthening (Otto, 1973). Guidelines for assessing strengths and needs are presented in Chapter 13.

Methods of Assessment

Assessment of patient and family should be ongoing. It need not take place in one or even two sessions; in fact, it is probably better to assess over several sessions and then reassess with each contact (Hymovich, 1979). People with chronic conditions require repeated contacts with the health care system, so more time is available for complete assessment than there is in an emergency, when assessment is limited only to pertinent areas. Over time, familiarity develops between nurse and client, so they are increasingly likely to be at ease and trust one another. As trust develops, clients are likely to share more about themselves and their concerns, enabling nurses to gain a better understanding of previous experiences leading to current strengths and needs. Clinical experience supports Strauss and colleagues' (1984) belief that chronically ill people are usually willing and eager to talk to interested personnel. Not all assessments are formal and much information can be gained during other contacts with the person and family, while one performs procedures, or in casual encounters. These casual encounters are "action interviews" (Strauss et al, 1984) or continuing conversations that take place over time.

Assessment generally begins with one or more of the individual family members and may be followed later by assessment of one or more of the subsystems (e.g., parent-child, spouse). Although assessment of the total family unit is uncommon, it can provide useful information about unique characteristics. The more specific and well-defined the strengths, needs, and current level of functioning, the easier it will be to plan and intervene appropriately. Because all systems are interrelated, assessment of one is likely to overlap with assessment of another; and because of the complex interrelation of stressors, coping strategies, strengths, and needs, placing information in neat categories is often difficult.

A number of instruments are available to assess components of individual and family functioning, and these are discussed in subsequent chapters. Criteria for selection of appropriate instruments for clinical practice include their appropriateness for the setting and type of client, reliability, and validity. Many instruments were developed for research, however, their clinical value has not always been documented. Most health-status measures in the field of chronic illness "emphasize the patient's ability to perform activities of daily living rather than whether the full range of work-related, social, and leisure activities are actually performed [nor do they] assess changes in a person's ability to perform activities over time" (Lubeck & Yelin, 1988, p. 459).

Assessment involves observing and interviewing the individual and family, and discussions with other health care professionals or relevant persons to increase insight and improve communication among the professionals. Galazka and Eckert (1984) suggest a home visit is required to gain a comprehensive understanding of the patient's perspective. Although the authors agree that first-hand information about the family's neighborhood and home would be helpful, home visits may not be feasible within the constraints of one's position. However, communication and cooperation between hospital and community agencies can facilitate obtaining and sharing such information.

Child assessment Assessment through observation is an important means of gathering information, regardless of the person's age. Interviewing and observing children may involve modifications relative to their age and cognitive development. For young children, much information may come from the child's parents or guardians. Observing the child at play and using play as an interview technique are effective means of assessment. Use of these techniques facilitates learning about the child's understanding and misconceptions, fears, coping strategies, strengths, and needs.

Guidelines for collecting and recording information based on the Contingency Model for Long-Term Care are discussed in the appropriate chapters. A copy of the entire assessment guide is in the Appendix. The guidelines presented in the following chapters cover information in greater detail than will be found in the Appendix. Information obtained for one part of the assessment may be the same as that acquired for another part. However, this redundancy has been deleted from the guide in the Appendix. As with any assessment, it is necessary to set priorities about what information needs to be collected at a given time. In-depth and detailed assessment is not required for every person, nor must all information be collected at a single visit. If detailed information is needed about a specific area, the information in the following chapters may be helpful. Patient and family needs are likely to change over time, thus necessitating periodic reassessment.

Intervention

Various strategies are available for health care professionals to use in helping patients and their families cope with chronic conditions. These interventions are planned to meet system needs while fostering self-care and maximizing the use of strengths. Intervention enables chronically ill individuals and their families to become more skillful in solving their problems, meeting their needs, and achieving their aspirations, by acquiring competencies that support and strengthen their level of functioning "in such a way that permits a greater sense of individual or group control over its own developmental course" (Dunst, 1987, p. 1).

The Nursing Process

Nursing involves a systematic problem-solving approach to the delivery of care based on knowledge, research, and client and professional perceptions of strengths and needs. The process is cognitive and behavioral, and the nurse uses background and experiential knowledge, including intuition, to assist individuals and their families. The nursing process involves identifying system characteristics and contingency variables, assessing strengths and needs, planning necessary interventions, implementing these interventions, and reassessing.

Nursing Strategies

Nursing intervention strategies are the methods used to reach desired goals. Selection of appropriate strategies is based on the assessed strengths and needs of nurse and client, and findings from re-

Table 3–2   Countercoping Tasks and Techniques of the Nurse

Task	Techniques
Clarification and control	Examine the problem forthrightly. Provide only reliable and accurate information.
Redefine and reduce problems to manageable size.	Consider feasibility and probable consequences of any action.
Collaboration	Share concern without sharing distress. Refer certain problems to the respected judgment of another. Veto or prevent hasty, ill-considered actions. Suggest various directions and proposals that reflect your understanding.
Directed relief	Encourage expression of pent-up feelings. Permit temporary avoidance, distraction, and respite. Look at familiar strategies that worked in the past. Allow yourself to ventilate doubt, misgivings, or confusion.
Cooling off	Modulate and mollify tendencies to emotional extremes. Encourage self-esteem and self-confidence. Emphasize rational, practical, prudent actions. At times be content to share silence and adopt a constructive resignation.

Source: Weisman, 1984.

search. Nursing interventions are selected according to the assessment, the intervention's associated research base, the feasibility of successful implementation, the acceptability of the intervention to the client, and the nurse's strengths (Bulechek & McClosky, 1985). Nurses need to be competent in three areas if they are to be successful in implementing interventions: "(1) Knowledge of the scientific rationale for the intervention; (2) the necessary psychomotor and interpersonal skills; and (3) ability to function within the setting to effectively utilize health care resources" (Bulechek & McClosky, 1985, p. 13).

Weisman (1984) employs the term *countercoping* to refer to tasks care givers use when they intentionally intervene to relieve client distress and solve problems. He identifies four major tasks, each involving four countercoping techniques that care givers can use to assist clients who are coping with chronic conditions. These tasks and techniques are listed in Table 3–2.

Categories of nursing intervention strategies discussed in this book are listed in Box 3–2. The strategies for establishing and maintaining trust and for providing support and guidance are discussed in

Chapter 13. Strategies for providing information and anticipatory guidance, facilitating stress reduction, fostering independence through self-care, facilitating access to resources, and collaborating with others are discussed in Chapter 12; those for modifying attitudes will be found in Chapter 9.

Box 3–2   *Categories of Nursing Intervention Strategies*

Establishing and maintaining trust
Providing support and guidance
Providing information
Providing anticipatory guidance
Modifying attitudes
Assisting with management of the illness
    Facilitating self-care
    Facilitating stress management
Facilitating access to resources
Collaborating with others

Nurses evaluate the impact a specific nursing intervention has on the individual and family. In many instances, several intervention approaches may be employed. Although we have tried to support suggested interventions with findings from research, we recognize that more research is needed and that nurses must continue to intervene before such documentation is available. We encourage nurses to be creative in trying new approaches while at the same time engaging in systematic efforts to document the effectiveness of such interventions, including the situations in which they are effective and ineffective.

References

Bulechek, G.M., & McClosky, J.C. (Eds.). (1985). *Nursing interventions: Treatments of nursing diagnoses.* Philadelphia: W.B. Saunders.

Dittmar, S.S. (1989). *Rehabilitation nursing: Process and application.* St. Louis: Mosby.

Dunst, C.J. (1987, Dec) What is effective coping? Paper presented at the biennial meeting of the National Clinical Infants Program Conference, Washington, D.C. Cited by Dunst, C.J., Trivette, C.M., Davis, M., & Cornwell, J. (1988). Enabling and empowering families of children with health impairments. *Child Health Care, 17*(2), 71–81.

Galazka, S.S., & Eckert, J.K. (1984). Diabetes mellitus from the inside out: Ecological perspectives on a chronic disease. *Fam Syst Med, 2*(1), 28–36.

Hymovich, D.P. (1979). Assessment of the chronically ill child and family. In D.P. Hymovich & M.U. Barnard (Eds.), *Family health care: Vol. 1. General perspectives* (pp. 280–293). New York: McGraw-Hill.

Lubeck, D.P., & Yelin, E.H. (1988). A question of values: Measuring the impact of chronic disease. *Millbank Q, 66*(3), 444–464.

Mechanic, D. (1986). *From advocacy to allocation: The evolving American health care system.* New York: Macmillan.

Otto, H.A. (1973). A framework for assessing family strengths. In A. Reinhardt & M. Quinn (Eds.), *Family centered community nursing* (pp. 87–94). St Louis: Mosby.

Pless, I.B., & Pinkerton, P. (1975). *Chronic childhood disorder—Promoting patterns of adjustment.* Chicago: Year Book Medical Publishers.

Schwenck, T., & Hughs, C.C. (1983). The family as patient in medicine. *Soc Sci Med, 17,* 1–16.

Shekleton, M.E. (1987). Coping with chronic respiratory difficulty. *Nurs Clin, 22*(3), 569–581.

Strauss, A.L., Corbin, J., Fagerhaugh, S. et al. (1984). *Chronic illness and the quality of life* (2nd ed.). St. Louis: Mosby.

Versluys, H.P. (1980). Physical rehabilitation and family dynamics. *Rehabil Lit, 41*(3–4), 58–65.

Weisman, A.D. (1984). *The coping capacity. On the nature of being moral.* New York: Human Sciences Press.

Whitehouse, F.A. (1953). Habilitation—concept and process. *J Rehabil, 19,* 4–7.

Whitehouse, F.A. (1976). The importance of habilitation philosophy. *J Rehabil, 42* (5), 2–14.

SECTION II
Systems

Systems are a major component of the Contingency Model of Long-Term Care, with the functioning of any one system being contingent upon the functioning of all other systems. The family and its individual subsystems form the core of the model, with the suprasystems (community, society) playing a role in family functioning when one of its members has a chronic condition. Subsystems may occur within the individual system (e.g. cardiovascular, cognitive), family system (e.g., parent-child, sibling, spouse), community system (e.g., health care, education), or social system (e.g., economic, political). All systems are important because they interact with, and are mutually influenced by, each other.

This section provides an overview of the individual, family, community, and societal systems. Chapter 4 covers the individual system and its identifying characteristics. Included in this chapter are theories of individual development relevant to the model (Erikson's psychosocial theory, Piaget's cognitive development theory, social learning theory, and developmental task theory) and the identifying characteristics of individuals (e.g., age, gender), likely to influence the impact of chronic conditions on families. Chapter 5 presents an overview of the family system and its identifying characteristics. This chapter describes characteristics of families likely to influence the impact of chronic conditions on families. Chapter 6 presents an overview of the community and societal suprasystems, and Chapter 7 provides additional information about the suprasystems and chronic conditions.

4 The Individual System

This chapter provides an overview of the individual system and its identifying characteristics. Theories of individual development relevant to the Contingency Model of Long-Term Care include Erikson's psychosocial theory, Piaget's cognitive development theory, social learning theory, and developmental task theory. Characteristics of individuals likely to influence the impact of chronic conditions include age, gender, and temperament.

Individuals, as systems, are made up of biologic, emotional, social, cognitive, and spiritual subsystems. Each subsystem may be affected by the presence of a chronic condition. Although the focus of this book is not on the biologic subsystem, it is an important component of nursing care and cannot be overlooked. Figure 4–1 represents subsystems of the individual and shows the relationships of the individual system to its suprasystems.

Individuals follow a general predictable pattern of development, yet each person also develops in a style uniquely personal. These individual differences are due partly to hereditary and partly to environmental influences. Although human development can be viewed from a variety of theoretic perspec-

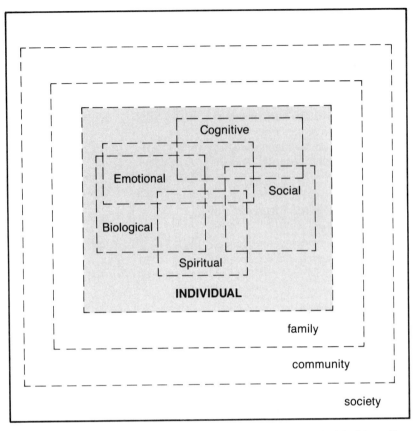

FIGURE 4–1 Individual Systems Component of the Contingency Model of Long-Term Care. The small boxes in the larger box represent subsystems of the individual. Broken lines indicate the openness of relationships between the individual system and its suprasystems.

tives, several are especially relevant to clinical practice and are reviewed briefly in this chapter. Since no single theory is useful in all situations, it is important to be aware of theories that can provide guidelines for clinical practice. Unless otherwise noted, discussion of the theories is taken from Hymovich and Chamberlin (1980). Guidelines for assessing individual systems from the perspective of these theories are also provided.

Theories of Individual Development

Psychosocial Theory

Erikson's theory of psychosocial development encompasses the life span and is an expansion of Freud's psychosexual framework. Its focus is on the autonomy of the ego and development of the personality through active involvement with the environment that occurs through the process of mutual regulation. Mutual regulation means that, as individual members grow and develop together, each person influences the development of the other. This interrelation of person and environment is consistent with systems theory.

Erikson's (1963) theory consists of eight stages, each with a psychosocial task to be mastered by the individual. Inherent in each stage is a developmental crisis, or turning point, when there is a period of increased vulnerability to, and heightened potential for, mastering the particular task. Erikson emphasizes the need for the person to actively cope with the tasks, not just pass through each phase. To move from one stage to the next, successful resolution of the previous developmental crisis is required. If resolution is not successful, later development becomes more difficult. Preparation for each stage begins in the previous stage and elaboration continues into subsequent ones. Choices at each stage represent opposite polarities to be balanced by the individual. For example, during the first stage of development the polarities are trust versus mistrust, whereas during adulthood, these polarities are generativity versus stagnation. Achievement at each stage may be hindered for the chronically ill person, and perhaps also for other family members, unless concerted efforts are made to foster their development. The polarities for each stage are listed in Table 4–1.

Cognitive Theory

Piaget's theory focuses on the cognitive aspects of development. Piaget (Piaget & Inhelder, 1969) assumes that personality evolves from a composite interrelation of affective and intellectual functions. His focus, however, is on the function of intellectual structures. The basic framework consists of a **schema** (organizational structure) and **adaptation.** Piaget views cognitive development as an integrated process involving maturation of the neurologic system, interaction with the physical world, and social communication. Initially, an infant's world is one of physiologic tensions, unorganized sensory capacities, and rudimentary motor patterns, devoid of objects and time. The formation of schemata that encompass internalized thought processes and overt motor behavior enables the child to organize and adapt to the environment. **Adaptation** takes place through the processes of assimilation and accommodation. **Assimilation** is the integration of new stimuli into already existing schemata. **Accommodation** is the modification of existing schemata, or the formation of new ones for stimuli that do not fit existing structures. For example, a child who has had many respiratory infections may be able to assimilate the diagnosis of cystic fibrosis into an existing schema for respiratory illness. On the other hand, a child diagnosed with diabetes may have to modify (accommodate) the existing schema for respiratory illness to include the new type of illness.

Development is an evolutionary process with a series of sequential stages and substages. Although Piaget suggests an approximate time frame for each stage, he notes there is no specific age at which a stage begins. Variability in timing is based on individual differences, cultural expectations, and experiences. Each of the theory's four stages is characterized by a different thought process. These stages and their characteristic thought processes, described in Table 4–2, have important implications for anyone communicating with youngsters.

During the **sensorimotor stage** (from birth to about age 2 years) infants learn through sensory and motor experiences. They assimilate and accommodate through actions and the sensations of tasting (everything goes into the mouth), touching, seeing, and hearing. Infants move from reflex behavior to a rudimentary understanding of the concepts of permanence, time, and space, and from motor communication to beginning language. Towards the end of this stage, they begin to differentiate between cause and effect.

The **preoperational** child (between approximately ages 2 and 7 years) is unable to differentiate between self and the world. The primary characteristics of this stage include (1) egocentrism (viewing

Table 4–1 Erikson's Developmental Tasks and Polarities

Infant	Establishing basic trust while overcoming mistrust
Toddler	Developing a sense of autonomy while overcoming feelings of shame and doubt
Preschooler	Developing a sense of initiative while overcoming feelings of guilt
School age child	Developing a sense of industry while overcoming a sense of inferiority
Adolescent	Developing a sense of identity rather than one of role confusion
Young adult	Developing a sense of intimacy with persons rather than a sense of isolation
Adult	Establishing a sense of generativity while avoiding stagnation
Older adult	Achieving a sense of integrity rather than one of despair

Source: Adapted from Erikson, 1963.

Table 4–2 Piaget's Stages and Characteristics of Cognitive Development

Age	Stage	Characteristics
Birth to 18 months or 2 years	Sensorimotor	Functioning depends on sensory and motor experiences (feeling, seeing, hearing, tasting). Self expression and communication are through motor activities.
1½ or 2 years to 7 years	Preoperational thought	Acquires language (symbolic thought, mental representations) Egocentrism (views world from own perspective) No concept of reversibility No concept of conservation Centering (concentrates on one detail rather than whole)
7 to 11 years	Concrete operational thought	Understands concepts of conservation, classification, serializing, reversibility in relation to concrete objects No longer egocentric
11 or 12 years to 15 years	Formal thought	Can reason on basis of propositions or hypotheses Can solve complicated abstract problems

Source: Adapted from Piaget & Inhelder, 1969.

the world from one's own perspective), (2) concreteness (preoccupation with external perceptual events), (3) magical thinking, (4) irreversibility (inability to conceptualize processes in reverse), (5) centering (focusing on a single part of an event rather than the whole), and (6) transductive reasoning (thinking moves from one particular to another, but the child cannot generalize). During this period children learn to use symbols such as language and mental representations. Young children operate mainly on the basis of immediate pleasure and pain, cannot plan ahead, and cannot choose present discomfort for promised relief later. They confuse wishes with reality, and their sense of past and future is not well established. Consequently they may think they will "outgrow" the disability or "catch" someone else's handicap.

Bibace and Walsh (1979) describe three subphases of understanding illness that are characteristic of the preoperational child. In the first phase, incomprehension, the child evades questions related to what, why, and how and gives answers that appear irrelevant. When asked what made her sick, a young preschooler responded, "The ghost makes you sick down the hole." In the second phase, phenomenonism, the child defines illness by a single external symptom usually related to something the child has seen or heard. Getting diabetes is "getting stuck with a needle." In the third phase, contagion, the

child explains illness by external objects, persons, or events that are either spatially or temporally near the immediate world of the sick person, but not actually touching the person. No explanation is given for causality other than proximity to the person, object, or event. For example, you can catch a cold by walking near someone.

When children reach the stage of concrete operations, there is clear differentiation of oneself and the world, and of the internal and external self. At this stage children focus on the concrete as opposed to the abstract. They become less egocentric and can understand the process of reversal, specify relationships among events, and classify events.

A systematic progression in understanding of illness-related concepts clearly parallels Piaget's stages of cognitive development from global to concrete to abstract (Perrin & Gerrity, 1981). There are two subphases of explanations about illness in the period of concrete operations (Bibace & Walsh, 1979). During the **first phase,** contamination, children cannot differentiate between mind and body, so bad behavior can be equated with illness in the same way that germs can. Illness is defined by multiple symptoms and can include "reference to bodily functions that are evident in external surface body parts or areas" (p. 293), such as a runny nose or pain from a cut. Children can draw a direct causal link between the source (e.g., bad behavior, germs) and its effect on the body. The cure is conceptualized as occurring when there is direct contact with the person, object, or event. Kindergarten children understand causes of illness to be magical or the result of disobeying rules (Perrin & Gerrity, 1981). The **second phase** is internalization, with illness described in a global way as being within the body. Illness occurs from swallowing or ingesting dirt, bugs, or germs. Rubbing medicine over a hurt, or kissing it, will make it go away. Fourth graders believe illness is caused by germs, but the complexity of how germs cause illness is not evident until the eighth grade (Perrin & Gerrity, 1981).

Development of concepts about illness may differ in healthy and chronically ill children (Perrin & Gerrity, 1981). Healthy children show a marked transition in understanding around age 11 or 12 years, but children with asthma or diabetes demonstrate an earlier spurt around age 9 years. Children with chronic conditions tend to have a more sophisticated understanding of the cause, treatment, and prevention of illness than do healthy children. Specifically, children with diabetes understand prevention better, whereas children with asthma have a better understanding of the recognition and causes of illness. Nurses and physicians may tend to overestimate what younger children understand and underestimate what older children understand (Perrin & Gerrity, 1981).

Once children reach the stage of **formal operations,** they are no longer bound by concrete reality. They learn to deal with abstract concepts and make hypotheses. They can understand and appreciate satires, proverbs, and analogies. Around age 15, cognitive processes are those of an adult.

There are also two stages of formal operational explanations of illness (Bibace & Walsh, 1979). In the first stage, physiological, illness is defined by internal physiologic structures and functions with multiple external symptoms, causes, and cures. Children become aware that personal actions contribute to illness and outcome and also perceive that they have some control over the illness. They are no longer bounded by the concrete and, therefore, are able to describe functions not visible externally, such as cells. In the final stage, psychophysiological, youngsters comprehend psychologic as well as physiologic causes of illness, such as worry causing a headache. By 12 or 13 years children begin to understand multiple causes of illness, that bodies respond differently to causative agents, and that there is an interaction between host and environment in causing illness (Perrin & Gerrity, 1981).

Learning Theories

Stimulus-response theories Learning theories place a heavy emphasis on the environment for shaping behavior. According to these theories behavior is learned by association with a stimulus. This process is considered to be the same at all ages, so there are no stages as with psychosocial and cognitive developmental theories. Reinforced behavior is strengthened, whereas punished or ignored behavior is weakened. **Stimulus-response (S-R) theory** is based on the concept of conditioning. Conditioning occurs when one or more stimuli (S) are repeatedly associated with one or more responses (R). In **classical conditioning (S-R)** a neutral stimulus is paired with a stimulus already known to elicit a response.

In **instrumental (or operant) conditioning (S-R-S),** the organism learns to manipulate the environment to produce the desired response. Skinner (1971) notes that many behaviors, called operants, which are "emitted" by the organism, cannot be attributed to a specific stimulus. Through S-R-S conditioning the probability increases that an emitted response will recur under the same conditions. The desired response is reinforced when it follows either presentation of a stimulus (positive reinforcer) or removal of an aversive stimulus (negative reinforcer). Rewarding behavior is similar to presenting a positive reinforcer or removing a negative reinforcer, whereas punishment is similar to removing a positive reinforcer or presenting a negative reinforcer. Giving a child praise (positive reinforcer) or refraining from nagging (negative reinforcer) are adult activities that may increase a child's good behavior. Showing a client his or her weight loss on a scale (positive reinforcement) but not commenting on no weight loss (negative reinforcement) are activities a nurse may use with adult clients. Restricting a child to the house (removal of positive reinforcer) or spanking (presentation of a negative reinforcer) are examples of punishment that are likely to decrease the child's misbehavior. An example of removing a positive reinforcer might be refusing to keep a promise because the patient's blood pressure has not decreased. On the other hand, blaming the person for not adhering to the regimen is the presentation of a negative reinforcer (See Table 4–3). It is also possible to extinguish behavior by ignoring unde-

Table 4–3 Reward and Punishment of
Behavior with Reinforcers

	Reinforcer	
	Positive	*Negative*
Reward	**present** (praise)	**remove** (stop nagging)
Punishment	**remove** (restrict to house)	**present** (spank)

sired behaviors. A variety of reinforcers may be rewarding to a person. However, what is reinforcing to one person may not be reinforcing for another, and what is reinforcing in one situation may not work in a different situation. Some rewards are concrete (candy, money) whereas others may be social (praise, hug). Some reinforcers, such as tokens or gold stars, may be exchanged at a later time for more concrete reinforcers. It is essential to tailor rewards to the individual.

Schedules of reinforcement can be either continuous (after every behavior) or intermittent. Intermittent reinforcement may be delivered according to a time interval (one reinforcement per given unit of time) or ratio interval (one reinforcement after a specific number of responses). Interval and ratio schedules can be either variable or fixed. A fixed-interval reinforcement might be letting a child watch television each evening after dinner, whereas a variable interval schedule would be praising a child every 2 to 10 minutes for remaining with an activity. A fixed-ratio schedule would be praising an adult each time she gets out of bed, whereas a variable-ratio reinforcer would be praising a patient every second to fourth time he walks down the hallway.

Behavior can be **shaped** by rewarding responses that come closer and closer to the desired behavior, until finally the desired behavior is reached and reinforced. Shaping the behavior of a person who is unwilling to walk may begin by first reinforcing sitting up in bed, then dangling legs over the bed, later standing, and eventually walking.

Social Learning Theory The learning theories of Pavlov and Skinner form the basis for social learning theory. From the perspective of social learning theory, much learning occurs vicariously through observation and imitation of others (Bandura, 1971), and reinforcement is based on subjective expectations of future consequences of one's actions (Rotter, Chance, & Phares, 1972). Childhood personality patterns develop primarily through imitation of parental models and other significant persons. Imitation, or modeling, is synonymous with what other theorists call identification. It involves the direct copying of certain behaviors, which leads to acquiring another person's mannerisms or style ("He acts just like his father") as well as accepting the other person's values and beliefs. Through this process, children develop a conscience, acquire sex-role behavior patterns, and learn to behave as adults. Clients and their families may learn techniques of their treatment through observation of the nurses working with them.

Intervention based on the social learning approach focuses on changing behavior and is built on the premise that people can change their behavior if they are committed to doing so. This time-limited, specific approach highlights one problem at a time. The process involves (1) mutual goal setting between client and professional, (2) analyzing behaviors and the conditions under which they occur, (3) identifying appropriate rewards and punishments, (4) giving feedback and evaluation of the program's success, and (5) revising goals or rewards as indicated in the evaluation (Henderson, Hall, & Lipton, 1979). Nursing intervention strategies based on social learning theories are described in more detail in Chapter 14.

Developmental Theories

Developmental theories are stage theories concerned with the maturation of the individual. Of the many developmental theories, the most relevant for the Contingency Model of Long-Term Care is the one related to developmental tasks. The concept of individual developmental tasks originated with Havighurst (1953, 1972) and was expanded to family tasks by Duvall (1977). The use of the term *task* implies that the person is an active participant, as noted in Erikson's theory. Tasks arise from three sources: physical maturation, cultural pressures, and personal values and aspirations. To a certain extent, tasks are culture bound because they are set by societal norms. Individuals take on tasks as a result of the expectations of others, discovery of their own changing capacities, and through observation of others. The person gains a new sense of self-awareness, perceives new possibilities, and feels ready to learn new ways of coping with a situation (taking on a new developmental task). Developmental tasks serve as guidelines that enable individuals and families to know society's expectations at any given developmental stage.

Developmental tasks and timing   The concept of developmental tasks implies timing; that is, individuals initiate actions because of their maturational and social development as well as their reactions to environmental pressures. Early tasks such as learning to walk arise from physical maturation, but bodily changes during puberty contribute to changes in self-identity.

Biological timing is important in the early years, but later change is tied to a social timetable, with individuals acting on aspirations and expectations arising from their interactions in a social environment. Social clocks prescribe the proper time sequence for activities such as leaving school, getting a job, marrying, and having children. Neugarten (1979) speaks of being "on schedule" or "off schedule" with biological timetables, and "early," "late," or "on time" with social schedules.

Individual Developmental Tasks   Individual developmental tasks are growth responsibilities arising at a particular stage in the person's life cycle. Persons who achieve the tasks successfully will feel satisfied, achieve approval from society, and be successful in accomplishing later tasks. For persons unable to accomplish them, the outcome is likely to be unhappiness, disapproval by society, and difficulty with later tasks (Duvall, 1977; Havighurst, 1972).

Individual developmental tasks are described in detail, especially for children in the United States, by Havighurst (1972). These tasks were later modified (Hymovich & Chamberlin, 1980) and incorporated under five general tasks for children and revised again so that they now encompass the adult life span. Specific tasks within these general ones vary at each stage of development. General individual tasks of children and adults are to (1) establish and maintain healthy growth and nutrition patterns; (2) develop and maintain control over one's body; (3) understand and relate to the physical world; (4) develop and maintain self-awareness and a satisfying sense of self; and (5) establish and maintain effective relationships with others.

Infants and young children learn to master developmental tasks related to early socialization, at-tachment, and separation: developing trust (infancy) and autonomy (preschool); settling into daily routines (eating, sleeping); developing large and small muscle control; learning to control impulses (share, wait); and mastering the basics of toilet training. The occurrence of chronic illness during these early years can interfere with mastering any of these tasks. For example, children requiring frequent hospitalizations, or siblings whose parents are with the chronically ill child, may have difficulty with attachment and separation. Learning to trust others can be inhibited when children suffer frequent assaults to their body integrity; and mastering muscle control may be complicated by various types of restraints or conditions, such as cerebral palsy.

School age children learn more complex physical and social skills and become contributing members to family functioning. They learn the basic skills of reading, writing, calculating, and problem solving. During these years, children come to terms with their sex-role identity, develop a sense of themselves as worthy persons, and develop inner moral controls.

According to Duvall (1977) the developmental tasks of adolescents include accepting and learning to effectively use their changing body, achieving a satisfying and socially acceptable sex role, developing more mature relationships with peers, achieving emotional independence from parents and other adults, learning to be adults, establishing an identity as socially responsible, developing intellectual skills and social sensitivities necessary for civic competence, and preparing for marriage and family life.

During the middle years, adults deal with the developmental task of establishing and maintaining intimacy versus developing a sense of isolation. To accomplish this goal involves other tasks, such as learning new skills, establishing oneself in the work setting, and forming intimate social relationships. The presence of a chronic condition may jeopardize social relationships. Tasks such as marriage, childbearing, child rearing, obtaining higher education, and employment may be affected in varying degrees. Work relationships may suffer also. Employers may be reluctant to hold a person's position, and the person may not have the energy to do the job. Temporary or permanent loss or disfigurement may lead to doubt, and wondering what he or she will be like can add to the person's isolation or sense of isolation.

During the later years of maturity, people deal with the task Erikson calls generativity while avoiding separation or self-absorption. At this time, chronically ill older adults may have to move into the homes of their children, which leads to their ambivalence toward the family.

A task of the older adult is to achieve ego integrity (Erikson, 1963). Characteristics of ego integrity are (1) cognizance of aging, reconciling past failures with present and future concerns; (2) acceptance of the inevitability of strife and the realization that everyone will die; and (3) a sense of growth and purpose in the future (Dietz, 1985). When a chronic condition afflicts an adult, there may be an identity crisis, especially if educational or occupational roles are affected.

Identifying Characteristics

Identifying characteristics are a complex set of variables that help define and describe each system. These characteristics transcend the typical demographic variables, for they play an important part in determining how one responds, adapts, and manages chronic illness. In addition, they affect one's general level of functioning. Variables in individual

responses to illness are numerous and include tolerance for pain, desire for self-care, and knowledge and understanding of the illness process. These identifying characteristics and other variables influence what people know, believe, and think about their condition, how it affects them, what symptoms they regard as serious, and what they should do about the symptoms. This section explores some ways these characteristics identify the individual system and may influence its level of functioning when a chronic condition is present. As depicted in Figure 4–2, identifying characteristics have the potential to influence stressors, coping strategies, strengths, needs, and level of functioning.

Age

Age influences perceptions of illness and physiologic as well as psychologic responses to a situation. It also influences life-style, social status, roles, and strengths. For example, a 9-year-old youngster might be a sibling, student, and good tennis player, whereas a 40-year-old adult might be a spouse, par-

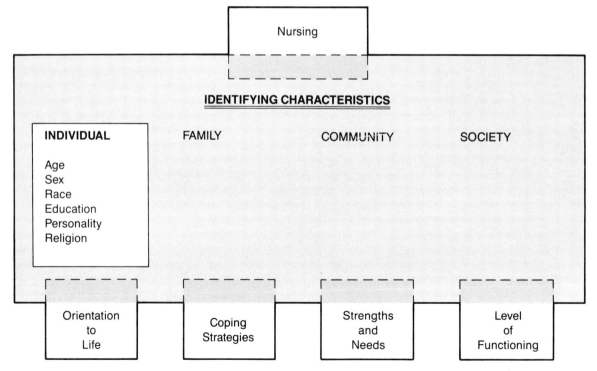

FIGURE 4–2 Relationship of Individual Identifying Characteristics to Other Variables of the Contingency Model of Long-Term Care. Each system has identifying characteristics that overlap with (broken lines) and are closely related to their orientation to life, coping strategies, strengths and needs, and level of functioning. Nursing care involves assessing identifying characteristics and using the information to plan and provide appropriate nursing interventions.

ent, wage earner, and respected local government representative.

Physiologic Responses Age affects the nature and type of physiologic condition one is likely to have. For example, age significantly predicts the incidence and severity of diabetes. Prevalence increases with age, with 70% of all diabetics being over 44 years of age (Jenny, 1984). Ninety-five percent of the patients with type I insulin dependent diabetes mellitus (IDDM) have onset under age 25 years whereas 85% of those with type II noninsulin dependent diabetes mellitus (NIDDM), are diagnosed after age 44 (Oleson, 1981). Degenerative diseases and disabilities such as osteoarthritis become more prevalent in middle age and increase over the life span (Mechanic, 1986). Premature infants may have respiratory distress syndrome whereas older children and adults will not. Older adults are predisposed to certain diseases not found in younger adults (Minaker & Rowe, 1985). For example, clinical manifestations of polycystic kidney disease are often not evident until the sixth decade of life. Pulmonary carcinoma is generally not manifested until middle or later life for individuals who smoked cigarettes in early life because it takes time to accumulate a carcinogenic dose of cigarette tobacco. On the other hand, diseases such as carcinoma of the breast may have a less virulent natural history in later life. Diseases such as hyperthyroidism, diabetes, and rheumatoid arthritis have different manifestations in younger and older adults. It is helpful to keep this in mind when listening to people talk of others they know with a similar diagnosis but a different trajectory. Knowing the age and background of the person you are talking with and the individual that person is talking about may help clarify the situation.

Psychologic Responses Children undergoing developmental transitions (e.g., starting school, puberty) are likely to have decreased ability to tolerate other stresses and frustrations that might occur with a chronic condition. Age may also influence the impact of a chronic condition on siblings of chronically ill children. However, findings are contradictory, as some studies report younger siblings may be more vulnerable than older (Lavigne & Ryan, 1979), whereas others report increased problems among older siblings (Gath, 1977). Undoubtedly, other variables besides age mediate the impact and need to be considered.

Some studies of adults with chronic physical conditions reveal poor mental-health and psychologic status in younger adults, but investigations with the elderly are less consistent. In one study, adults with cancer and the poorest mental health scores were women under age 40 years undergoing treatment and not fully capable of normal activity (Cassileth et al, 1986). Younger family members also had greater depression, poorer emotional ties, and more loss of control than did older relatives. Three alternative explanations regarding the relationship of age to chronic illness were proposed (Cassileth et al, 1986): (1) Chronic conditions come as a greater shock to younger individuals. (2) Increasing age may exert a positive influence on one's ability to deal with life stress. (3) Age represents a major risk factor for psychologic distress. Regardless of the possible explanation, evidence suggests that age is an important mediator in the impact of chronic conditions and should be considered in planning care.

Other studies also note developmental differences in adult psychosocial functioning. Patients with cancer under age 50 years were found to experience more frequent and more severe psychologic problems than did those over age 70 (Edlund & Sneed, 1989; Ganz, Schag, & Heinrich, 1985). The research may indicate that older patients used more denial than did the younger. Furthermore, the later years see changes in life-style and social status (e.g., retirement); illness and death among friends and significant others; and often relocation of self, children, or grandchildren. Depression is common among the elderly experiencing the loss of loved ones through death and loss of home. Losses of autonomy, independence, and decision making accompany other life-style and social-status changes (e.g., retirement).

Aging is a psychosocial as well as a biologic process. Unique social, health, and economic issues over the life span influence personal development, coping resources, and physical functioning. Mechanic (1986) notes the importance of differentiating between age and cohort (generation) in considering the health and welfare of the elderly. Health outcomes of past cohorts can be used only with caution because those who are currently in their 70s and 80s have different life expectancies and needs than those who were that age 10 or 20 years ago.

Cognitive abilities and education level Age influences psychosocial responses to chronic conditions. For example, developmental differences in thinking among children and adults influence comprehension of illness and other life events. These differences are based on cognitive stage of development rather than merely on chronological age.

Chronological age is not synonymous with developmental level, so it is important to distinguish between age, and the cognitive, social, and emotional levels of development of children and adolescents. For example, a child may be age 8 years chronologically but functioning at 11 years cognitively and only 5 or 6 years emotionally and socially.

Cognitive abilities and educational level may differ from expectations based on a person's age. Although children can be expected to follow Piaget's stages of cognitive development, they will not all do so at the same chronological age. It is difficult during periods of transition from one stage to the next to know how much the child understands.

Many children function adequately, but their scholastic achievement may suffer. A significant number (20% to 40%) of children with chronic conditions have scholastic achievement lower than that of healthy children, despite average or better intellectual ability. Academic problems may be related to the child's difficulty in completing assignments, inflexible teachers, or school missed due to illness or the need to attend the clinic or hospital. Scholastic achievement may be affected indirectly if parents or teachers expect less of the child. Side effects of medications, such as drowsiness, may contribute to learning difficulties. Drugs associated with lower scholastic achievement include phenytoin taken for at least 2 years for epilepsy, and methotrexate. In addition, radiation therapy to prevent central nervous system complications of childhood leukemia also contributes to problems with scholastic achievement, with children acquiring leukemia at younger ages being more seriously affected than those who get the disease at a later age.

Not all adults reach the level of formal operations. Therefore it cannot be assumed that all individuals will understand complex or abstract notions. Educational and cognitive level affects one's capacity to learn.

Gender

Gender is another identifying characteristic that may influence response to chronic conditions. Much of the difference in sex-linked mortality is related to life-style factors such as smoking, violence, and heavy drinking. For example, most diseases prevalent among women are not life threatening, whereas those seen in men, such as cardiovascular disease, are life threatening. Women have a longer longevity than men by about 7 years, but they report more illnesses and use more medical services than do men (Mechanic, 1986). Levy (1981) noted that the decline in physical abilities is more rapid in women than in men.

Gender differences are noted in parents' response to either an actual or threatened loss (Cook, 1983; Miles et al, 1984; Trout, 1983) and differences in adult physiologic and psychosocial adaptation to selected chronic conditions (Pollack, 1986). As with age, findings regarding the impact of a child's chronic condition on siblings are mixed, with some reporting increased risk for male siblings, others reporting the opposite (Ferrari, 1987; Seligman, 1983), and some reporting an interaction of age and sex (Breslau, 1982). Other studies suggest that same-sex pairs of siblings in which one is disabled are at greater risk than are opposite-sex pairs (Ferrari, 1987).

Gender of the ill person and others in the family may influence the roles they assume in the family. The role of the male spouse is controversial. For example, Horowitz (1982) found that males tend to be less involved in direct care of family members, whereas King and colleagues (1986) found that husbands do provide direct care to their ill wives. Fitting and Rabins (1986) found that male care givers suffered fewer psychologic reactions than did female care givers.

Gender has also been found to influence attitudes. For example, in several studies, females were found to have more favorable attitudes toward handicapped persons than did males (Fiedler & Simpson, 1987; Newman & Simpson, 1983).

Personality Characteristics

The extent to which personality characteristics have an impact on health and chronic illness is equivocal. Some characteristics that have been studied as they pertain to chronic conditions are discussed in this chapter. Personality characteristics may be one of the variables that predispose people to appraise situations differently and therefore to have differing emotional responses to them (Cohen, 1979). For example, persons with low self-esteem are likely to interpret many situations as stressful and therefore have difficulty coping, leading to increased depression or anxiety. People who use repression as a defense mechanism may prolong stressful events by not confronting them.

Traits are "generalized dispositions to thoughts, feelings, and behavior and endure over substantial periods of time" (Costa & McCrae, 1980, p. 90). Interestingly, the concept of enduring personality traits has found little support in research. Current data suggest that personality traits are not stable across situations or over time and do relatively little to determine how a person will behave in a given situation. According to Mechanic (1986), it is probably more realistic to speak of predispositions or orientations that may vary with certain situations rather than traits. Although it may be useful to know how people generally respond to situations, one should note that they may not necessarily respond to their current stressors in the same manner. Since personality characteristics may only be predispositions, the potential exists to help individuals change ways of coping with certain situations, thereby strengthening their coping resources.

Among the personality characteristics thought to have bearing on adaptation to chronic conditions are temperament, hardiness, introspection, dispositional optimism, and locus of control. These characteristics are discussed in the following sections.

Temperament Individual differences in behavioral styles have been noted in infancy. Thomas, Chess, and Birch (1970) identified nine **temperament** qualities that characterize a child's individuality: (1) level and extent of motor activity, (2) regularity (rhythmicity) of daily schedule, (3) response to new objects, (4) adaptability to change, (5) sensitivity to stimuli, (6) intensity of response, (7) general mood (e.g., friendly, unfriendly, pleasant, unpleasant), (8) attention span, and (9) persistence in activity. Children with certain clusters of these temperament characteristics tend to have typical behavior patterns. For example, **easy children** were observed to have regular biological rhythms, positive mood, rapid adaptability, low or mildly intense reactions, and a positive approach to new situations. **Difficult children,** on the other hand, had irregular biological rhythms, a predominantly negative mood, slow adaptability to change, and intense negative or withdrawal reactions to new situations.

Temperament characteristics have important implications for children's interactions with their parents (Rutter & Hersov, 1977). Children who are extremely active, difficult to console and have irregular sleeping and waking patterns are likely to be criticized and scapegoated by their parents. When parents are under stress, they are likely to have problems with and "pick" on a child with a difficult temperament. Eight of the nine temperament di-

mensions were found to have highly significant associations with behavioral symptomatology (Wertlieb et al, 1987). These temperament orientations are high activity level, low adaptability, withdrawal from new stimuli, distractibility, high intensity, unpleasant or unhappy mood, a lack of persistence, and an irregular or unpredictable behavioral style. Temperament also appears to be differentially related to internalizing and externalizing behavioral symptomatology. Withdrawal was more relevant to internalizing problems, whereas high activity, high distractibility, and a low threshold of stimulation were more relevant to externalizing problems. These findings lend further empirical support to the notion that temperament is relevant to socioemotional functioning and the outcome of stress reactions, at least in school age children (Lerner & East, 1984).

Hardiness **Hardiness** may represent one aspect of a person's resistance to stress (Bigbee, 1985). The concept of hardiness was deductively derived from existential psychology (Kobassa & Maddi, 1981). Kobassa (1979) suggests that people who do not become ill when faced with serious stressors have a constellation of characteristics she calls hardiness. This concept, currently being studied by a number of nurse researchers, refers to a set of attitudes toward challenge, commitment, and control that mediate one's response to stress (Kobassa, 1979, Kobassa & Maddi, 1981). Hardy individuals view change as a challenge, are deeply involved and committed to various areas of life, and believe they can influence events. Antonovsky (1979) suggested a similar concept, coherence, as fostering adjustment to stress. Coherence involves a view of the world as comprehensible, manageable, and meaningful.

It has been hypothesized that a hardy personality style may play a role in decreasing the potential negative effects of life stressors (Lambert & Lambert, 1987), but more research is needed to support this. According to Pollack (1986), hardiness may have a direct effect on a chronically ill person's ability to cope or use social support. Preliminary studies of hardiness in relation to chronic conditions are relatively recent and their value in working with people who have chronic conditions remains to be seen.

Introspection **Introspection** is a person's tendency "to think about oneself and one's motivations and feelings" (Mechanic, 1986 p. 108). Introspection may be one of the many personality inclinations or predispositions that interact with perceptions of a stressful event and the ability to cope with it. Evidence suggests that introspective persons tend to report psychologic and physical distress, be upset by stressful life events, and have negative self-evaluations. They are likely to use medical, psychiatric, and other helping services. Introspection also may be associated with qualities such as sensitivity, empathy, creativity, and artistic expression.

Dispositional Optimism **Dispositional optimism,** one's tendency to judge expectations optimistically rather than pessimistically, may be a factor determining how well people respond to stress (Scheier, Weintraub, & Carver, 1986). Optimism was found to be positively associated with the following: problem-focused coping, especially when the situation was perceived as controllable; use of positive reinterpretation; seeking social support; and acceptance/resignation when the situation was perceived as uncontrollable. Optimism was negatively correlated with denial/distancing. That is, the more optimistic the people were, the more they were likely to reinterpret the event in a positive way, seek social support, and become resigned to it; they were also less likely to use denial or distancing. Patterns of association between optimism and emotion-focused coping were more variable. These findings suggest that optimism may facilitate coping even when an event cannot be controlled but is something the person gets used to. Pessimists tended to focus on stress, ventilate feelings, and adopt coping strategies that implied disengagement from the goal with which the stressor was interfering. Perhaps optimists do better than pessimists because their strategies are likely to be problem focused and therefore "pay off."

Locus of Control **Locus of control** is a psychologic construct that refers to the extent a person believes his or her own actions influence events in the world (Rotter, 1966). Internally controlled people believe events are contingent on their own actions, that is, are under personal control. Externally controlled people believe events are unrelated to their own behavior and, therefore, beyond their control, i.e., events are in the hands of fate, luck, chance, or powerful others.

Stress is a transient state, so its intensity is influenced by the immediate situation: A person's state at the stressful moment is more likely to determine response than is the enduring trait. For example, a person with Type A characteristics usually has an internal locus of control, but when an event is sufficiently stressful locus of control may change to exter-

nal. Studies suggest that internal locus of control is significantly related to metabolic control of adolescents with diabetes (Hamburg & Inoff, 1982) and renal disease (Hudson et al, 1986).

Health locus of control is a dimension of one's locus of control and pertinent to understanding families of children and adults with chronic conditions. Health locus of control refers to the extent to which people believe their health is a function of their own control or of external control. Health locus of control may be related to compliance. As compared with healthy adults, chronically ill adults consistently state lower internal beliefs and higher beliefs in control by chance and powerful adults (Wallston & Wallston, 1981). Studies of health locus of control in adults and children suggest that it varies with age (internality increases with age), socioeconomic status (SES) (internality increases with higher SES), and gender (greater in females than males), and the nature of the child's condition (Carraccio, McCormick, & Weller, 1987; Perrin & Shapiro, 1985).

Assessment

Table 4–4 provides an overview of areas to cover while assessing the individual system's identifying characteristics. More detail regarding assessment is provided in this Section.

Cognitive Abilities and Educational Level

Relevant for chronically ill or disabled children is the child's grade in school. Appropriate grade level for age was found to be more predictive of overall academic, social, and family functioning than was information from a neurological examination (Hodgman et al, 1979). Close monitoring of the child's school functioning and family life is necessary for early identification of cognitive and emotional problems (Rubinstein, 1984).

Equally important for nursing intervention is the cognitive and educational level of adults. Although individuals may have completed a certain grade level, they may in actuality be functioning either above or below that level. One way to be certain they fully comprehend what you are saying is to seek feedback through nonthreatening questioning.

Personality Characteristics

Not all people who experience stressful life events become ill. However, it is still unclear which person-

Table 4–4 Assessment of Identifying Characteristics

System	Useful Information

Individual
  Chronically ill person
  [Use interviews, Checklists, PPIINFO]
  Other family members
	Age
	Sex
	Educational level
	  Grade in school
	  Last grade completed
	Occupation
	Race
	Religion
	Personality characteristics
	  Introspection
	  Hardiness
	  Locus of control
	  Dispositonal Optimism
	  Temperament
	Developmental level
	  Emotional
	  Cognitive
	  Social
	Health status
	  Past
	  Current

Strengths	Needs

ality traits are most useful for predicting health outcomes or may modify the associations between stress and disease (Elliott & Eisdorfer, 1982). It may be helpful to assess an individual's personality traits if such information will facilitate planning and providing care.

Temperament The Carey Infant Temperament Questionnaire (Carey & McDevitt, 1978) is used clinically to assess maternal perceptions of their 4-through 8-month-old infants' temperament. The scale is based on the infant temperament characteristics described by Chess and Thomas (1976). The questionnaire contains 95 six-point Likert-type items (1 = almost never through 6 = almost always) arranged in nine subscales and takes about 25–30 minutes to complete. The infants can be categorized into one of five clusters: (1) difficult, (2) slow to warm up, (3) intermediate high (difficult), (4) intermediate low (easy), and (5) easy. Total test interitem correlations ranged from .76 to .83 (Carey & McDevitt, 1978). Test-retest reliability was .66 to .81 for a 3 1/2-week interval.

Additional temperament questionnaires are available for older children. The Toddler Temperament Scale is for children age 1 to 3 years. Two Behavioral Style Questionnaires, one for 3- to 7-year-olds and one for 8- to 12-year-olds, are also available. The Dimension of Temperament Survey (DOTS) (Lerner et al, 1982) is a 34-item instrument to assess temperament of individuals from age 3 to 22 years. It contains the following dimensions: activity attention span, approach-withdrawal, distractibility/adaptability, rhythmicity, and reactivity.

Locus of control Locus of control has been measured in adults by means of the Rotter Internal-

External (I-E) Locus of Control Scale (Rotter, 1966) and in children with the Nowicki-Strickland Children's Locus of Control Scale (NSLC) (Nowicki & Strickland, 1973). The NSLC is a 40-item instrument with yes or no responses to questions such as, "Do you have a choice in deciding who your friends are?" or "Do you believe that wishing can make good things happen?"

The Multidimensional Health Locus of Control (MHLOC) scale (Wallston, Wallston, DeVillis, 1978) has been used to measure health locus of control in adults. This instrument measures the extent to which people believe their health is a result of their actions or those of more powerful others, such as medical personnel, or to fate, luck, or chance.

The Children's Health Locus of Control scale (Parcel & Meyer, 1978) is a 20-item instrument with moderately high internal consistency reliability, moderate test-retest reliability, and evidence of concurrent validity. Children age 5 to 12 years respond yes or no to statements such as, "I can do things to keep from getting sick" or "Good health comes from being lucky."

Summary

This chapter identified characteristics of individuals likely to influence or be influenced by chronic conditions. Individual characteristics include the person's age, gender, and personality characteristics. These variables provide guidelines for data collection during initial and ongoing assessments of the patient and family. The reader is cautioned to recall that each individual system is unique, and while certain generalities are possible, they may not be true for any given person. To provide high quality, meaningful care, it is important to carefully identify in both individuals with chronic conditions and their families in both the characteristics that make them unique.

References

Antonovsky, A. (1979). *Health, stress, and coping.* San Francisco: Jossey.

Bandura, A. (1971). *Psychological modeling.* Chicago: Aldine-Atherton.

Bibace, R., & Walsh, M.E. (1979). Developmental stages in children's conceptions of illness. In G.C. Stone, F. Cohen, N.E. Adler (Eds.), *Health psychology—A handbook* (pp. 285–301). San Francisco: Jossey-Bass.

Bigbee, J. (1985). Hardiness: A new perspective on health promotion. *Nurse Pract, 10*(11), 51–56.

Breslau, N. (1982). Siblings of disabled children: Birth order and age-spacing effects. *J Acad Child Psychiatry, 10,* 85–96.

Carey, W.B., & McDevitt, S.C. (1978). Revision of the infant temperament questionnaire. *Pediatrics, 61,* 735–739.

Carraccio, C.L., McCormick, M.C., & Weller, S.C. (1987). Chronic disease: Effect on health cognition and health locus of control. *J Pediatr, 110,* 982–987.

Cassileth, B.R., Lusk, E.J., Brown, L.L., Cross, P.A., Walsh, W.P., & Hurwitz, S. (1986). Factors associated with psychological distress in cancer patients. *Med Pediatr Oncol, 14,* 251–254.

Chess, S., & Thomas, A. (Eds.). (1976). *Annual progress in child psychiatry and child development.* New York: Brunner/Mazel.

Cohen, F. (1979). Personality, stress, and the development of physical illness. In G.C. Stone, F. Cohen, N.E. Adler (Eds.). *Health psychology—A handbook* (pp. 77–111). San Francisco: Jossey-Bass.

Cook, J. (1983). A death in the family: Parental bereavement in the first year. *Suicide Life Threat Behav, 13*(1), 42–61.

Costa, P.T., & McCrae, R.R. (1986). Still stable after all these years: Personality as a key to some issues in adulthood and old age. In P.B. Baltes & O.G. Brim, Jr. (Eds.), *Life-Span development and behavior* (pp. 65–102). New York: Academic Press.

Dietz, K.A. (1985). Middlescence. *Cancer Nurs, Suppl 1,* 25–27.

Duvall, E.M. (1977). *Marriage and family development.* Philadelphia: Lippincott.

Edlund, B., & Sneed, N.V. (1989). Emotional responses to the diagnosis of cancer: Age-related comparisons. *Oncol Nurs Forum, 16*(5), 691–697.

Elliott, G.R., & Eisdorfer, C. (Eds.) (1982) *Stress and human health.* New York: Springer.

Erikson, E.H. (1963). *Childhood and society* (2nd ed.). New York: Norton.

Ferrari, M. (1987). The diabetic child and well siblings: Risks to the well child's self-concept. *Child Health Care, 15*(3), 141–148.

Fiedler, C.R., & Simpson, R.L. (1987). Modifying the attitudes of nonhandicapped high school students toward handicapped peers. *Except Child, 53*(4), 342–349.

Fitting, M. et al. (1986). Caregivers for dementia patients: A comparison of husbands and wives. *Gerontologist, 26*(3), 248–252.

Ganz, P., Schag, C., & Heinrich, R. (1985). The psychosocial impact of cancer on the elderly: A comparison with younger patients. *J Am Psychiatr Soc, 33*(6), 429–435.

Gath, A. (1977). The impact of an abnormal child upon the parents. *Br J Psychiatry, 130,* 405–410.

Hamburg, B.A., & Inoff, G.E. (1982). Relationships between behavioral factors and diabetic control in children and adolescents: A camp study. *Psychosom Med, 44,* 321–339.

Havighurst, R.J. (1953). *Human development and education.* New York: Longmans, Green.

Havighurst, R.J. (1972). *Developmental tasks and education.* New York: David McKay.

Henderson, J.B., Hall, S.M., & Lipton, H.L. (1979). Changing self-destructive behaviors. In G.C. Stone, F. Cohen, N.E. Adler (Eds.). *Health psychology—A handbook* (pp. 141–160). San Francisco: Jossey-Bass.

Hodgman, C.H., McArarney, E.R., Meyers, G.H., Iker, H. (1979). Emotional complications of adolescent grand mal epilepsy. *J Pediatr, 95,* 309–312.

Horowitz, M.J. (1982). Psychological. processes induced by illness, injury, and loss. In T. Millon, C. Green, & R. Meagher (Eds.), *Handbook of clinical health psychology.* New York: Plenum.

Hudson, J., Fieldly, D., Jones, S., et al. (1986). Adherence to medical regime and related factors in youngsters on dialysis. *Br J Clin Psychol, 23,* 49–59.

Hymovich, D.P., & Chamberlin, R.W. (1980). *Child and family development: Implications for care.* New York: McGraw-Hill.

Jenny, J.L. (1984). A comparison of four age groups' adaptation to diabetes. *Can J Pub Health, 75,* 237–244.

King, F.E., Figge, J., & Harmon, P. (1986). The elderly coping at home. A study of continuity of nursing care. *J Adv Nurs, 11*(1), 41–46.

Kobassa, S.C. (1979). Stressful life events, personality and health: An inquiry into hardiness. *J Pers Soc Psychol 37,* 1–11.

Kobassa, S.C., & Maddi, S.R. (1981). Personality and constitution as mediators in the stress-illness relationship. *J Health Soc Behav, 11,* 368–378.

Lambert, V.A., & Lambert, C.E. (1987). Coping with rheumatoid arthritis. *Nurs Clin North Am, 22*(3), 551–558.

Lavigne, J., & Ryan, M. (1979). Psychological adjustments of siblings with chronic illness. *Pediatarics, 63,* 616–627.

Lerner, J.V., & East, P.L. (1984). The role of temperament in stress, coping and socioemotional functioning in early development. *Infant Ment Health J, 5*(3), 148–159.

Lerner, R.M., Palermo, M., Shapiro, A., et al. (1982). Assessing the dimensions of temperamental individuality across the life span: The dimensions of temperament survey (DOTS). *Child Dev, 53,* 149–159.

Levy, S.M. (1981). The psychosocial assessment of the chronically ill geriatric patient. In C.K. Prokop & L.A. Bradley (Eds.), *Medical psychology: Contributions to behavioral medicine* (pp. 119–137). New York: Academic Press.

Mechanic, D. (1986). *From advocacy to allocation: The evolving American health care system.* New York: Macmillan.

Miles, M., Spicher, C., & Hassanein, R. (1984). Maternal and paternal stress reactions when a child is hospitalized in a pediatric intensive care unit. *Issues Compr Pediatr, 7,* 333–342.

Minaker, K.L., & Rowe, J. (1985). Health and disease among the oldest old: A clinical perspective. *Milbank Mem Fund Q, 63*(2), 324–349.

Neugarten, B.L. (1979). Time, age and the life cycle. *Am J Psychiatry, 136,* 887–894.

Newman, R.K., & Simpson, R.L. (1983). Modifying the least restrictive environment to facilitate integration of severely emotionally disturbed children and youth. *Behav Disord, 4*(2), 103–112.

Nowicki, S., & Strickland, B.R. (1973). A locus of control scale for children. *J Consult Clin Psychol, 40,* 148–154.

Oleson, C. (1981). *Diagnosis and management of diabetes mellitus.* Philadelphia: Lea & Febiger.

Parcel, G.S., & Meyer, M.D. (1978). Development of an instrument to measure children's health locus of control. *Health Educ Monogr, 6,* 149–159.

Perrin, E.C., & Gerrity, S.P. (1981). There's a demon in your belly: Children's understanding of illness. *Pediatrics, 67*(6), 841–849.

Perrin, E.C., & Shapiro, E. (1985). Health locus of control beliefs of healthy children, children with a chronic physical illness, and their mothers. *J Pediatr, 107*(4) 627–633.

Piaget, J., & Inhelder, B. (1969). *The psychology of the child.* New York: Basic Books.

Pollack, S.E. (1986). Human responses to chronic illness: Physiologic and psychosocial adaptation. *Nurs Res, 35,* 90–95.

Rotter, J.B. (1966). Generalized expectancies for internal versus external control of reinforcement. *Psychol Monogr, 80,* 1–28.

Rotter, J.B.. Chance, J.E., & Phares, E.J. (1972) *Applications of a social learning theory of personality.* New York: Holt, Rinehart and Winston.

Rubinstein, B. (1984). When a child has a serious illness: Psychiatric aspects of chronic handicaps. In E. Aronowitz & E.M. Bromberg (Eds.), *Mental health and long-term physical illness* (pp. 45–65). Canton, MA: Prodist.

Rutter, M., & Hersov, L. (Eds). (1977). *Child psychiatry.* Oxford: Blackwell Scientific.

Scheier, M.F., Weintraub, J.K., & Carver, C.S. (1986). Coping with stress: Divergent strategies of optimists and pessimists. *J Pers Soc Psychol, 51*(6), 1257–1264.

Seligman, M. (1983). *The family with a handicapped child: Understanding and treatment.* New York: Grune & Stratton.

Skinner, B.F. (1971). *Beyond freedom and dignity.* New York: Knopf.

Thomas, A., Chess, S., & Birch, H. (1970). The origin of personality. *Sci Am, 223*(2), 102–109.

Trout, M. (1983). Birth of a sick or handicapped infant: Impact on the family. *Child Welfare, 62*(4) 337–348.

Wallston, K.A., & Wallston, B.S. (1981). Health locus of control scales. In H. Lefcourt (Ed.), *Research with the locus of control construct. Vol. 1.* New York: Academic Press.

Wallston, K.A., Wallston, B.S., & DeVillis, R. (1978). Development of the multidimensional health locus of control (MHLOC) scale. *Health Educ Monogr, 6,* 161–170.

Wertlieb, D. et al. (1987). Temperament as a moderator of children's stressful experiences. *Am J Orthopsychiatry, 57*(2), 234–245.

5 The Family System

This chapter provides an overview of the family system and its identifying characteristics. The family system is a core component of the Contingency Model of Long-Term Care. Relevant concepts for use when one is working with chronically ill persons are discussed. These concepts are from family systems, developmental, and interactional theories. The family system will be affected by a member's chronic condition and, in turn, will have an effect on the person with the condition.

Family systems are composed of individual members (individual systems) and subsystems of paired positions, such as husband-wife, parent-child, and siblings. Leavitt (1982) defines the family as a human group with significant emotional bonds that usually lives together in the same household. We are defining **family** as a system of interdependent interacting individuals who are related to one another by marriage, birth, adoption, or mutual consent, who may or may not reside in the same household. The whole of the family system is greater than the sum of its individual parts (Beavers, 1977). Thus, while individual family members perceive and respond to events in unique ways, the family unit as a whole may respond in a somewhat different manner. For example, a mother who knows she is dying may not tell her children. The children, however, may have overheard people talking about their mother's impending death but do not tell their mother. The children may talk about their mother's impending death when they are together but not when they are with their parents.

Three theoretical approaches have relevance to understanding the family and planning comprehensive care when a member has a chronic condition. These approaches are the systems approach, interaction approach, and developmental approach. Selected concepts from these frameworks are identi-

57

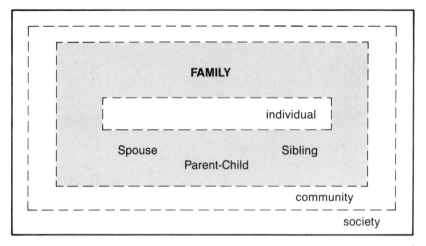

FIGURE 5–1 Family Systems Component of the Contingency Model of Long-Term Care. The broken lines indicate the openness of the family system with its individual subsystems and its suprasystems.

fied for their relevance to nursing practice. Unless otherwise noted, the following discussion is taken from Aldous (1978), Duvall (1977), and Hymovich and Chamberlin (1980). Figure 5–1 depicts the family system in relation to other systems in the model: It is composed of individual members in paired relationships (spouse, sibling, parent-child) with one another and interacting with its suprasystems (community, society).

Systems Approach

Systems theory involves patterns of living among the people who make up the system. Systems have boundaries that separate the individual system from the rest of the environment and control the flow of information, energy, and matter between the system and the surrounding environment (von Bertalanffy, 1968). The boundary of a family system reflects the family's psychic energy and internal processes.

According to family-systems theory, illness in one family member affects all family members (Kerr & Bowen, 1988; Minuchin, 1974). Any long-term illness can generate considerable anxiety within a family system and alter communication patterns, roles, and relationships among family members (Benoleil & McCorkle, 1978; Cassileth & Hamilton, 1979; Kerr & Bowen, 1988). Family-systems theory suggests that families are in a dynamic state of change, constantly responding to events outside the family

(Minuchin, 1974). Thus, families having a member with a chronic condition change over time as they try to cope with alterations over the course of the illness.

The family can be conceptualized as a system of interdependent interacting individuals related to one another by marriage, birth, adoption, or mutual consent. This broad definition includes a variety of family forms, including single persons living together, communal families, and nuclear, extended, and multigenerational families. To be certain of the composition of a given family, one needs to ask the person to identify the family members. Generally, the family shares a common residence. Living systems are open systems; and as a living system, the family is constantly exchanging energy and information with its environment. The family is an integrated system of interdependent functions, structures, and relationships, a unique and complete entity. Four characteristics of the family system are relevant to clinical practice using the Contingency Model of Long-Term Care: (1) interdependence, (2) boundary maintenance, (3) adaptability to change and change initiation, and (4) task performance (Aldous, 1978).

Interdependence

Families are made up of positions of individual family members and subsystems. Each position (husband-father, wife-mother, son-brother, daughter-sister) is behaviorally, physically, and emotionally interdependent with the others in varying degrees, depending upon the stage in the life cycle (Aldous, 1978). Interdependence involves both cooperation and conflict. Family subsystems are composed of paired positions (e.g., spousal, parental, sibling) in which the behaviors associated with one position assume someone is occupying the other position. Subsystems may be formed by sex, generation, function, or interest (Goldenberg & Goldenberg, 1980). In some families, one or more positions may be unfilled, as in a family with only one child (no sibling subsystem) or a family that has experienced divorce (no spousal subsystem) or death of a member. The spousal subsystem defines the marital relationship and serves as a role model to the children about the nature of intimate relationships. The parental subsystem is involved in child-rearing functions such as nurturance, guidance, and discipline. The sibling subsystem exposes children to learning patterns of negotiation, cooperation, and competition. Siblings spend more time together than any other family subsystem (Bank, 1981; Sutton-Smith & Rosenberg, 1970). Because the family is a system, a change in one family member affects all other members. Thus, a chronic condition in any member will have an impact on all other members. For example, the diagnosis of diabetes in a child may necessitate alterations in the family eating schedule to accommodate the child's routine. The presence of a debilitating illness in one spouse may mean the other has to take on an additional job or leave a job to remain home, and the children may have to forgo some outside activities or remain quiet when home. When one parent is ill, the other may spend so much time with the spouse that children may be deprived of both parents. √

Not all interactions affect the other subsystems. For example, parents disagree about issues that children may be completely unaware of, while siblings engage in activities of which parents may be unaware. Only role changes that reach a certain threshold will influence other subsystems (Hill, 1976). A parent may be ill and unable to work for a day or two with no effect on the sibling subsystem. When the condition is chronic and interferes with household tasks or family finances, the children will feel the effects.

Boundary Maintenance Families create and maintain boundaries that set them apart from other systems. Boundaries can be interpreted as rules that determine who participates in each subsystem and the tasks and communication patterns associated

with each subsystem (Minuchin, 1974). Boundary permeability varies, with some family systems being closed (close-knit), and other's more open (loose-knit). Family systems interact to varying degrees with other social systems, such as the occupational, educational, religious, economic, health care, and legal systems. In turn, these community systems have an impact on family functioning. For example, the religious system influences philosophy of life; the legal system affects responsibilities of the family, community, and state; and the health system influences services available for the care of those who are chronically ill.

Open-system families have many social relationships and interact with social institutions, such as religious, school, and health institutions. These families have greater access to social networks and outside resources and have more energy for problem solving and life pursuits than families not very open to the outside. Although it is rare to find families that are completely closed systems, many families have restricted networks and little social interaction. Consequently, little energy comes into the system to strengthen the family. Such families are vulnerable during periods of crisis and ongoing stressful situations because they lack social support and expend energy to maintain their boundaries. See Table 5–1 for characteristics of healthy and vulnerable families.

Families create their own histories as they have

Table 5–1 Characteristics of Healthy and Vulnerable Families

Healthy Families	Vulnerable Families
Open system 　Permeable boundary 　Many social 　　relationships and 　　interactions	Closed system 　Tight boundary 　Few social 　　relationships and 　　interactions
Negentrophic 　Receives energy from 　outside	Entrophic 　No energy received 　　from outside
Strong structure	Weak structure
Strong social supports	Weak social supports
Access to resources	Restricted access to 　resources
Receptive to change	Unreceptive to change
Free communications	Poor communications
Respect for family 　members	Lack of respect for 　family members

new experiences and interpret them according to their own frame of reference (Aldous, 1978). Shared intimacies and family rituals, such as Sunday brunch or Thanksgiving at Grandmother's, bring families together in habitual ways and contribute to their solidarity.

Minuchin (1974) identified two variations of family boundary functions: enmeshment and disengagement. The boundaries of an **enmeshed family** are somewhat permeable and diffuse, with minimal differentiation between its subsystems (members). Family members speak for each other and overreact to even minor stressors. When confronted with a chronic condition, the enmeshed family becomes overwhelmed and immobilized. It may be difficult to identify who is in charge in the family because all members seem "overly involved with the patient" (Gray-Price & Szczerny, 1985, p. 62).

Members in a **disengaged family** function separately and autonomously rather than interdependently. They have little sense of belonging to the family and rarely communicate about their feelings. Subsystem boundaries are rigid, so only high levels of individual stress lead to support (Minuchin, 1974). Because family members have little experience communicating with one another, they may have difficulty establishing relationships outside the family. Thus, mobilizing disengaged families is often difficult for health care providers (Gray-Price & Szczerny, 1985).

Adaptability to Change and Change Initiation

Families are adaptable to internal and external change. They can usually change in response to the information they receive and can initiate change. Information flows between members within the family and between the members and outsiders. In systems theory, this transmission of information is conceptualized as a feedback process. Families develop patterns for communicating information and interpreting information they receive.

Chaotic families, or those that are seriously disturbed, are entropic and have few interactions with the outside world (Beavers, 1976). Because chaotic families are impermeable and do not acknowledge the perceptions of others, they do not change readily. The less competent the family becomes, the more rigid the boundaries become, with fewer and fewer messages getting through. Commu-

nications are characterized by parallel discussions and repetitive patterns of interaction. Members talk at and through each other and are insensitive to cues. There is only noise and no signal (substance) in their messages.

Well-functioning families can hear and acknowledge each other's verbal and nonverbal communications. Parents support each other in a respectful manner, although they do not always have to agree with one another. There is respect for the uniqueness of others, freedom in communication, and skill in negotiation. These families are receptive and open to the communication of others.

Task Performance

Family roles may be defined by sex, age, function, or membership in a subsystem. Members are assigned certain rights and responsibilities that define their roles. Associated with these roles are specific functions or tasks to be carried out. Each family member, and the unit as a whole, is expected to perform certain tasks (Aldous, 1978). When a chronic condition is present, role functions may shift among the family members. Some changes may be temporary, whereas others may be permanent, depending upon the characteristics of the condition. Role transitions can be sources of stress to the family members because such changes involve reorganization of family interactions (Gray-Price & Szczerny, 1985). As roles change, shifts in the division of labor occur. Children may be required to fulfill household chores previously performed by an ill parent (role reversal) (Korer & Fitzsimmons, 1985). Increased chores and responsibilities reduce recreation time for these children. Family schedules may change to accommodate the patient's required rest and exercise periods. Spouses may experience frustrations and disappointment and fear trying to accommodate role changes. In addition, both may be prevented from carrying out the role of nurturing parent.

Although illness itself is stressful, role transitions within the family may be equally stressful. The family is a social system whose structure is founded on a contracted network of interactions and obligations (Dow, 1965). Therefore, impairment in any family role requires alterations in reciprocal roles (MacVicar & Archbold, 1976), with the likelihood of increasing family stress and crisis (Livsey, 1972). Even if the ill or hospitalized person is able to maintain or fulfill part of his or her role expectations, illness reduces role performance, making role compliance variable and unpredictable. Until high role complementarity is achieved and actual role performance becomes consistent and stable, familial stress remains (Glasser & Glasser, 1970).

Interactional Approach

The interactional perspective views the family as an ever changing "unity" of personalities. Concepts such as role, position, adaptation, and communication are components of this approach. The family is viewed as a relatively closed system of interaction. According to this approach, people live in a symbolic as well as a physical world and are stimulated by and stimulate others through symbols. Relevant to assessment and intervention is the notion that interaction cannot be completely understood by objective means but must be viewed through the perceptions of the persons involved in the interaction. As noted in Chapter 1, the Contingency Model of Long-Term Care assumes that perceptions influence the way people behave. People behave according to the facts as they perceive them, not as they are perceived by others. Consequently, knowledge of their subjective perceptions is important to the nurse.

Emphasis is on the interpersonal relationships of family members as they communicate. These interaction patterns develop over time; interaction is always a dynamic process involving the continuous testing one has of another's role (role taking). Healthy communication patterns involve openness and honesty among family members.

In the course of a lifetime, each person occupies a variety of roles. **Role** is a behavioral term defined as a "set of activities that are expected of a person by virtue of his or her occupancy of a particular position in social space" (Kahn & Antonucci, 1980, p. 261). Roles require proximity and interactions; they are prescribed (expectations) and proscribed (prohibitions). Role stresses include conflict, ambiguity, overload, underutilization, and responsibility for others (Coehlo, Hamburg, & Adams, 1974; Lazarus & Launier, 1978). Many roles change in content and style with respect to age. For example, a child who is the recipient of care from a parent as a youngster may become a care giver to that parent in adult life. Roles involve opportunities and resources as well as expectations and demands. A young man paralyzed in an accident can become an inspiration and role model for another. He may participate in wheel chair sports, graduate from college, and visit hospitalized individuals in his spare time.

Role clarity is essential to adequate role performance (Hardy, 1978; Sarbin & Allen, 1968). Role clarity involves having knowledge of the goals of role performance and role boundaries in relation to occupants of counter roles. When crises occur, role clarity may diminish, leading to personal disorganization. Role-taking ability promotes role transition (Meleis, 1975), while inability to understand the experiences and perceptions of the person in the counter role results in anxiety (Rudy, 1980).

Developmental Approach

The developmental approach attempts to synthesize compatible concepts of other frameworks to view the family as it changes over time. As with the interaction framework, the family is viewed as a "unity" of interacting personalities and as a semiclosed system (Hymovich & Chamberlin, 1980). Important components of this framework are the family life cycle, positions, roles, norms, and developmental tasks.

Family Life Cycle

Inherent in the developmental approach is the concept of the family life cycle, based on the recognition of successive phases and patterns over the family life span (Duvall, 1977, p. 140). The family life cycle may be divided into few (e.g., expanding, contracting) or many stages. Duvall (1977) suggests an eight-stage cycle, whereas Rodgers (1973) identifies a 24-stage cycle that takes into account the overlapping nature of stages in family life. Although we recognize the limitations in Duvall's eight stages, we find it useful for obtaining information about families that can guide intervention. The child-rearing stages are based on the age of the oldest child in the family. They are listed in Table 5–2.

Family Developmental Tasks

Tasks are functional requirements expected of a system at various stages in its development. Family developmental tasks arise from demands placed on the family by societies, in addition to the demands on family members, to accomplish their individual tasks. Family tasks can be conceptualized as any of the functions considered necessary for family continuation at a particular stage of development (Aldous,

Table 5–2 General Family Developmental Tasks and Examples of Specific Tasks

Stage in life cycle	General Tasks				
	Meet basic physical needs of family	Assist members develop potential	Provide emotional support, and communicate effectively	Maintain organization, and management	Function within the community
Married couple	Find, furnish, maintain first home Establish mutually satisfying way of supporting selves	Become established in occupation(s) Plan for possible children	Establish mutually acceptable personal, emotional, sexual roles Maintain motivation, morale	Allocate responsibilities	Interact with in-laws, relatives, community
Childbearing	Adapt housing arrangements Meet present, future costs of childbearing	Facilitate members' role learning	Communicate with one another Maintain motivation, morale	Assume mutual responsibility Develop family rituals, routines	Relate to relatives, others
Preschool stage	Supply adequate space, facilities, equipment	Rear, plan for children Motivate family members	Maintain mutually satisfying intimate communication	Assume more-responsible roles	Relate to relatives Tap outside resources
School-age stage	Provide for children's activities, parents' privacy	Further socialization of family members	Upgrade communication in family Develop morally, build family morale	Reassign role responsibilities	Establish ties with life outside family
Teenager stage	Provide facilities for widely different needs Work out ever-changing financial problems	Widen horizons of teens, parents	Keep marriage relationship in focus Bridge communication gap between generations Maintain ethical, moral stance	Reassign role responsibilities as appropriate	Keep in touch with relatives
Launching young adults	Rearrange physical facilities, resources to meet expenses	Come to terms with selves as husband, wife	Maintain open systems of communication within family, between family, others Reconcile conflicting loyalties, philosophies of life	Reallocate responsibilities among grown, growing children	Widen family circle through release of young adult children, recruitment of new

Table 5–2 General Family Developmental Tasks and Examples of Specific Tasks   *Continued*

Stage in life cycle	General Tasks				
	Meet basic physical needs of family	**Assist members develop potential**	**Provide emotional support, and communicate effectively**	**Maintain organization, and management**	**Function within the community**
Middle-aged parents in an empty nest	Provide for comfortable, healthful well-being Allocate resources for present, future needs	Develop patterns of complementarity Undertake appropriate social roles	Assure marital satisfaction Affirm life's central values	Establish new routines	Enlarge family circle Participate in life beyond the home
Aging family members	Make satisfactory living arrangements as aging progresses Adjust to retirement income Safeguard physical, mental health	Keep active, involved	Maintain love, sex, marital relationships Find meaning in life	Establish comfortable routines	Remain in touch with other family members

Sources: Duvall, 1977; Hymovich & Chamberlin, 1980.

1978). These functions are (1) physical maintenance of family members, (2) socialization of family members, (3) maintenance of members' motivation to perform roles, (4) maintenance of control within the family and between the family members and outsiders, and (5) addition and release of family members. Although individual tasks change from stage to stage, family functions, except for the fifth, remain essentially the same at each stage.

Based on these functions, the developmental tasks families have to accomplish are to (1) meet the basic needs of the family for food, health care, shelter, and money; (2) assist each family member develop his/her own individual potential; (3) provide emotional support and communicate effectively with all family members; (4) maintain and adapt family organization and management to meet changing needs; and (5) function within the community (Hymovich & Chamberlin, 1980).

Family Identifying Characteristics

Each family has certain characteristics in common with other families, yet the way in which these characteristics are combined makes each family unit unique. The relationship of family identifying characteristics to other components of the model is depicted in Figure 5–2. The model shows that each system has identifying characteristics that overlap with the system's orientation to life, coping strategies, strengths and needs, and level of functioning.

Developmental Stage

The family life cycle is a useful frame of reference for looking at family life because it emphasizes the dynamics of interaction as they shift over time. Duvall's (1977) eight stages of the life cycle are used

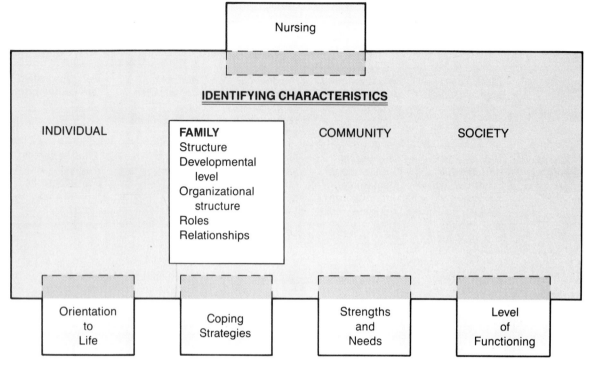

FIGURE 5–2 Relationship of Family Identifying Characteristics to Other Variables of the Contingency Model of Long-Term Care.

within the Contingency Model of Long-Term Care. However, it is recognized that these stages may need to be modified because of the particular family form with which you are working. The relationship of family tasks for these eight stages to Hymovich and Chamberlin's (1980) five general family tasks is depicted in Table 5–2.

Organizational Structure

Family structure varies from the traditional nuclear family to single-parent, three-generation, dual-career, blended, and communal family forms. It is not uncommon for people to move from one form to another during the life cycle. Family size and composition influence level of functioning. For example, size determines the number of interactional systems within the family. So that a family of three will have three interactions, a family of five would have 10, and a family of six would have 15. Family members have individual interests and needs, thus making different demands on the other family members. The relation between number of family members and economic resources available to the family also influences family functioning in many areas, including

potential educational opportunities or access to health care.

Family Roles and Relationships

Coordination of family members' emotional and adaptive response is needed for a family to cope effectively with a chronic condition (Barbarin, Hughs, & Chesler, 1985). The ages of the family members provide some general information about potential role responsibilities and obligations.

Sociocultural Characteristics

Illness behavior may relate to cultural background. Different cultures interpret symptoms differently, use different vocabulary to express symptoms, and vary in readiness to act on symptoms (Rosenstock & Kirscht, 1979). Each culture has different norms for behavior when health disturbances are present. For example, Americans of Irish and Italian descent interpret and respond to symptoms differently (Zola, 1973). Sociocultural factors influence life-style (smoking, drinking, diet, risk taking), attitudes, and perceptions of life and health (Mechanic, 1986).

Cultural e... tutes a far... members, ... tient care...

A cult... ences indiv... dividual de... tural ones... (Philp & D... normality a... problems as... which prese... without suc...

Awaren... ences betw... families with... establishing ... ship. Differe... lead to a mu... and the fam... may affect h... males are kn... breast cancer... (Satariano, B...

This secti... family identif... garding asses... appears in Ch... formation reg... strengths, nee... vided in follow...

Identifying (

Family organiza... ...in a genogram. Other data can be obtained by having the client or family member complete a questionnaire or by interview. Family characteristics include developmental level, assessed by determining the ages of the children and size. Family size determines the number of interactional systems in the family. Family characteristics and suggested assessment methods are listed in Table 5–3.

Family Relationships and Communication

Even if it is not possible to assess family members other than the patient, it remains important to

...ather information about family relationships. Patient or care-giver (e.g., child's parent) perceptions ...f relationships and communication provide information regarding available support. With this knowledge, nurses can gauge whether information, assistance with emotional responses, provision of resources and equipment, and teaching will be sufficient, or whether a stronger support system is needed. Information regarding boundary permeability, role flexibility, quality of relationships, communication patterns, tolerance for differences, and perceptions of events is useful. Guidelines for obtaining this information appear in Table 5–3.

velopmental Tasks

...ough Hymovich and Chamberlin's overall family ...elopmental tasks cut across the life cycle, specific ...s are to be accomplished at each stage in the life ...e. The general tasks and examples of specific ...s at each stage appear in Table 5–2.

entially Useful Assessment ruments

...ly system data can be obtained through a combination of interviewing, observing, and using available assessment instruments. Although many instruments have been used for research, little evidence documents their use in clinical nursing assessments. The instruments described below are discussed because of their usefulness in research and potential usefulness with individual families. The difficulty in using some instruments to base nursing interventions with individual families is their relatively low reliability. Internal consistency reliability of .75 or higher may be adequate for new instruments or group data but is low for clinical practice with any one family.

The Dyadic Adjustment Scale (DAS) The Dyadic Adjustment Scale (DAS) (Spanier, 1976, 1987) is a 32-item, self-administered, paper-and-pencil scale measuring marital satisfaction. The DAS has four subscales (cohesion, five items; consensus, 13; satisfaction, 10; affectional expression, four). It has high internal consistent reliabilities (alpha) for the total scale (.96), Dyadic Consensus scale (.90), Dyadic Satisfaction scale (.94), and Dyadic Cohesion scale (.86). The reliability of .73 for the Affectional Expression scale suggests caution in using for individual assessment. The DAS shows acceptable con-

Table 5–3   Guide for Assessment of Family-System Identifying Characteristics

Characteristics	Assessment

Structure
[Can use interviews, checklists,
genograms, PPIINFO]
	Family composition
	  Names
	  Ages
	  Sex
	  Relationship
	Marital history
	Marriages
	Separations
	Deaths
	Education
	  Grade level (in school or completed)
	Race
	Cultural background

Meet the basic needs of the family.
[Can use interviews, checklists]
	Home
	  Structure
	  Location
	  Outdoor access
	  Sleeping arrangements
	  Adaptations for person with chronic condition
	Health care
	  Where
	  For whom
	  For what
	    prevention, crisis
	  How paid for
	Finances
	  Income
	    sources
	    stability
	    who contributes
	    who supported
	  Insurance
	  Major expenses
	  Cost of illness
	Clothing
	Food
	  Basic four
	  Special diets
	Satisfaction with
	  Housing
	  Health care
	  Financial situation
	  Nutritional needs

Maintain and adapt family organization
and management.
[Interviews, checklists]
	Role of each member
	  Role flexibility
	Occupation
	  Type of employment
	  Work schedules (full-time, part-time)

Table 5–3 Guide for Assessment of Family-System Identifying Characteristics   *Continued*

Characteristics	Assessment
Assist each family member develop his/her own potential. [If possible assess each member, using appropriate developmental tasks.]	Extent to which each family member is accomplishing tasks Satisfaction with each member's development Development prior to illness Changes in development since diagnosis

Provide emotional support and communicate effectively with all family members.
[Interviews, observation]
	Relationships between family members
	Preexisting family functioning
	    Communication patterns
	    How decisions are made
	    Feelings of closeness
	    Power structure
	How family members get along with one another
	Support systems within family

Maintain and adapt family organization and management to meet changing needs.
[Interviews, observation]
	Roles of each member
	Role flexibility
	Daily schedule
	    Change since diagnosis
	Tasks to be accomplished
	    Who helps with tasks
	    Change since diagnosis

Function within the community
[Interviews, home visit, ecomap]
	Resources available (e.g., health care, recreation, educational, vocational)
	Organizations belong to (e.g., religious, volunteer, PTA, condition-related groups)
	Day-care arrangements
	Leisure activities outside home:
	    Where
	    Frequency
	Contacts with
	    Extended family
	    Friends/neighbors
	Available support system

Strengths	Needs

struct validity with other measures of marital satisfaction (.86 to .88). Scores range from 0 to 151, with higher scores representing better adjustment to the marriage.

The Family Adaptability and Cohesion Evaluation Scales-Version 3 (FACESIII) The Family Adaptability and Cohesion Evaluation Scales-Version 3 (FACESIII) (Olson, Portner, & Lavee, 1985, 1987), a 20-item self-report scale with a seventh grade reading level, is based on the Circumplex Model of Marital and Family Systems. The model relates to the importance of cohesion and adaptability in family functioning. Adaptability (Change) items measure the extent to which the family is adaptable and subject to change on the following dimensions: leadership, discipline, child control, roles, and rules. Cohesion items measure emotional bonding, supportiveness, family boundaries, shared time and friends, and shared activities. The instrument's construct validity has been demonstrated. Each item has a five-point response option.

The scale's authors recommend administering to as many adolescent and adult family members as possible and having them complete it twice, first in response to the instruction to "Describe your family now" and then to "Ideally, how would you like your family to be?" Perceptions and ideal scores of various family members can be charted in a family profile for interpretation. Internal reliability was .71 for the 10-item cohesion scale, .62 for the 10-item adaptability scale, and .68 for the entire scale. Although these reliabilities are somewhat low for use with individual families, the instrument can be useful for group data.

The Family Environment Scale (FES)   The Family Environment Scale (FES) (Moos & Moos, 1987) is a 90-item, true-false, self-report questionnaire measuring social and environmental characteristics of the family. The authors indicate the FES contains 10 subscales, of which three are relationship dimensions (cohesion, expressiveness, conflict), five are personal growth dimensions (independence, achievement orientation, intellectual-cultural orientation, active-relational orientation, moral-religious emphasis) and two are system maintenance dimensions (organization, control). However, these factors have not been confirmed by factor analysis. There are three parallel forms of the FES: The Real Form (Form R) measures perceptions of families of origin or orientation. The Ideal Form (Form I) measures preferred family environment. The Expectations Form (Form E) measures expectations of engaged couples or adolescents about to enter a foster home. Internal consistency reliability estimates for the 10 subscales varied between .61 (independence) to .78 (cohesion, moral-religious orientation, intellectual-cultural orientation). Test-retest reliability for 8 weeks ranged between .68 for independence to .86 for cohesion; for 12-month interval the range was .52 (independence) to .89 (moral-religious orientation). This scale has discriminant and predictive validity. As with the FACES III, the reliability coefficients mean the instrument is less useful with individual families than for group data.

The Parent Perception Inventory: General Information (PPIINFO)   The Parent Perception Inventory: General Information (PPIINFO) (Hymovich, 1990) is a paper-and-pencil questionnaire that provides information about number and ages of children, race, religion, age, employment status, educational background, health status, marital status, and family income. This instrument was developed for research but has recently been modified for clinical use.

Genograms   **Genograms** are tools for recording selected family information. A genogram is a drawing of a family tree that contains information about family members over at least three generations. It provides a graphic representation of a family and allows the health care provider to clearly and quickly understand family structure. In addition to family structure, family information (e.g., critical events) is recorded and relationships are delineated. Genograms can help clinicians think systematically about how events and relationships may be related to patterns of health and illness (McGoldrick & Gerson, 1985).

To construct a genogram, various symbols are used. Some are depicted in Box 5–1. Family members are represented by boxes or circles, according to gender. The index person, or patient, is represented by double lines. Birth and death dates are indicated above the figure, and age at death is indicated inside the figure. Marriage, separation, stillbirth, and divorce dates are also indicated. Children are indicated by figures from left to right, oldest to youngest.

After the structure has been drawn, demographic information is added as well as functional information and critical events. Demographic information includes age, birth date, death date, location, occupation, and level of education. Functional information includes data about medical, emotional, and behavioral functioning, such as drug or alcohol abuse, absenteeism, and military service. Critical events are recorded in the margin and include losses, successes, job changes, moves, and other significant happenings that give a sense of the family history.

Ecomaps   An **ecomap** is an assessment tool to diagram relationships between a family and its suprasystems (Hartman, 1978). It accomplishes this by mapping the major suprasystems that are part of the family environment, such as school, friends, ex-

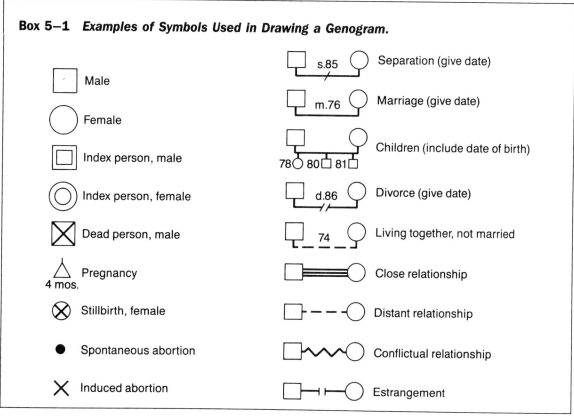

Box 5–1   *Examples of Symbols Used in Drawing a Genogram.*

Male

Female

Index person, male

Index person, female

Dead person, male

Pregnancy
4 mos.

Stillbirth, female

Spontaneous abortion

Induced abortion

s.85   Separation (give date)

m.76   Marriage (give date)

Children (include date of birth)
78○ 80□ 81□

d.86   Divorce (give date)

74   Living together, not married

Close relationship

Distant relationship

Conflictual relationship

Estrangement

Source: McGoldrick & Gerson, 1985.

tended family, and the health care system. By highlighting the nature of these relationships, the ecomap illustrates the flow of resources to and from the family, as well as unmet needs, providing an understanding of family stresses and available supports (Hartman, 1978). Hartman (1979) suggests that as the worker and family join together to create the ecomap, family members are likely to feel comfortable and less defensive in providing information. The nurse can observe family interaction while creating the ecomap if several family members are involved in the process.

A large circle is drawn in the center to depict the family. Within the circle, the family members are indicated with symbols, squares for the males and circles for the females. They are joined to form a family tree, similar to part of the genogram. Connections are drawn to the suprasystems to show the flow of relationships between family members and significant persons or systems in the external environment. An example of an ecomap is depicted in Box 5–2 containing part of an ecomap of the Mitchel family. Mrs. Mitchel has multiple sclerosis. An ex-

ample of the interpretation is as follows: Richard's extended family provides resources to the family, but there is essentially no reciprocity as there is with Anita's extended family. Joe's relationships with work and Beth's relationships at school are strained. Anita's experiences with the regional health clinic are stressful.

Summary

This chapter presented an overview of the family system, its identifying characteristics, and guidelines for the family assessment. The family is a core component of the Contingency Model of Long-Term Care. Relevant family theories (systems, developmental, interactional theories) were discussed. The family system is composed of individual members (individual systems) and subsystems of paired positions. The **family** was defined as a system of interdependent interacting individuals who are related to one another by marriage, birth, adoption, or mutual consent, who may or may not reside in the same household.

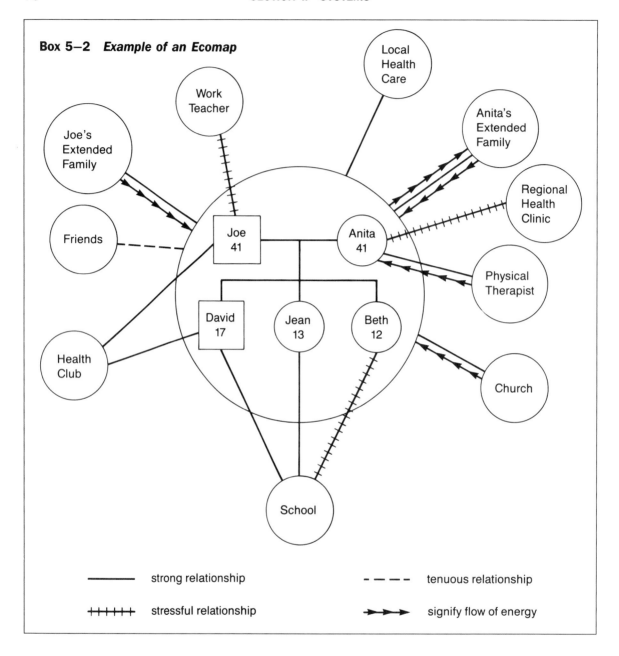

Box 5–2 *Example of an Ecomap*

Local Health Care

Work Teacher

Joe's Extended Family

Anita's Extended Family

Regional Health Clinic

Friends

Joe 41

Anita 41

Physical Therapist

Health Club

David 17

Jean 13

Beth 12

Church

School

——————— strong relationship   – – – – tenuous relationship

+++++ stressful relationship   ➤➤➤ signify flow of energy

References

Aldous, J. (1978). *Family careers: Developmental change in families.* New York: Wiley.

Anderson, J. (1986). Ethnicity and illness experiences: Ideological structures and the health care delivery system. *Soc Sci Med, 22*(11), 1277–1283.

Bank, S. (1981). *Sibling bond.* New York: Basic Books.

Barbarin, O.A., Hughs, D., & Chesler, M.A. (1985). Stress, coping, and marital functioning among parents of children with cancer. *J Marr Fam, 47,* 473–480.

Beavers, W.R. (1976). A theoretical basis for family evaluation. In J.M. Lewis et al., *No single thread: Psychological health in family systems* (pp. 46–82). New York: Brunner/Mazel.

Beavers, W.R. (1977). *Psychotherapy and growth: A family systems perspective.* New York: Brunner/Mazel.

Benoleil, J.Q., & McCorkle, R. (1978). A holistic approach to terminal illness. *Cancer Nurs, 1,* 143–149.

Cassileth, B.R., & Hamilton, J.N. (1979). The family with cancer. In B.R. Casselith (Ed.), *The cancer patient, social and medical aspects of care* (pp. 233–247). Philadelphia: Lea & Febiger.

Coehlo, G.V., Hamburg, D.A., & Adams, J.E. (Eds.). (1974). *Coping and adaptation.* New York: Basic Books. (1974).

Dow, T. (1965). Family reaction to crisis. *J Marr Fam, 27,* 363–366.

Duvall, E.M. (1977). *Marriage and family development.* Philadelphia: Lippincott.

Glasser, P.H., & Glasser, L.N. (Eds.). (1970). *Families in crisis.* New York: Harper & Row.

Goldenberg, I., & Goldenberg, H. (1980). *Family therapy: An overview.* Monterey, CA: Brooks/Cole.

Gray-Price, H., & Szczerny, S. (1985). Crisis intervention with families of cancer patients: A developmental approach. *Top Clin Nurs, 7*(1), 58–70.

Hardy, M.E. (1978). Role stress and role strain. In M.E. Hardy, & M.E. Conway (Eds.), *Role theory: Perspectives for health professionals* (pp. 72–109). New York: Appleton-Century-Crofts.

Hartman, A. (1978). Diagrammatic assessment of family relationships. *Soc Casework, 59,* 465–476.

Hartman, A. (1979). *Finding families: An ecological approach to family assessment in adoption.* Beverly Hills, CA: Sage.

Hill, R. (1976). Social theory and family development. In J. Cuisenier & M. Segalin (Eds.), *The family life cycle in European societies.* The Hague: Mouton.

Hymovich, D.P. (1990). *Overview of the Parent Perception Inventory.* Unpublished manuscript.

Hymovich, D.P., & Chamberlin, R.W. (1980). *Child and family development: Implications for care.* New York: McGraw-Hill.

Kahn, R.L., & Antonucci, T.C. (1980). Convoys over the life course: Attachment, roles and social support. In P.B. Baltes & O.G. Brim (Eds.), *Life-span development and behavior* (pp. 253–286). New York: Academic Press.

Kerr, M.E., & Bowen, M. (1988). *Family evaluation: An approach based on Bowen theory.* New York: Norton.

Korer, J., & Fitzsimmons, J.S. (1985). The effect of Huntington's chorea on family life. *Br J Soc Work, 15,* 581–597.

Lazarus, R.S., & Launier, R. (1978). Stress-related transactions between person and environment. In L.A. Pervin & M. Lewis (Eds.), *Perspectives in international psychology* (pp. 287–327). New York: Plenum.

Leavitt, M.B. (1982). *Families at risk: Primary prevention in nursing practice.* Boston: Little Brown.

Livsey, C. (1972). *Physical illness and family dynamics. Adv Psychosom Med, 8,* 237–251.

MacVicar, M., & Archbold, P. (1976). A framework for family assessment in chronic illness. *Nurs Forum, 15*(2), 180–194.

McGoldrick, M., & Gerson, R. (1985). *Genograms in family assessment.* New York: W.W. Norton & Co.

Mechanic, D. (1986). *From advocacy to allocation: The evolving American health care system.* New York: Macmillan.

Meleis, A.L. (1975). Role insufficiency and role supplementation: A conceptual framework. *Nurs Res, 24,* 264–271.

Minuchin, S. (1974). *Families and family therapy.* Cambridge, MA: Harvard University Press.

Moos, R.H., & Moos, B.S. (1987). Family environment scale. In N. Fredman, & R. Sherman (Eds.), *Handbook of measurements for marriage and family therapy* (pp. 82–86). New York: Brunner/Mazel.

Olson, D.H., Portner, J., & Lavee, Y. (1985). FACES III: Family adaptability and cohesion evaluation scales. In D. Olson, H. McCubbin, H. Barnes, A. Larsen, M. Muxen, & M. Wislon (Eds.), *Family inventories* (rev ed.) St. Paul, MN: Family Social Science, University of Minnesota.

Olson, D.H., Portner, J., & Lavee, Y. (1987). Family Adaptation and Cohesion Evaluation (FACES III). In N. Fredman, & R. Sherman (Eds.), *Handbook of measurements for marriage and family therapy* (pp. 180–185). New York: Brunner/Mazel.

Philp, M., & Duckworth, D. (1982). *Children with disabilities and their families.* London: NFER-Nelson.

Rodgers, R.H. (1973). *Family interaction and transaction: The developmental approach.* Englewood Cliffs, NJ: Prentice-Hall.

Rolland, J.S. (1987). Family systems and chronic illness: A typological model. *J Psychother Fam, 3*(3), 143–168.

Rosenstock, I.M., & Kirscht, J.P. (1979). Why people seek health care. In G.C. Stone, F. Cohen, N.E. Adler (Eds.). *Health psychology—A handbook* (pp. 161–188). San Francisco: Jossey-Bass.

Rudy, E.B. (1980). Patients' and spouses' causal explanations of a myocardial infarction. *Nurs Res, 29,* 352–356.

Sarbin, T., & Allen, V. (1968). Role theory. In G. Lindzey & E. Aronson (Eds.), *The handbook of social psychology* (Vol. 1, pp. 488–567, 2nd ed.). Reading, MA: Addison-Wesley.

Satariano, W.A., Belle, S.H., Swanson, G.M. (1986). The severity of breast cancer at diagnosis: A comparison of age and extent of disease in black and white women. *Am J Pub Health, 76*(7), 779–782.

Spanier, G.B. (1987). Dyadic adjustment scale. In N.

Fredman, & R. Sherman (Eds.), *Handbook of measurements for marriage and family therapy* (pp. 52–58). New York: Brunner/Mazel.

Spanier, G., & Cole, C. (1974). Toward clarification and investigation of marital adjustment. *Int J Sociol Fam, 6,* 121–146.

Sutton-Smith, B., & Rosenberg, B.G. (1970). *The sibling.* New York: Holt, Rinehart & Winston.

von Bertalanffy, L.V. (1968). *General systems theory.* New York: George Braziller.

Zola, I.K. (1973). Pathways to the doctor—From person to patient. *Soc Sci Med, 7,* 677–689.

6 Systems: Community and Society

This chapter provides an overview of the family suprasystems, community and society, and issues facing these systems. The suprasystems have an impact on family functioning and are important aspects of family life when someone has a chronic condition. The **community system** is composed of the family's neighborhood, health, recreational, educational, social, and political institutions that affect its functioning. **Society** is the larger political, economic, and social system under which the other systems (individual, family, community) function. Figure 6–1 illustrates the relationship of these suprasystems to one another and to the individual and family systems. Figure 6–2 illustrates the relationship of the suprasystems' identifying characteristics to other components of the model.

To fully understand families undergoing stress, it is important to attend to the "multiple interdependent levels of the social system: individual, dyadic, familial, social network, community, and cultural/historical" (Riegal, 1976). The social system and institutions outside the family system influence how the individual and family adjust to stress (Walker, 1985). For example, a community's lack of hospice care for a dying patient may interfere with patient and family desires to have the person remain home. Conversely, individuals can have an impact on society, as evidenced by the role disabled individuals are playing in effecting change by sit-ins and other means of making their needs known to society.

Chronic conditions by their very nature are prolonged. Most chronically ill people spend relatively short periods in the hospital or with their health care providers. In the future, even fewer people will be in the hospital and more will be cared for at home, thus placing greater demands on the family and community. Since each community is unique, the demands placed on it can also be expected to be unique, and the ways these needs are managed can be expected to differ.

73

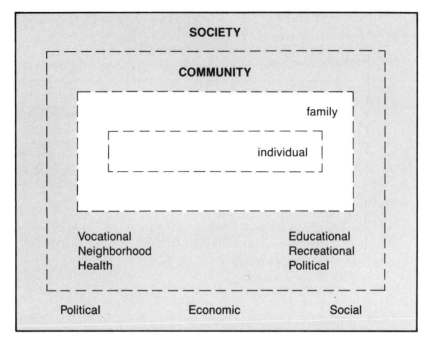

FIGURE 6–1 Community and Societal Systems Component of the Contingency Model of Long-Term Care. The broken lines denote the openness of the systems to one another; the unbroken line delimits the boundaries of the systems component of the model.

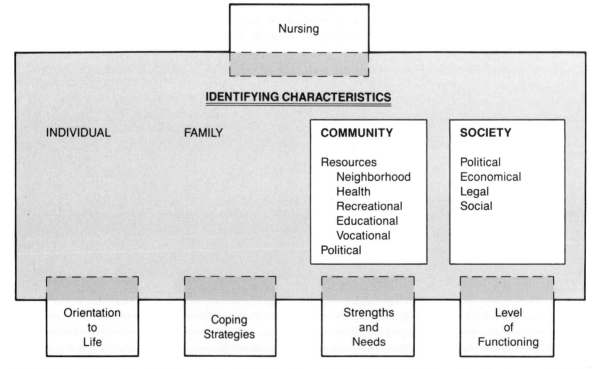

FIGURE 6–2 Relationship of the Suprasystems' Identifying Characteristics to Other Variables of the Contingency Model of Long-Term Care.

Community System

Observations show that few communities know how or are prepared to meet most needs of the growing population of those with chronic disabilities. Only a small number of people have adequate continuing care, and for the majority such care is weak or nonexistent. The predominant response of the health care system remains episodic care. The numbers and life expectancy of children and adults with chronic or disabling conditions is increasing, placing a tremendous burden on all systems to assess and reassess the options for improving care to this population.

Community Services and Resources

Community services and resources include places, people, and information. The types of services needed for chronically ill children and adults and their families are discussed more fully in Chapter 7. Nursing assessment and interventions are also discussed in that chapter.

Society

Society is the large political, economic, and social system under which the other systems (individual, family, community) function (See Figure 6–1). The nurse's role in relation to the society was mentioned in Chapter 1 and is discussed again in Chapter 7.

Health Care System

The health care system is a subsystem of the larger society (Miller & Stokes, 1978). It occupies a specific structural position within the system and is the mixture of resources a society commits to the health concerns of its population. The health care system commits personnel (manpower), knowledge, economic resources, physical facilities, and services to the social system. The target of any particular health system is a population of defined scope, such as a town, city, or region.

The health care system in the United States is made up of many thousands of agencies at the local, state, and federal levels. Unfortunately, the health care system and its many subsystems have many problems, including fragmentation, lack of commu-

nication, insufficient or duplicated services, and unequal distribution of care.

Nursing systems and family systems adapt to one another through the mutual exchange of materials and information. This process involves getting needed materials and information from the environment, giving materials and information to the environment, leaving in the environment materials and information that are not needed, and keeping essential materials and information within one's boundaries (Bredemeier, 1961). At the individual system level nurses and family members interact, allowing the assessment and intervention process to take place. Through this process, the nurse acting as a client advocate then interacts with the health care system to provide necessary and appropriate information and references to families in need.

Through this system knowledge and technology reach those with chronic conditions and their families. Rettig (1982) describes the diffusion pathway of new knowledge and technology. The primary diffusion pathway is from a specialty group in a tertiary medical center to members of that same specialty in other tertiary centers. The secondary diffusion pattern occurs later within the same specialty but moves from the tertiary centers to community hospitals. If the information has an expanding range of applications, another diffusion pattern or set of patterns occurs. This is from the primary specialty group to an adjacent specialty group within the tertiary center, and then to community hospitals. For example, initially an innovative technique in open-heart surgery is shared among cardiac surgeons within medical centers. Once perfected, this technique will then be adopted at the community hospital level. If the information has an expanding range of applications, another diffusion pattern or set of patterns occurs. This is from the primary specialty group to an adjacent specialty group within the tertiary center, and then to community hospitals. Diffusion from hospitals to settings such as homes depends on the physical characteristics of the technology and incentives from others, especially third-party insurers.

Issues Affecting the Health Care System

A number of issues face all health care professionals working with chronically ill individuals and their families. Among them are ethical, economic, delivery-of-care, legislative, and public-policy issues. Each issue is highlighted briefly in this section.

Ethical Issues

Although ethical issues are prominent in the care of chronically ill individuals of any age and in any setting, detailed discussion of these issues and the dilemmas they present is beyond the scope of this book. "Ethical dilemmas occur both at the nurse-patient-family level of interaction in hospital and home settings and at the policy making level of institutions and communities" (Aroskar, 1980, p. 658). It is important to keep abreast of these issues and be aware of one's own beliefs and their influence on ethical decisions. Among the numerous ethical issues are those pertaining to treatment of severely impaired newborn infants, treatment of youngsters without parental consent, research involving children, euthanasia, refusal of treatment by parent or child, unconscious individuals, those dependent on unusual life-support measures, and scarce resources.

McCullogh (1984, p. 67) identifies two basic questions in our moral lives: "What sort of person ought I to be?" and "What are my duties and obligations to others?" He goes on to say that health care professionals must also ask, "What are my obligations to patients, to their families, and to the community I serve?" The question families must ask is, "What is my obligation to my family member who is the patient?" The question communities must ask themselves is, "What are our obligations as communities to these patients, to their families, and to the health care professionals and institutions that seek to serve their needs?" Each question has important implications for health care professionals working with the chronically ill and their families.

Three principles have emerged in relation to the health care setting. Each principle generates different obligations that often conflict with one another (see Table 6–1). The principle of beneficence requires us to assist others in advancing their interests and goods (e.g., health, relief of pain and suffering, amelioration of illness, prolongation of life) without causing unnecessary harms (e.g., disease, unnecessary pain and suffering, handicapping conditions, premature death). The principle of respect for autonomy requires the health care professional to make decisions and take actions based on the beliefs and values of their individual patients, rather than

from goods and harms as in the first principle. The principle of justice applies at the level of society's relationship with patients, families, and health care providers and helps in negotiating differences among these groups. An important notion related to justice is that all persons should be treated fairly. Unfortunately, people disagree about what is considered fair. Justice requires us to benefit society while at the same time benefitting those who are least well off. Chronically ill persons are less well off than those who are healthy, and danger exists that in providing for the larger society, the interests of the chronically ill may be sacrificed. The principles of beneficence and respect for autonomy apply to relationships among patient, provider, and family, whereas the principle of justice is applied to the community system.

Pain   McCullough (1984) discusses three ethical principles related to five topics important to those who care for the chronically ill. The first topic, pain in chronic illness, is difficult to deal with from a moral or ethical perspective. Although health professions have operated on the belief that temporary pain is acceptable for improved health (e.g., from surgery and treatments), pain associated with chronic illness is often prolonged, and although it can be managed is rarely eliminated. Life, though prolonged, has its quality diminished by pain. A moral dilemma may arise from using pain medication to the point of patient addiction. The principle of beneficence presents a conflict because both addiction and pain are serious disabilities. If the princi-

Table 6–1   System Level and Provisions of Ethical Principles

Principle	Level	Provisions
Beneficence	Individual	Assist others in advancing their interests and goods without causing unnecessary harm
Respect for autonomy	Individual	Make decisions and take actions based on beliefs and values of individual patients
Justice	Community	Treat all persons fairly

ple of autonomy is brought into the situation, the patient decides, based on information about the risks and benefits of the choices. Another pain-related issue concerns the decision to continue living with the pain or decide that death is an acceptable alternative.

> Respect for the patient's autonomy is one of the major grounds on which health care professionals and institutions should determine their responses to moral problems in pain management. They should not rely simply on the beneficence model and take decisions away from the patients as if they were simply *technical* decisions. (McCullough, 1984, p. 72)

Nurses have an ethical obligation to ensure that people receive the necessary information and emotional support to make an informed decision (Davis, 1981). They can help patients think through these matters. It may help patients to bring their family into the decision making and to talk with other patients who have had to make decisions. The nurse is then obligated to provide the appropriate care required on the basis of the final decision. Family members need nonjudgmental support as they try to identify their own ethical position and the consequences of their ethical decisions.

The Elderly   Two moral principles apply to the health care of the elderly with chronic illness. These principles are the obligations (1) not to compound the elderly's losses unnecessarily and (2) to sustain the elderly's own moral authority to make personal decisions (Christiansen, 1978). To follow these principles, health care professionals need to develop patience and tolerance, as it often takes the elderly longer to make decisions. Using family and community resources is one way to help them make decisions about management of their chronic illness. Family members can often help nurses understand what their chronically ill elderly relative is like now and was like in the past (e.g., feisty, passive). Community members can take responsibility for the broader education of others by debunking the myths of aging.

Diminished Competence   Another important ethical and moral issue relates to appropriate treatment for a person with diminished competence and the time to stop treatment for someone dying. McCullough (1984) recommends consideration of three

basic strategies. The first is to treat the person with reversible diminished capacity to restore autonomy so that the patient can make decisions about future care. Second, for the person with irreversible diminished capacity, treatment decisions should be based on that person's values, beliefs, and past autonomy. Third, when patients have irreversible diminished capacity but no known value history (e.g., stranger, young children), health professionals are obligated to provide treatment until the "harms of treatment outweigh the goods that are to be achieved" (p. 78).

Living Wills   The fourth topic concerning chronic illness is living wills. Living wills are a way for patients whose capacity may become diminished to express autonomy prior to a serious medical condition. Unfortunately, the language of these wills is vague and does not provide clear guidance. It is wise to establish the values and desires of those who are chronically ill and have living wills before the course of their illness worsens to the degree that they can no longer participate in decisions. Issues such as being on a respirator should be discussed with the patient and documented on the record (McCullough, 1984).

Resource Allocation   The principle of justice can help in dealing with the allocation of scarce health care resources to the chronically ill. At issue here is the amount of our gross national product that should be allocated to health care, and how these resources should be allotted justly and fairly to those with chronic illness (McCullough, 1984). According to the principle of distributive justice, these decisions should be based on categories of people who are most vulnerable rather than on a case-by-case basis as is current practice.

Economic Issues

Rising costs have made health care unaffordable for many Americans. Approximately 15 million Americans have inadequate health coverage and 33 million more have no medical insurance (Andreoli & Musser, 1985). As economic and regulatory pressures increase, people with chronic health problems are experiencing reduced funding of health-related programs. People with chronic illnesses are large consumers of health care, accounting for 58% of all short-term hospital stays. Zook and Moore (1980) reported that 87% of hospital costs are spent on only 13% of the chronically ill. Swint (1982) reported that the net future commitment of society to the maintenance and care of individuals with chromosomal abnormalities alone will be over $3 billion per year. The Bureau of the Census (U.S. Department, 1986) estimated that because of the limiting effects of arthritis, it is an extremely costly disease, with 26.6 billion work days lost and $4.8 billion in wages lost per year. In addition, $5 billion are spent on medical costs and another $1 billion on insurance and disability aid each year.

Financial Burden The financial burden of chronic illness includes both direct and indirect costs. Direct costs, those related to the illness itself, include hospital and physician expenses, diagnostic studies, treatments, and medications. Health insurance pays for a substantial portion of direct costs but does not cover all of them. Most policies, including catastrophic coverage, require a percentage of the expenses to be paid by the insured. In 1978, 90% of the respondents in a Gallup Poll indicated they had health insurance and 59% had catastrophic coverage as well (Schroeder, 1981). Many individuals with long-term health problems are then forced to pay for their expenses out-of-pocket or to "spend down" until they become eligible for Medicaid. Nearly everyone who is chronically ill faces the frustration of the financial burden. In addition, there is greater governmental support for institutionalized aged and handicapped than for family members who wish to keep a relative at home.

There are two major approaches to valuing the monetary impact of chronic disease on individuals. "The human capital approach values worsening health as the net present value of change in individuals expected lifetime earnings or productivity (adjusted by age and sex) resulting from disease and disability. The cost of illness is the difference between what individuals would earn in future years, discounted to present values, in the presence or absence of illness" (Lubeck & Yelin, 1988, pp. 445–446). Although it is possible to obtain data for direct cost expenditures, it is extremely difficult to estimate indirect costs.

Indirect costs of chronic illness include expenses for illness-related items such as special diets or equipment and vocational rehabilitation. Other costs are time lost from work, travel expenses, telephone calls, and insurance. In addition, family members, and even friends, can incur costs when they provide assistance to the chronically ill person. The person with the chronic condition may have to leave the work force temporarily or permanently, and many times the care giver loses time from work to take a family member to appointments. Out-of-pocket expenses are rarely reimbursed and can be costly for families. Estimating indirect costs is difficult, but data show them to be three to five times higher than direct costs (Hatunian et al, 1980; Meenan & Yelin, 1981). Involvement of informal care givers minimizes the demand for formal services in the community but also limits our ability to determine the actual indirect costs of the illness.

In 1980, based on expenditures for hospital and nursing home care, professional services, and medications, circulatory system diseases were identified as the most costly category of physical illness. These were followed by digestive system diseases, injuries and poisonings, respiratory system diseases, cancer, musculoskeletal and connective tissue diseases, nervous system and sensory organ disorders, and endocrine, nutritional, and metabolic disorders (Mechanic, 1986).

The cost of some chronic illnesses is staggering. Since 1972 the government has been paying for dialysis for all persons with kidney failure at a cost of $2 billion a year. The majority of the nearly 100,000 patients receive dialysis at clinics where Medicare pays about $125 per treatment per patient (Campbell, 1990). In 1986 the overall direct and indirect costs of respiratory illness were estimated to be $40.9 billion.

An estimated one quarter of all functionally restricted, community-based elderly (1.1 million persons) receive some level of formal care services, costing $99 million per month (National Long-Term Care Survey, 1982). These are out-of-pocket expenses for over three quarters of those who receive such services. The average out-of-pocket payments increase with age and disability. For persons 85 years of age and older who have extreme limitations in activities of daily living, this cost peaks at $466 per month (Manton & Soldo, 1985).

The economic costs of prenatal diagnosis are substantial (Paucker, 1982). For example, amniocentesis with ultrasound examination, obstetrician fees, genetic counseling, and cytogenetic studies cost about $550 in 1982. Third-party payers vary in their coverage of such procedures, so parents must weigh the short-term costs of the procedure versus the long-term costs of raising a chronically ill, handicapped, or retarded child. It is anticipated, however, that the tremendous costs of some technological advances will be reduced in the future (Johnson,

1983). On the other hand, some technologies will be so expensive in the future that they may not be affordable at all (Stocking & Morrison, 1978).

At present, greater governmental support exists for institutionalized people than for family members who wish to keep the person at home (Kahn & Antonucci, 1980). Inadequate access to home health services is a major problem because Medicare pays for those who have short-term rehabilitation needs but not for those with long-term needs (Harrington, 1988). There is an urgent need to restructure the health care system to reduce the economic burden of chronic illness on society, while still being responsive to the needs of the patient and family. One example of this attempt to reduce the cost of long-term health care was the study by Brooten and her colleagues (1986). They demonstrated the feasibility of early discharge of very low birth weight infants from the hospital by providing home supervision by hospital based clinical specialists. The infants received safe, practical, and less costly care, with a mean savings per infant of $18,560.

The rising costs of health care place a tremendous burden on society to find alternative approaches to financing care. Both the public and private sectors are trying to contain costs (Mechanic, 1986). Medicaid eligibility has been severely limited, and premiums, coinsurance, and deductibles increased. Reimbursement by diagnostic-related groups (DRGs) means hospitals are paid a flat fee based on the patient's classification, rather than on the actual cost of the care. The mandate for peer review in organizations has led to stricter reviews of hospital utilization and surgical admissions. Some states have preferred provider agreements (PPOs) that reimburse prenegotiated prices for recipients of state aid. Major employers have begun establishing their own health care plans for employees, providing incentives for employees to use less medical care, and increasing cost sharing on health insurance plans. Most insurance companies are designed to help those who are acutely ill, and often have policy clauses excluding preexisting conditions. Such exclusions are likely to limit mobility (often for higher paying jobs) because they would leave people without insurance for a period of time, if not permanently. For example, a father could not take a position offered because it meant moving to a company whose insurance would not cover his son's illness. "It's a shame, but I'm limited to this dead-end job. I can't afford to take care of all his medical bills and keep any kind of living for the rest of us without the insurance. We were lucky I had the policy when he was born. We couldn't have survived without it."

Several programs are trying to meet the needs of clients faced with financial burdens. On Lok, a demonstration program in San Francisco, and the Social Health Maintenance Organization (SHMO) are attempts to overcome the fragmentation of financing and categorical services currently being provided (Mechanic, 1986). The SHMO provides for hospital, nursing, and home health services, as well as meals, transportation, and counseling for the elderly within a single system. The Loeb Center in New York has demonstrated that a hospital based extended care facility can provide cost-effective care to long-term patients at half the cost of inpatient hospital care (Alfano, 1988). In addition to the financial burden of chronic conditions, the psychosocial burden on the family must be considered. Caring for the ill or disabled person at home takes a toll on the family member who is responsible for providing that care.

Delivery-of-Care Issues

Delivery-of-care issues include the cost of providing services, their accessibility, the availability of needed resources, and the effectiveness of the services. To be considered are who receives care, who provides care, what services are available, how care is distributed, and the cost-effectiveness of care. Present information does not adequately identify the handicapped and the benefits and effectiveness of existing programs. Community services are generally varied, uncoordinated, and not particularly responsive to the person's total needs. There may be insufficient services, gaps, or overlaps in what is available. Prevention, case findings, and referral services are often neglected or underdeveloped. The range of services needed for a given family may not be available within a reasonable distance from the family's home. Where total gaps exist, such as lack of a school for a partially-sighted child, the family may have to move to another community. Within the school systems, children may lack adequate support services, such as occupational or physical therapy, special diets, or transportation.

There is marked unevenness in accessibility to services and the level of services. Eligibility rules vary across the country. Rural youth and preschoolers are especially shortchanged. Regional programs can be problematic to families who must travel long distances. Outreach programs are one approach to bringing some services closer to the person's home.

Patients and their families are frequently seen by a variety of professionals, each involved with only one aspect of the person's or the family's care. Some families receive most or all of their care from specialists, others from primary-care providers, while others have a combination of specialty and primary care. Still others go to emergency rooms when health care is needed. Often the result is fragmented care, with overall emphasis on the person's impairment, and insufficient attention to other aspects of person and family development and functioning (Kahn & Antonucci, 1980).

Institutional rules and regulations affect families in various ways (Kahn & Antonucci, 1980). For example, nursing home regulations usually require the segregation of men and women, thus separating spouses from each other. Regulations discourage remarriage among the elderly by reducing or eliminating Social Security benefits for remarriage. Social Security regulations prevent older people from continuing to work and thereby maintain important supportive relationships.

Legislative and Public Policy Issues

The implications of new technologies need to be thought about relative to health service logistics (Stocking & Morrison, 1978). New procedures and techniques often are adapted in practice before their effectiveness is thoroughly examined. In addition, resource allocation and choice of priorities are not clearly thought out before procedures such as liver transplants are introduced. Part of the dilemma is public pressure and the feeling of physicians that they are morally obligated to try a new technology or treatment that shows any promise. Unfortunately, the adoption of a new technology may mean insufficient funds for new buildings or staff, or for increased emphasis on health education and prevention.

Decisions about allocating resources for a technology involve assembling necessary data about cost-effectiveness. It is also necessary to consider the impact of future developments as well as current ones. An example of the approach to making such decisions is the hierarchy of things to consider when deciding about the effectiveness of computed tomography (CT) scanners. Stocking and Morrison (1978, p. 22) suggest the following hierarchy for making such decisions: technological capability followed by diagnostic accuracy, diagnostic impact (in replacing other procedures), therapeutic impact (change in disease management), and patient outcome with respect to morbidity and mortality.

Summary

An overview of the community and societal systems was presented in this chapter. The **community system** is composed of the family's neighborhood, health, recreational, educational, social, and political institutions that affect its functioning. **Society** is the larger political, economic, and social system under which each of the other systems (individual, family, community) function. Issues facing the health care system are related to ethical dilemmas, economics, delivery of care, legislation, and public policy. Nurses play a significant role in helping clients and families achieve a balance within the health care system, between their medically defined and self-defined illness needs.

References

Alfano, G.J. (1988). A different kind of nursing. *Nurs Outlook, 36*(1), 34–37, 39.

Andreoli, K.C., & Musser, L.A. (1985). Trends that may affect nursing's future. *Nurs Health Care, 6*(1), 47–51.

Aroskar, M.A. (1980). Anatomy of an ethical dilemma: The theory. *Am J Nurs, 80*(4), 658–660.

Bredemeier, H. (1961). *Transactional analysis and social systems.* New Brunswick, NJ: Urban Studies Center, Rutgers University.

Brooten, D. et al. (1986). A randomized clinical trial of early hospital discharge and home follow-up of very-low-birth-weight infants. *N Eng J Med, 315,* 934–939.

Campbell, R.H. (1990, January 9). Dialysis cost curbs to hit home. *Philadelphia Inquirer.* pp. 10, 13.

Christiansen, D. (1978). Dignity and aging: Notes on gerontologic ethics. *J Humanistic Psychol, 18,* 41–54.

Davis, A.L. (1981). Dilemmas in practice: A newborn's right to life vs. death. *Am J Nurs, 81,* 1035.

Hatunian, N., Smart, C., & Thompson, M. (1980). Economic costs of cancer, motor vehicle injuries, coronary heart disease and stroke: A comparative analysis. *Am J Pub Health, 70*(12), 1249–1257.

Harrington, C. (1988). Quality, access, and costs: Public

policy and home health care. *Nurs Outlook, 36*(4), 164–166.

Johnson, J.L. (1983). It's dangerous to ignore the impact of medical technology advances. *Mod Health Care, 13*(1), 100.

Kahn, R.L., & Antonucci, T.C. (1980). Convoys over the life course: Attachment, roles and social support. In P.B. Baltes & O.G. Brim (Eds.), *Life-span development and behavior* (pp. 253–286). New York: Academic Press.

Lubeck, D.P., & Yelin, E.H. (1988). A question of values: Measuring the impact of chronic disease. *Milbank Mem Fund Q, 66*(3), 444–464.

McCullough, L.B. (1984). Ethical issues in long-term physical illness. In E. Aronowitz & E.M. Bromberg (Eds.), *Mental health and long-term illness* (pp. 67–82). Canton, MA: Prodist.

Manton, K.G., & Soldo, B.J. (1985). Dynamcis of health changes in the oldest old: New perspectives and evidence. *Milbank Fund Q, 63*(2), 206–285.

Mechanic, D. (1986). *From advocacy to allocation: The evolving American health care system.* New York: Macmillan.

Meenan, R., & Yelin, E. (1981). The impact of chronic disease: A sociomedical profile of rheumatoid arthritis. *Arthritis Rheum, 24*(3), 544–549.

National Long-Term Care Survey. (1982).

Miller, M.K., & Stokes, C.S. (1978). Health status, health resources, and consolidated structural parameters: Implications for public health care policy. *J Health Soc Behav, 19*(2), 263–279.

Paucker, S.P. (1982). Prenatal genetics diagnosis by amniocentesis: The human problem. In B.J. McNeil & E.B. Cravalho (Eds.), *Critical issues in medical technology* (pp. 317–324). Boston: Auburn House.

Rettig, R.A. (1982). The end-stage renal disease workshop: Introduction. In B.J. McNeil & E.G. Cravalho (Eds.), *Critical issues in medical technology* (pp. 271–287). Boston: Auburn House.

Riegel, K.F. (1976). The dialectics of human development. *Am Psychol, 31,* 689–700.

Schroeder, S. (1981). National health insurance: Always just around the corner? *Am J Pub Health, 71*(11), 289–291.

Stocking, B., & Morrison, S.L. (1978). *The image and the reality.* Oxford, England: Oxford University Press.

Swint, J.M. (1982). Antenatal diagnosis of genetic disease: Economic considerations. In B.J. McNeil & E.B. Cravalho (Eds.), *Critical issues in medical technology* (pp. 325–342). Boston: Auburn House.

U.S. Department of Commerce Bureau of Census. (1986). *Statistical abstract of the U.S.* Washington, DC: Government Printing Office.

Walker, A.J. (1985). Reconceptualizing family stress. *J Marr Family, 47,* 827–837.

Zook, C., & Moore, E. (1980). High cost users of medical care. *N Eng J Med, 302*(18), 966–1002.

7 Suprasystems and Chronic Conditions

by
Margaret Grey, DrPH, FAAN

A chronically ill individual has an obvious and measurable effect on those closest, particularly the family. The presence of a chronic condition, however, represents a challenge in adaptation that reaches far beyond individual physiologic changes to alterations in the manner in which an individual interacts with the environment (Larkin, 1987). In the aggregate, chronic conditions have a significant measurable impact on the community and the society in which the individual lives, and in turn, that society has an effect on the chronically ill person.

Although usually described as a personal experience, a chronic condition is also important to consider from a broader perspective. Data from the National Ambulatory Medical Care Survey of 1980, for example, show that 66% of all visits to medical specialists are for chronic problems (Gortmaker & Sappenfield, 1984). Thus, just in the amount of care required and provided, chronic conditions affect the community and the society at large. The social impact of chronic illness is important from the standpoint of the availability of community supports in planning care, to the need for care providers for the chronically ill to be involved in social issues engendered by chronic conditions.

Stressors Faced by Communities and Society

It has been said that the humanity of a society is measured by how well it cares for its neediest citizens. Chronically ill individuals are among the neediest. Communities and society at large both affect and are affected by the presence of chronic conditions. Social networks, productivity at work, cultural expectations of role, financial burden, and access to care are all part of this reciprocal effect between the community and those with chronic conditions.

Social Networks

Chronic conditions affect the availability of social support, a prime purpose of a social group. Social relationships are frequently interrupted and may disintegrate under the stress of a chronic illness. Chronic conditions may involve disfigurement, inability to maintain employment, and the need for additional rest. Each factor can reduce the individual's ability to develop and maintain social supports. Loss of social relationships, of course, may lead to further problems engendered by social isolation (Strauss et al, 1984). See Chapters 10 and 13 for further discussion of social support.

Management of a chronic condition affects the manner in which individuals spend their time. In a study of families living with multiple sclerosis, Weinert (1975, quoted in Tilden & Weinert, 1987) found that these families spent significantly more time each week than did a comparison group on health-related activities and significantly less time on leisure activities. The families having a member with multiple sclerosis perceived society's response to those with long-term illness as more negative than did other families. Thus, a chronic condition may constrict the involvement of family members in community activities.

The ability to be productive is highly valued in American culture. Presence of a chronic condition may affect an individual's ability to work. Data from the National Health Interview Survey show that in 1986 about 10% of the population between ages 45 and 64 had a chronic condition that limited their ability to work or perform major activities (Division of Health, 1986). Viney and Westbrook (1981) found that the inability to work was not related to the severity of the condition per se, but rather a function of perceived severity and psychologic response to the situation. However, Kinchloe (1986) reported that all chronically ill patients, regardless of diagnosis, wanted to be productive. Thus, conflict exists between desire for a productive life-style and perceived impact of the condition. The inability to work creates important effects on the community, such as the need to provide material support for the chronically ill individual and the loss of that individual's productive financial contribution to society (Nelson-Walker, 1981).

Cultures also impose a set of expectations on chronically ill individuals about their behavior; this has been labeled the "sick role." Sick role behavior is activity undertaken by those who consider themselves ill for the purpose of getting well (Kasl & Cobb, 1966). Such expectations may vary within communities, and they may be important in determining the impact of the condition. The classic study in this area was reported by Zborowski (1952), who described ethnic variations in the response to pain and its significance. Suchman (1964) found that ethnocentric and socially cohesive groups included more persons who knew little about disease and who were more dependent when ill. Further, cohesive group structures, such as ethnically similar neighborhoods, may have considerable influence on a member's illness behavior, which may either assist or retard treatment (Geersten et al, 1975). Thus, in certain communities, there may be a differential need for certain services, such as outreach workers or transportation.

Physical Barriers

Many conditions involve some limitation in mobility. Nelson-Walker (1981) surveyed households in one county and identified 1,051 handicapped people, 46.9% of whom reported impairment in mobility. He extrapolated the findings to suggest that 238 of every 10,000 people consider themselves handicapped by some significant limitation. Such physically disabled people are prevented from integrating fully into the community because barriers may hinder their ability to move about freely. Architectural barriers may prevent people with limitations in mobility to gain access to buildings, parks, and housing, and in some communities, to voting as well (Weiss, 1988). Lack of access to public transportation further reduces disabled people's ability to participate in the social and work environment. Access for persons with disabilities is mandated by the Urban Mass Transportation Act of 1964 and Section 504 of the Rehabilitation Act of 1973 (Smith & Riggar, 1988). Section 504 provides that no otherwise qualified handicapped individual shall be excluded from participation in any program or activity receiving federal financial assistance. The goal of barrier-free design is to allow autonomous functioning of the handicapped person (Kliment, 1978). In other words, any handicapped person should be able to participate without help in everyday activities such as acquisition of goods and services, living and employment, leisure, entertainment, and schooling. The cost of change can be staggering. The Department of Transportation estimated that it would take more than $10 billion over 50 years to retrofit the rapid transit systems of New York City, Philadelphia, Boston, Cleveland, and Chicago alone. On the other hand, Bowe (1981) suggests that removal of architectural barriers will cost approximately $20 billion over 10 years, but that the cost of removing barriers would cost the country far less than inaccessibility does now. He estimates the cost of lost revenue and expenses to maintain dependency in excess of $200 billion per year. Thus, spending $20 billion to improve access is trivial compared to over $1 trillion in lost wages and expenses for the disabled over the next 10 years.

Financial Considerations

Considerable economic cost is associated with chronic conditions, as well as the social and physical costs to communities. Some chronically ill individuals are consumers of highly technological and expensive services. Zook and Moore (1980) found that chronically ill patients were among the top five high-cost consumers of general hospitals. Expenses for hospital care in 1983 were nearly $175 billion (Gibson et al, 1984). Further, these individuals have recurring expenses for medical, nursing, physical, and social services, as well as for special therapies and counseling, at a total cost of over $150 million in 1983 (Gibson et al, 1984). Such a financial burden often falls to the community when family resources cannot meet the demand.

Only about 10% of children are chronically ill. They, however, use more physician services and are hospitalized more than are other children. Fox (1984) reported that children with severe disabilities have an average of 21.8 physician visits per year, compared with four visits per year for children without chronic problems. The chronically ill are admitted to the hospital almost 30 times more often and, when admitted, stay in the hospital nearly twice as long.

The cost for such care for adults and children is huge, and expenses are not one-time expenses but recur and may increase as the problem worsens. Those with chronic conditions are likely to incur catastrophic debts because the services needed are often not covered by private insurance and may be unavailable from public programs. Fox and Newacheck (1990) reported from a survey of firms offering health insurance to their employees that the chronically ill have access to increased coverage of lower-cost alternatives to hospitalization and to improved lifetime benefits, but they also have increased cost-sharing requirements. Thus, while these people may have access to an increasing array of services, they and their families, and thus the community, are forced to bear an increasing proportion of the cost. As noted above, a chronic condition may affect the ability of either the ill person or the care giver to work. Therefore, the condition itself may interfere with eligibility for private insurance.

Worse, often those who are sickest and have the greatest need for health services are also those whose health care needs are inadequately financed. Many who are chronically ill have no insurance coverage. According to Butler and colleagues (1985), 10% of all children with functional limitations have no insurance coverage at all, and almost 20% of disabled children are from families with incomes below the poverty level. Fully three fifths of disabled adults of working age are at or below the poverty level (Bowe, 1981). Clearly, these families cannot afford the necessary care and are more likely to rely on charity and public programs than are more affluent families. In addition, some authors (Berkowitz & Rubin, 1978; Bowe, 1981) have suggested that the public and private insurance systems perpetuate dependency and potential for poverty by spending about 1/60 of the amount spent on dependent care for promoting independence.

The result of patchwork coverage for care of the chronically ill is that the expense is eventually borne by society at large. As the gap grows between the expenses covered by private insurers and those not covered, the resulting difference is often absorbed by the care providers (*Philadelphia Inquirer*, 1990). When care providers cannot absorb the cost, then the community suffers with a loss of essential services or larger debt. When communities cannot meet the cost of care, then hospital beds may be closed or community services such as visiting nursing may be cut back. In any case, the impact is felt not only by the chronically ill, but also by the entire community.

Legal/Political Stressors

Even when families have the resources to pay for care, that care should be available. Chronically ill individuals need comprehensive, ongoing care. Families with an ill member need access to specialized health care. Recent data suggest that this care may be difficult to find and obtain (Hobbs, Perrin, & Ireys, 1985). In addition, the chronically ill rarely receive adequate primary health care services. Should they be among the fortunate few who receive good care for their condition, they may receive little or no primary health care.

The discrepancy between the need for care and available care is worse for many chronically ill adults. The rapid decline in mortality across the life span seen in the 20th century is likely to have an impact on morbidity and disability in the elderly, and therefore, on their need for health services as well (Estes & Lee, 1986). A large number of adults, up to 10% of the total population and more than half of the chronically ill population, have more than one chronic condition (Rice & LaPlante, 1986). Multiple conditions are more likely to occur in the elderly, and the presence of more than one chronic condition leads to a multiplication of management problems, both in health care facilities and at home (Strauss & Corbin, 1988). Further, the American health care system is organized around an acute care framework such that those with multiple problems will require care in multiple settings. In addition, the poorest Americans suffer most from disabling chronic illness and are the least well insured (Davis & Rowland, 1987).

Although it is true that public programs have improved access to health care for the poor over the past 20 years, eligibility standards for Medicaid and copayments for Medicare impinge on these benefits (Butler, Rosenbaum, & Palfrey, 1987). For example, the proportion of low-income Americans insured by Medicaid fell from 63% to 46% between 1975 and 1983 (Rosenbaum & Johnson, 1986). The health

care system thus gives priority to those who are insured and require critical acute care rather than to prevention and chronic care. This acute care perspective also emphasizes technology and downplays less technologic modes of care and the social and psychologic aspects of care. The result is a fragmented approach to care that does not provide the continuity required by individuals and families with chronic conditions.

The chronically ill require a large number of supportive services, which may include genetic counseling, special schooling, home care, and respite care. These services may be provided, if available, in various ways but are almost universally not reimbursable (Perrin & Ireys, 1984). Home care is a case in point. In 1980 and 1981, Medicare home health benefits were increased, and since then there has been a rapid growth in the home care industry, with a compound annual growth rate of over 20%. In addition, the advent of diagnostic related groups (DRGs) as a method of containing hospital costs resulted in early hospital discharge for many patients (Vladeck, 1985). Unfortunately, the regulations have not kept up with the need, and many chronically ill persons who need extended home care services cannot get them. Other services, such as special schooling and respite care, are not reimbursable under either public or private insurance programs.

Schooling is a particular issue for chronically ill children, and thus for communities. Public Law 94-142, the Education for All Handicapped Act, provided that communities must provide free, appropriate public education in the least restrictive environment for all children between the ages of 6 and 21 years. To the maximum extent possible, these children are to be educated with their nonhandicapped peers and must have "individualized education programs" outlining their special educational curricula and related services necessary to meet their unique needs. In 1983, the law was amended to expand the age of eligibility to include birth through age 5 years. More than 4 million children receive services under this legislation (Willian & Jones, 1987). The result of this legislation on communities has been expensive in both planning and implementation costs, estimated to be about $35,000 per child. The funding source for such services remains unclear, since they may be viewed as either education or health services.

Furthermore, data from a variety of sources demonstrate that chronically ill children miss an average of twice as much school as their healthy peers

(Fowler, Johnson, & Atkinson, 1985; Weitzman, 1986; Weitzman, Walker, & Gortmaker, 1986). Fowler and colleagues (1985) reported that children with chronic health conditions missed about 16 days of school per year, whereas the average for the state of North Carolina was less than seven days. Absence from school poses educational and social threats for all children by interfering with academic performance and peer relationships. In one study, (Fowler, Johnson, & Atkinson, 1985) performance on the National Achievement Scale was significantly lower for the absentees than for their classmates. Frequent absenteeism is also associated with higher dropout rates (Weitzman, 1986). Such statistics are of concern to communities because they reflect the decreased potential for chronically ill individuals to contribute to society through work.

In summary, chronic illness in the community causes significant stress to that community and the society. Such stressors include the productivity of the citizens, physical barriers, financial strains, and political issues.

How to Assess Community Strengths and Deficits

Just as health care providers assess the strengths and deficits of individuals, so can the characteristics of communities and societies be defined. The word *community* is derived from the Latin *communitas*, as the root of community. A community is composed of the individuals and households who live and work there, as well as the buildings, historical traditions, power structures, and social values and customs. To define and assess a community, one needs to know precisely who and where the individuals and households are, how they live and behave in ways that influence their health, where and when they seek care for their ailments, and how they perceive and finance their care. A population is a class or group of people that is more clearly definable than a community, in which all the inhabitants of a given country or area are considered together. A denominator is defined as one number that is used to divide another; in community assessment, the denominator is the population base (Strelnick, 1987).

Defining a community is an ongoing dialectical process between the assessor and the human environment. Communities may be defined by preexisting boundaries (e.g., school districts, catchment areas) or by historical neighborhood traditions (e.g.,

Chinatown). Communities may also be defined by common experiences, problems, or exposures, as in the relationship of the gay community to the population at risk for AIDS. In such a case, when problems are defined as being identified as characteristics of people rather than of social, geographic, or cultural phenomena that transcend their aggregate as individuals, then the population is the appropriate level of focus. The presence or absence of the relevant problem or characteristic defines the population.

A community is a whole entity that functions because of the interdependence of its parts or subsystems. Table 7–1 identifies eight community subsystems and a central community core that must be assessed to understand a community and the resources available therein for the chronically ill. Such a model can be used to assess a community regardless of size, location, resources, or population characteristics; the process remains the same.

Community Core

The community core is that which is essential, basic, and enduring; it is its people. The first stage of community assessment is to learn about the people in the community—their history, characteristics, values, and beliefs. Table 7–1 lists the components of community core data. Some of this information is available in community materials found in libraries, historical societies, and health departments. Information about values, beliefs, religion, and the like is obtained by personal contact with the people in the community.

Physical Environment

Assessing the physical environment gives an indication of the nature of the community. For the most part, information on the environment can be obtained by observation of such items as the type and condition of structures, including the degree of handicapped accessibility, evidence of community problems such as homelessness, signs of decay, and the layout of the community. Other important information about the environment includes climate and topography. Such information might be found in the library, historical society, or weather bureau.

Health and Social Services

It is particularly important for the nurse working with the chronically ill to be familiar with all of the

Table 7–1 Subsystems for Community Assessment

Community Core

History
Demographics (age, sex, racial and ethnic distribution)
Household types
Marital status
Vital statistics (births, deaths, causes of death)
Values, beliefs, religions

Physical environment	**Education**
Climate	Educational status
Terrain	Educational sources
Natural boundaries	
Resources	
Housing	
Recreation	**Economics**
Facilities	Financial characteristics
	Labor force characteristics
Communication	**Politics, government**
Formal (newspaper, radio, telephone)	Organization
Informal (sources, dissemination)	Politically active groups
Safety, transportation	**Health, social services**
Protection services	Extra- or intra community
Air quality	
Private transportation	
Public transportation	

Source: Adapted from Anderson & McFarlane, 1988.

local service agencies. This analysis should include services inside the community and outside the community that are used by the people of interest. Health services should include all hospitals and clinics, home health care agencies, extended care facilities, public health services, and private practices. This information might be obtained from the local chamber of commerce, planning board, or telephone directory.

Social service agencies may offer counseling and support, clothing, food, and shelter, or answer other special needs. Information on such agencies might be obtained from sources listed previously as well as from philanthropic concerns like the United Way. For both health and social services, it is important to know the services provided, the resources available, the characteristics of the users, and the accessibility of the facility or agency.

Economics

The economic subsystem is the wealth of the community, including the goods and services available to the community and the costs and benefits of improving patterns of resource allocation. Both financial and labor-force characteristics need to be assessed. Census data help in compiling this information, providing figures on median household income in the community, the proportion of households below the poverty level, those receiving public assistance or headed by females, and individual per capita income.

Assessing the economic subsystem also includes determining employment within the community. Information about the percentage of community employment, occupations, and union membership can be obtained, respectively from Department of Labor statistics, census records, and local union offices. In assessing an industry in relationship to the chronically ill, it may be important to know the number of handicapped or disabled employees, the health services available, the safety of the work environment, and employee benefits. Such information would be obtainable from the employee relations officer in the industry.

Safety and Transportation

Those who are chronically ill need to live in a safe environment and be able to get to needed treatment facilities. Safety services include fire, police, emergency, and sanitation. Environmental factors such as air quality are important for those with chronic obstructive lung disease. Availability of heat, hot water, and electricity are important: An elderly person on a fixed income may have difficulty paying a large heating bill in an unusually cold winter, and provision for emergency support should be available. Similarly, many electric companies provide emergency service for ventilator dependent patients at home in the event of a cutoff in service. Information about safety services may be obtained from the local offices for planning, fire, and public safety.

Transportation may be public or private. It is important to know the proportion of the community with transportation disability. Local and state highway departments can provide information about bus service, roads, interstate highways, and air and rail service.

Politics and Government

It is relatively easy to determine the political structure of a community by examining community records. Such information may be important for identifying important persons to lobby for change. In all communities, however, there are other less-visible groups who influence decision making at the government level. A community services directory should list appropriate agencies, but only discussion with agency individuals will suggest the level of their involvement in community decision making.

Communication

Formal communications include newspapers, radio and television stations, postal service, and the number of residences with telephones. Such information is important for working with chronically ill individuals and families because of the importance of communication in social networks and support. Informal sources of communication include bulletin boards, newsletters, and neighborhood flyers. It is also important to determine how people in the community receive information (e.g., word of mouth, mail, radio, television).

Education

As noted, the provision to educate ill children is mandated by law. Thus, the assessment of community educational facilities is important to understanding the availability of services and must include the type of schools, size of enrollment, funding (publicly supported and/or tuition supported), and available services. In many communities, the school nurse is in a particular school only one day per week. In regard to chronically ill children, one day per week may not provide enough nursing care, and other support will need to be obtained.

Recreation

Indoor and outdoor facilities and their accessibility should be considered. The availability of play areas convenient to the community, health clubs and swimming pools, barrier-free theaters and auditoriums, and special olympics and other programs for the disabled may all be important to the welfare of those with chronic conditions.

Analysis

Once the characteristics of the community are known, the provider analyzes the information and determines the adequacy of the community for the needs of the clients. Community analysis helps to identify community health needs, strengths, and patterns of use.

The first step in analyzing the community data is to categorize them. Traditional categories include demographic characteristics (e.g., age, sex, ethnicity), geographic characteristics (e.g., area boundaries, neighborhoods), socioeconomic characteristics (e.g., income, occupations, education), and health resources and services (e.g., hospitals, emergency services, clinics, counseling). These data are then summarized. If the nurse discovers gaps in the data, they may be filled through further research, but usually the analyst proceeds, aware that the information gap can affect the analysis.

Finally, the nurse aims to synthesize the data by focusing on the strengths and inadequacies of the community to meet the needs of the people. This process is sometimes referred to as community diagnosis. Note that the services required will vary by the types of people and problems found in the community. If the community tends to be transient, with many young working families, the need for elderly care, for example, may be secondary to needs for women's and children's services. Thus, the nurse assesses community needs and determines the availability of services to meet the needs. A community diagnosis perhaps important in working with the chronically ill might include, for example, "Inadequate hospice care for cancer patients related to the overused public health agency and visiting nurse service and manifested by overuse of inpatient facilities for the terminally ill." Further examples of this process in action may be found in Box 7–1 and Box 7–2.

Role of the Nurse

Assessment and analysis of the community help to provide the nurse with the information necessary to help families meet their developmental tasks (Du-

Box 7−1 *Example of Community-based Practice with a Child*

John N. is an 8-year-old boy newly diagnosed with diabetes mellitus. He and his parents have learned the basics of management, including insulin injections and methods of monitoring control. He is medically stable, having recovered from the ketosis that brought him to care, so he is ready for discharge from the acute care institution. Several issues face this family: John's mother is nervous about managing his diet and insulin at home; the school is concerned about John's capability of participating fully in school activities; and John's father is concerned about the costs of John's care.

The nurse can and should advocate for this family in a variety of ways. First, ongoing support for the parents needs to be made available. Such support could come from the visiting nurse, if she or he is knowledgeable about management of type I diabetes, or from the clinical specialist or nurse practitioner in the diabetes service that provides follow-up care. Referral to a dietician who can work with the family to accommodate personal needs and preferences may be necessary. Prior to his discharge from the hospital, John and his family need to be provided information on how to deal with school personnel and others who have concerns about his participation in activities. In some cases, the nurse or the visiting nurse will need to go with the family to ensure that the child gets the appropriate follow-up in the community. Finally, the family needs to know all the financial options available to support the day-to-day management costs, which for type I diabetes can run to over $50 per month. In addition, there is the cost of follow-up care, such as routine visits to the specialist ($100, four times per year) and laboratory tests ($25, four times per year). John's family needs to know how much of these costs, if any, will be covered by their health insurance, and whether there are special state programs for the medically indigent to help them deal with these costs. Further, the nurse should be in contact with the legislators to know what the current thinking is regarding funding for such long-term care.

Box 7−2 *Example of an Elderly Person Requiring Community Services*

Mrs. Brown is a 68-year-old female who was admitted to the hospital with a right cardiovascular accident (CVA) in addition to her previous history of hypertension, hypercholesterolemia, glucose intolerance, and partial tongue resection associated with a carcinoma. She lives with her husband in a housing complex for the elderly. She is to be discharged home with her husband following acute care and rehabilitation hospitalization. She has some recovery of strength in her left arm, so she can use that arm for gross assistance with activities of daily living. She is independent at meals, requires moderate assistance with dressing, and minimal assistance with bathing. She does require help with housekeeping and minimal help with wheelchair mobility. Her speech is 75% intelligible in conversation.

At home, she is to have medical follow-up by her primary care provider and a rehabilitation physician, as well as physical, speech, and occupational therapy. A referral is made to the Visiting Nurse Service, specifically to monitor her diabetes and to check the skin integrity periodically. The nurse assesses that Mrs. Brown has multiple health care needs, including coordination of services; physical, speech, and occupational therapy; transportation; financial assistance with Medicare/Medicaid and supplementary programs; and homemaker services to provide respite care for her husband. Coordination of services is necessary for several reasons—not having appointments scheduled at conflicting times, allowing adequate time for rest, and coordinating transportation services. The 10-day inpatient hospitalization and 30 days in the rehabilitation center had exhausted the majority of the Brown's private insurance coverage, so help from a social worker with Medicare and supplemental programs was needed for Mrs. Brown to receive all the necessary services.

Despite the fact that Mrs. Brown made a good recovery at about 2−2½ months postdischarge, the nurse observed how difficult it was to coordinate all the transportation efforts to

Box 7-2   *Example of an Elderly Person Requiring Community Services Continued*

various services—PT, OT, follow-up appointments, and the social worker. She tried to find a way for some services to be obtained in the home, but to no avail, because she could not demonstrate that Mrs. Brown required them as individual services to be done in the home. Therefore, insurance would not cover the cost of home care. This gap in financial coverage resulted in less than adequate service for this family. The nurse contacted various legislators to see if there was a way to finance such care. Eventually, she found herself lobbying for alterations in the way home care services are financed.

vall, 1977). Aquilera and Messick (1968) presented a paradigm for crisis intervention that is useful in understanding the effect of balancing factors in the presence of a stressful event, such as a chronic condition. Although their paradigm is intended for interpreting crisis situations with individuals, it is equally helpful in understanding the balance between the person who is chronically ill and the society at large.

Realistic perception is vital in the reacquisition of emotional equilibrium that may be disturbed by a stressful event. When there is distorted perception, there is no relationship between the event and the feelings of stress. It is therefore important that communities understand the nature of chronic conditions and the potential for impact on the community. Realistic perception can be promoted by the attitudes and knowledge of the persons in the environment, particularly nurses, physicians, and significant family members. While not diminishing the seriousness of the condition, the family and those in the community should be provided with factual knowledge and assistance in problem solving.

Another balancing factor in the paradigm is adequate situational support. Situational support helps to solve the stressful event, and it includes the availability of services in the community. Each family must be assessed to determine the available coping mechanisms or intermediate problem-solving methods and services in the community that are available to them. It is the responsibility of the nurse to ensure that families have access to the necessary situational support.

A critical task for families is that of physical maintenance, which includes providing food, clothing, shelter, and health care for its members. Families with an ill member need access to specialized health care that may be difficult to find and obtain (Hobbs, Perrin, & Ireys, 1985). Other family decisions may be influenced by the need for this access to care. For example, the ability of the family to travel for work or pleasure and the ability to provide for the finances of physical maintenance may be impaired by the burden of caring for an ill person (Vance et al, 1980).

In an optimally functioning family, financial, space, and time resources are allocated according to family members' needs. A person who is disabled may have a disproportionate need for family resources, leaving fewer available for other family members. As noted before, concerns about finances are often paramount for these families. For example, routine day-to-day management of a child with diabetes can cost an average of $50 per month, including insulin, syringes, and glucose strips. For families in which the chronically ill member is dependent on others to accomplish activities of daily living, the time demanded by the condition can be substantial and may interfere with time available for other activities (Haggerty, Roghmann, & Pless, 1975). Such support for the activities of daily living may require community help, which may or may not be available.

In families with preexisting contraints on time and resources, such as single-parent families, the difficulties of allocation can be increased exponentially. Families living in areas where support services are scarce may find that the majority of time is spent travelling to the needed services (Hobbs et al, 1985).

Another developmental task of families is the determination of individual roles in support, management, and care of the home and family members. The increased burden of care for the chronically ill person usually falls to one individual, most frequently the wife (Brody, 1981) or mother (Stein & Jessop, 1984). Many families have reported that the work of dealing with a chronically ill child is not equitably shared, with most responsibility falling to the mother. Further, other studies (Sabbeth & Leventhal, 1984; Silbert, Newberger, & Fyler, 1982) have shown that familiy members who share the work and the worry report that sharing is a source of strength, and mothers of chronically ill children report concern with fatigue when the work of caring for the child is not shared. A disabled child may also influence the parent to enter or leave the work force and may limit employment mobility. Shifts in the division of labor in the family may also affect the adjustment of others in the family. Concerns like these may require the availability of respite care so that the health of the care giver is not negatively affected.

Another family developmental task involves the relationship of family members to the larger society, including work, school, church, friends, and extended family (Duvall, 1977; Hymovich & Chamberlin, 1980). In some cases, the volume of care associated with a chronic condition may isolate the family. Where conditions like muscular dystrophy and spina bifida are present, difficulties with mobility may keep the family home and isolated. Fear of infection and other problems may also keep the family from involvement in the larger community. Whatever the reason, lack of social support beyond the family limits the available mechanisms for sharing the burden of caring (Burr, 1985).

As noted previously, school provides a long-term relationship for the child with the community. Chronic illness may severely impact the child's participation in school. A number of studies (Fowler, Johnson, & Atkinson, 1985; Weitzman, 1986; Weitzman, Walker, & Gortmaker, 1986) document that chronically ill children miss more school than do their healthy peers. In addition, for some children, school performance, adjustment, and illness are interrelated (Grey, 1988). Communities are assigned the task of educating their young people, and nurses must advocate for chronically ill children to ensure that they receive an adequate, appropriate education.

Policy Implications

Beyond the responsibility to provide direct services to these families, and to ensure the availability of services in the community, health professionals also have a responsibility to advocate for public policies favorable to families with chronically ill members (Burr, 1985). Several areas of public policy need to be addressed. One critical area for families is the availability of financial resources for meeting the direct and indirect health care expenses for the chronically ill. The financial burden of a chronic condition in a family is remarkable and will affect the ability of the family to carry out its developmental tasks. Policies that limit access to financial support to those with certain conditions or to families who meet specific income guidelines may need to be reexamined. The availability and distribution of health care resources should also be examined, in terms of both quality of available services and psychological and financial effects on families with limited resources. This omission has broad implications for overall health, and must be addressed.

Families burdened by chronic illness also need services beyond traditional biomedical services. They need to receive information to improve their understanding of the disease, its cause, and treatment, and requirements for day-to-day management. In addition, they need access to social and health resources such as homemaker services, visiting nurses, and respite care. Such services are difficult at best to find, and their availability needs to be addressed through policy change as well as providers' understanding of their necessity.

The need is also urgent to find alternative methods of providing care for the chronically ill. Such methods must not only be responsive to the needs of the patient and family, but they must also begin to reduce the economic burden of chronic illness and disability on society. Strauss and Corbin (1988) documented the inability of the current acute-care-focused health care system to deal effectively with the long-term care issues engendered by chronic illness. They note that, in general, the acute care providers prepare the person to go home, but then largely neglect him or her until the next crisis returns the person to the acute care setting. Five major points must be addressed to deal with the overwhelming problems of chronic conditions: (1) Long-term care must involve more than that offered in acute care facilities. (2) Clinical care should be supplemented by services that will meet the rehabilitative, psychologic, economic, social and other needs of the ill. (3) There should be a shift in funding patterns so that such other services can be greatly expanded. (4) Funding for the poor requires special attention because they bear the burden of the health care system's failings. (5) Funding arrangements to cover potential economic catastrophe for all ill or disabled Americans are imperative (Strauss & Corbin, 1988, pp 35–36).

An attempt to restructure the system is a program at the University of Maryland (Taylor, Ryan, & Mandrell, 1986), which involves a transition unit for adult patients facing premature hospital discharge. Patients and families have the option of requesting admission to the transition unit in the chronic care hospital. Patients are initially evaluated by a nurse practitioner to assess eligibility, and once they are enrolled in the program, their self-care abilities and independence in daily living are assessed weekly. If additional help is needed, the person is referred to community services.

Once the referral is made to the community, the nurse is often faced with myriad services, many not designed to provide the necessary care. A patient with a recent stroke, for example, may need help from sources including visiting nursing, rehabilitation, and respite care for the spouse, as well as ongoing medical and health supervision. Such services, if available, are often uncoordinated, so the family may see the visiting nurse on Monday and Friday, go to the physical therapist on Tuesday and Thursday, and then have to work in medical visits to specialists—all this with a patient who has had a stroke and is nonambulatory. It is clearly nurse's responsibility to assume the role of care coordinator and intervene with community agencies either to acquire as many services as possible in the home or to help the family schedule services to allow ample time and ample rest periods. To succeed requires a working knowledge of all agencies involved, obtained through the community analysis, and the commitment in time and energy to advocate for these patients. The community health nurse, "street-wise" and well versed in services available, can serve as a client advocate and vital link between family and community resources.

Further, the nurse must get involved in the political process in order to effect change in the care provided for the chronically ill. Politicians need to know the issues and the measures to be taken. Nurses working with the chronically ill should get to know their local, state, and federal legislators. Many legislators have a staff member whose major responsibility is health-related legislation. Let the staff know who you are and your area of expertise. Suggest changes that should be made. When a particular piece of legislation is coming up for a vote, make sure the legislator knows your opinion and why you hold it. Nurses must become vocal in the political

process, or the acute care focus of the health care system will not be changed. Recently, the U.S. Congress attempted to pass legislation regarding funding for catastrophic illness. Although legislation is necessary for this population, the bill in question put the burden of payment on those most likely to be affected, the elderly. Outcries from providers and the elderly by telephone, telegram, and personal visit forced the Congress to repeal the legislation. This is the type of action nurses need to take concerning all relevant legislative issues.

Summary

Chronic conditions have a significant, measurable impact on the community and the society in which the individual lives. In turn, that society has an effect on the chronically ill person. These effects are important from a number of standpoints, such as the availability of community supports in planning care, to the need for involvement by care providers for the chronically ill in social issues engendered by chronic conditions. Social networks, productivity at work, cultural expectations of role, financial burden, and access to care all have this reciprocal effect with the community and the chronically ill.

The process of community assessment and analysis is the nurse's tool for understanding the community and its reciprocal impact on the chronically ill. Assessment of the community includes information on the community core: the physical environment, communications, recreation facilities, safety and transportation, education, economics, politics and government, and health and social services. Analysis and community diagnosis give the nurse an understanding of the adequacy of the community to deal with the needs of the chronically ill. The nurse's role in helping families deal with these issues is to ensure access to appropriate services so that the family can meet its developmental tasks, and to advocate for policy change to increase the availability of essential services.

References

Anderson, E.T., & McFarlane, J.M. (1988). *Community as client: Application of the nursing process*. Philadelphia: Lippincott.

Aquilera, D.C., & Messick, J.M. (1978). *Crisis intervention: Theory and methodology*. St. Louis: Mosby.

Berkowitz, M., & Rubin, J. (1978). *The costs of disability:*

Estimates of program expenditures for disability, 1967–1975. New Brunswick, NJ: Bureau of Economic Research.

Bowe, F. (1981). *Rehabilitating America: Toward independence for disabled and elderly people.* New York: Harper & Row.

Brody, E. (1981). "Women in the middle" and family help to older people. *Gerontologist, 21,* 471–480.

Burr, C.K. (1985). Impact on the family of a chronically ill child. In N. Hobbs & J.M. Perrin (Eds.), *Issues in the care of children with chronic illness* (pp. 24–40). New York: Springer.

Butler, J.A., Budetti, P., McManus, M.A., Stenmark, S., & Newachek (1985). Health care expenditures for children with chronic illness. In N. Hobbs & J.H. Perrin (Eds.), *Issues in the care of children with chronic illness* (pp. 827–863). San Francisco: Jossey-Bass.

Butler, J.A., Rosenbaum, S., & Palfrey, J.S. (1987). Ensuring access to health care for children with disabilities. *N Eng J Med, 317,* 162–165.

Davis, K., & Rowland, D. (1987). Uninsured and underserved: Inequities in health care in the United States. In H. Schwartz (Ed.), *Dominant issues in medical sociology* (2nd ed.) (pp. 513–629). New York: Random House.

Division of Health Interview Statistics. (1986). *Data from the National Health Interview Survey.* Washington, DC: Department of Health and Human Services.

Duvall, E.M. (1977). *Marriage and family development.* Philadelphia: Lippincott.

Estes, C.L., & Lee, P.R. (1986). Health problems and policy issues of old age. In L.H. Aiken & D. Mechanic (Eds.), *Applications of social science to clinical medicine and health policy* (pp. 335–355), New Brunswick, NJ: Rutgers University Press.

Fowler, M.G., Johnson, M.P., & Atkinson, S.S. (1985). School achievement and absence in children with chronic health conditions. *J Pediatr, 106* (5), 683–687.

Fox, H.B. (1984, September). *A preliminary analysis of options to improve health insurance coverage for chronically ill and disabled children.* Paper prepared for the Division of Maternal Health, Department of Health and Human Services, Washington, D.C.

Fox, H.B., & Newacheck, P.W. (1990). Private insurance of chronically ill children. *Pediatrics, 85* (1), 50–57.

Geersten, R., Klauber, M.R., Rindflesh, M., et al. (1975). A reexamination of Suchman's views on social factors in health care utilization. *J Health Soc Behav, 16,* 226–237.

Gibson, R.M., Levit, K.R., Lazenby, H., & Waldo, D.R. (1984). *Bureau of data management and strategy: National health expenditures, 1983* (HCFA Publication No. 03177). Health Care Financing Administration, Washington, DC: U.S. Government Printing Office.

Gortmaker, S.L., & Sappenfield, W. (1984). Chronic childhood disorders: Prevalence and impact. *Pediatr Clin North Am, 31* (1), 3–18.

Grey, M. (1988). Stressful life events, absenteeism, and the use of school health services. *J Pediatr Health Care, 2,* 121–128.

Haggerty, R., Roghmann, K.J., & Pless, I.B. (1975). *Child health and the community.* New York: Wiley.

Hobbs, N., Perrin, J.M., & Ireys, H.T. (1985). *Chronically ill children and their families.* San Francisco: Jossey-Bass.

Hymovich, D.P., & Chamberlin, R.W. (1980). *Child and family development: Implications for care.* New York: McGraw-Hill.

Kasl, S.V., & Cobb, S. (1966). Health behavior, illness behavior, and sick role behavior. *Arch Environ Health, 12* (2), 246–266.

Kinchloe, M. (1986). The energizing effect of purposeful, creative activity. *Nurs Forum, 18,* 269–277.

Kliment, S.A. (1978). Removing environmental barriers. In R.M. Goldenson (Ed.), *Disability and rehabilitation handbook* (pp. 110–119). New York: McGraw-Hill.

Larkin, J. (1987). Factors influencing one's ability to adapt to chronic illness. *Nurs Clin North Am, 22* (3), 535–542.

Nelson-Walker, R. (1981). *Planning, creating and financing housing for handicapped people.* Springfield, IL: Charles C Thomas.

Perrin, J.M., & Ireys, H.T. (1984). The organization of services for chronically ill children and their families. *Pediatr Clin North Am, 31* (1), 235–257.

Philadelphia hospitals face serious shortage of cash. (1990, January). *Philadelphia Inquirer,* p. 1.

Rice, D., & LaPlante, M. (1986, October). The burden of multiple chronic conditions: Past trends and policy implications. Paper presented at the annual meeting of the American Public Health Association, Las Vegas, NV.

Rosenbaum, S., & Johnson, K. (1986). Providing health care for low income children: Reconciling child health goals with child health financing realities. *Milbank Mem Fund Q, 64,* 442–478.

Sabbeth, B.F., & Leventhal, J.M. (1984). Marital adjustment to chronic childhood illness: A critique of the literature. *Pediatrics, 73,* 762–768.

Silbert, A., Newberger, J., & Fyler, D. (1982). Marital stability and congenital heart disease. *Pediatrics, 69,* 747–750.

Smith, E.R., & Riggar, T.F. (1988, April/May/June). Accessible transportation: Human rights versus costs. *J Rehabil,* pp. 13–17.

Stein, R.E.K., & Jessop, D.J. (1984). General issues in the care of children with chronic physical conditions. *Pediatr Clin N Am, 31,* 189–198.

Strauss, A., & Corbin, J. M. (1988). *Shaping a new health care system.* San Francisco: Jossey-Bass.

Strauss, A.L., Corbin, J., Fagerhaugh, S., Glaser, B.G.,

Maines, D., Suczek, B., & Weiner, C.L. (1984). *Chronic illness and the quality of life* (2nd ed.). St. Louis: Mosby.

Strelnick, A.H. (1987). The community-defining process in COPC. In P.A. Nutting (Ed.), *Community-oriented primary care: From principle to practice* (pp. 35–39). (HRSA Publication No. HRS-A-PE 86-1). Washington, DC: U.S. Government Printing Office.

Suchman, E.A. (1964). Sociomedical variations among ethnic groups. *Am J Sociol, 70,* 319–331.

Taylor, G., Ryan, J., & Mandrell, H. (1986). The transition unit: The bridge between acute and long-term care. *Maryland State Med J, 35,* 913–915.

Tilden, V.P., & Weinert, C. (1987). Social support and the chronically ill individual. *Nurs Clin North Am, 22* (3), 613–620.

Vance, J.C., Fazan, L.E., Satterwhite, B., & Pless, I.B. (1980). Effects of nephrotic syndrome on the family: A controlled study. *Pediatrics, 65,* 948–955.

Viney, L.L., & Westbrook, M.T. (1981). Psychological reactions to chronic illness-related disability as a function of its severity and type. *J Psychosom Res, 25,* 513–523.

Vladeck, B. (1985). The static dynamics of long-term health policy. In M. Lewin (Ed.), *The health policy agenda* (pp. 2–19). Washington, DC: American Enterprise Institute.

Weiss, D.V. (1988, April/May/June). Work with local election officials to make polling places accessible. *J Rehabil,* pp. 8–9.

Weitzman, M. (1986). School absence rates as outcome measures in studies of children with chronic illness. *J Chron Dis, 39* (10), 799–808.

Weitzman, M., Walker, D.K., & Gortmaker, S. (1986). Chronic illness, psychosocial problems, and school absences. *Clin Pediatr, 25* (3), 137–142.

Willian, M.K., & Jones, J.M. (1987). Implementing early childhood intervention: Overcoming boundaries between health and education. *George Washington University National Health Policy Forum,* Issue Brief No. 470, Washington, D.C.

Zborowski, M. (1952). Cultural components in responses to pain. *J Soc Issues, 8,* 16–30.

Zook, C., & Moore, F. (1980). The high-cost users of medical care. *N Eng J Medicine, 302,* 996–1002.

SECTION III
Contingency Variables: Time and Orientation to Life

This section contains two chapters related to the contingency variables time and orientation to life. Chapter 8, Time, provides background information regarding the concept of time, its meaning to persons with chronic conditions, and factors influencing time perception. Suggestions for nursing assessment and selected nursing interventions are included in the chapter.

Chapter 9, Orientation to Life, differentiates between values, attitudes, and beliefs of each system in the Contingency Model of Long-Term Care. Pertinent attitudes of relevance to nursing include spread, stigma, anxiety, and labeling. Health beliefs and their measurement are also discussed in this chapter. Spiritual orientation is viewed as the core of one's being. Nursing interventions to modify attitudes and to support spirituality are discussed.

8 Time

Systems evolve over time, each one having a past, present, and future. Events taking place within systems are not static but transact with one another in a dynamic and continuous process of change. Viewing systems from a developmental perspective also implies change over time. Although nurses interact with an individual or family system in the present, the system's functioning cannot be understood without some notion of its past or some idea of its anticipated future. "Each person brings to the present moment his or her own unique causal past" (Watson, 1988, p. 47).

The temporal dimension of a system is important because all social activities require and may, therefore, be inhibited by the expenditure of time; and within its own culture, each system perceives time differently and manages it differently. Chronic conditions evolve over extended periods and stressors of varying intensity and duration often change over time. The relation of time to other variables in the Contingency Model of Long-Term Care is illustrated in Figure 8–1. The model shows time as an underlying factor that must be considered during interaction with clients. Although time moves forward, past experiences are relevant to current stressors, orientation to life, coping strengths and needs, and level of functioning; and these variables will, in turn, impact on future functioning and experiences. Figure 8–2 illustrates the forward direction of time by the wide arrow. The small unidirectional arrow indicates past influences on the present, which is the point of reference for interaction. For example, the woman whose mother has severe congestive heart failure will take her mother to the emergency room immediately when she complains of tightness in the chest and shortness of breath because the last time it happened her mother had pulmonary edema. The double arrow indicates that what happens in the present or happened in the past will influence the system's future; and future system goals may be determined by current decisions. For example, the job decisions made today by a 58-year-old woman with rheumatoid arthritis are based on her plans for the future. Since she wants to retire in the South, she decided to seek a transfer there rather than to Colorado. She hopes to have to move just once and begin to make friends prior to retirement.

This chapter provides an overview of the concept of time as it pertains to the Contingency Model of Long-Term Care. Time is defined, objectively and subjectively, and various aspects of time are explored in detail. The relation of chronic illness and hospitalization to time is examined, and selected aspects of the nurse's role in assessment and intervention are discussed.

Definition of Time

Time may be defined objectively as "clock time," that is, "what the clock measures"; or subjectively, as "a set of mental schemata and concepts that individuals and cultures have developed for various purposes" (Gorman & Wessman, 1977, p. 217). Within the context of the Contingency Model of Long-Term Care, time is defined as "an indefinite,

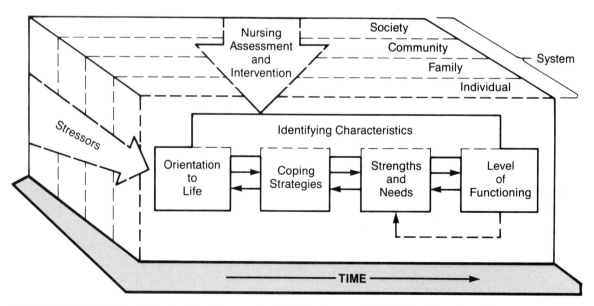

FIGURE 8–1 Relationship of Time to Other Components of the Contingency Model of Long-Term Care. Time is an underlying dimension that permeates all aspects of long-term care.

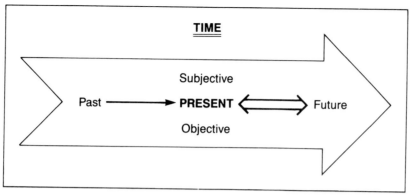

FIGURE 8–2 Time Component of the Contingency Model of Long-Term Care. The wide arrow depicts time as moving forward; the small unidirectional arrow indicates past influences on the present, which is the point of reference for interaction; the double arrow indicates that what happens in the present, or happened in the past, will influence the system's future; system goals for the future also are determined by present decisions.

unlimited duration in which things are considered as happening in the past, present, or future" (Guralnik, 1984, p. 1489). Although time is used commonly as a noun in everyday language, it is really not an "object"; it is probably an internal *process of judgment* rather than the primary object of judgment itself.

The Concept of Time

Time is an elusive and difficult concept to grasp. According to Ornstein (1969), time

. . . is one of the continuing, compelling, and universal experiences of our lives, one of the primary threads which combine in the weave of our experience. All of our perceptual, intellectual and emotional experiences are intertwined with time. We continually *feel* time passing but where does it come from? We continually experience it but we cannot taste it, smell it, hear it or touch it. (p. 15)

Concepts related to time include its (1) sequence, (2) duration, (3) rate, (4) rhythm, (5) recurrence, (6) routine, and (7) synchronization (Pastorello, 1982). To measure the temporal process, we determine its rate by standardized clocks and calendars. Piaget (1971, pp. 61–62) distinguishes between *temporal order,* the simple succession of events, and *temporal duration,* the length of the interval between events. Leach (1961, p. 133) noted that time may be observed in one of three ways: as a line (going on and on), a wheel (going around and around), or a pendulum (going back and forth).

Time viewed as a pendulum is considered to be discontinuous, as in day and night, winter and summer. See Figure 8–3.

According to Hendricks (1982), time has four dimensions. The **ecological dimension,** routed in nature, provides a basic calendar for regulating behavior by linking time to changes, such as wet and dry, cold and warm. The **individual dimension** refers to a person's subjective construction of time, and the **social dimension** is related to normative determinations as to when events such as mealtimes or holidays take place. The **ideational dimension** refers to historical and mythical temporality that relate the past, present, and future to traditions and

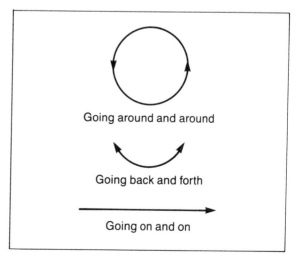

FIGURE 8–3 Ways of Observing Time

significant historical events that have been given meaning in the culture.

People with chronic illness talk about their disease in relation to these dimensions of time, as evidenced by the following examples. The man with osteoarthritis says he is stiffer in the spring when it's cold and damp. A grandmother with Parkinson's disease says time passes slowly since she hasn't been able to do her needlepoint. They are referring to the ecological and individual dimensions respectively.

The widower with chronic obstructive pulmonary disease (COPD) who says he gets depressed during the holidays because he's lonely and the man with a spinal cord injury who recalls diving into the swimming pool the day John F. Kennedy was shot are talking about the social and ideational dimensions respectively.

Time is connected with the observation of events. Since events occur in an irreversible process, people develop a sense of direction of time from their perception of events. This sense of time gives an element of organization to events, helping us regulate our actions by noting cues in time (Riegel, 1977). Many nursing activities follow clock time. However perception of the time it takes to engage in an activity may be quite different from the actual time taken. When very busy, we are likely to ask, "Where did the time go?" When bored, we may think that time is standing still. When working with patients who are depressed or difficult to talk with, time seems like an eternity. When we are in the room of a happy person, however, time may seem to fly by. Patients may have different perceptions of the amount of time it takes to change their dressings, have their catheters irrigated, or have their tube feedings.

Time can be treated as a primary organizer for activities and a way of handling priorities and categorizing experience (Hall, 1983). For example, decisions about preoperative teaching, anticipatory guidance, and giving medications whenever necessary (PRN) are based on appropriate timing. Treatments and medications are generally scheduled for specific times, as are many appointments and meetings. Scheduled times enable us to plan our activities for days, weeks, or even months.

Time can be a feedback mechanism for how things are going, such as finding it took 2 hours to complete a task that should take only 1 hour. It can also be a means for judging competence, effort, or achievement, such as a person's progress during rehabilitation, a medication to take effect, how long it takes to put on a brace, improvement rate in speech and motion after a stroke, or the number of months it takes a child to learn to tie a shoelace.

Many studies have demonstrated correlations between individual temporal orientations and personality characteristics. Some temporal orientations may be personality traits, whereas others are states: A person awaiting results of diagnostic tests may perceive time as dragging, when ordinarily that person perceives it as hurrying.

Scheduling of Time

Much temporal organization of modern social life is based on systematically forcing activities into somewhat rigid temporal patterns (Zerubavel, 1982). This is done by establishing "temporal regularity," a fundamental process underlying schedules. Zerubavel (1982) views temporal regularity as a routine association of events or activities with four dimensions:

Rigid sequential order

Rigid sequential order refers to the ordering of events by sequence. Many events and activities cannot take place simultaneously, so they must be temporally segregated. Examples of rigid sequence are taking insulin before eating breakfast, and having nothing to eat (NPO) prior to surgery.

Fixed duration

Events occur on a regular basis measured against the uniform rate of the clock, i.e., on "clock time." For example, a nurse may give medications at 9 a.m. and 1 p.m. and do treatments at 10 a.m. and 2 p.m. Other examples include the 60-minute lecture, 8 a.m. rounds, 20-minute warm soaks, and dinner served between 5 p.m. and 7 p.m.

Standard location in time

Many social events are associated routinely with a time of the day (breakfast, bedtime), day of the week (school, church), part of the year (spring cleaning, vacation), or period in a person's lifetime (confirmation, bar mitzvah). These periods have become perceived as natural and inevitable "containers." Rigid scheduling is probably a key characteristic of social life in the modern West and may be part of chronic illness care, e.g., postural drainage before breakfast, medication at mealtime, or irrigating a foley catheter every 4 hours.

Uniform rate of occurrence

Uniform rate of occurrence refers to the "rhythmic structure of social life" (e.g., annual celebration of birthdays, anniversaries, and holidays; monthly meetings). These regular uniform rates of recurrence can be identified even within relatively unstructured informal relations, such as physician visits every 3 months. Such notions as "too often" or "hardly ever" suggest the temporal spacing of "casual" visits, telephone calls, and exchanging letters between friends.

Temporal regularities provide individuals with normative prescriptions and standards that save questions, such as how long they ought to stay, what they should do next, and when they should pray. In general, people feel uncomfortable without rigid temporal constraints. Hospital visitors, for example, may wonder how long they should remain. If constraints are not imposed externally, people tend to impose them on themselves to function efficiently (Zerubavel, 1982).

Biological Time

Evidence suggests that biologic rhythms, such as temperature regulation and sleep-wake cycles, do exist, but no organ is known to regulate them. Biologic rhythms are thought to be unique to the individual (Hall, 1983). A striking phenomenon is the way in which biologic activities are structured in accordance with social time (sociotemporal), rather than any biologic order (biotemporal). For example, resting on weekends or having dinner at 6 p.m. is more a social notion than a biological imperative (Zerubavel, 1982). A first stage of socialization is imposing a convention schedule on one's internal biological clock. Daily conflicts between parents and children over mealtime and bedtime exemplify this aspect of socialization.

Systems and Time

Discrepancies are likely to occur when systems interact with one another: e.g., when a family system is concerned with present functioning, while members of the health care system are concerned with future goals. These differences may lead the family to believe their concerns and problems have been negated. By assessing the importance an individual places on the present and future and emphasizing goals in keeping with the person's time orientation,

discrepancies can be minimized. Making short-term goals for those who are present oriented, and long-term goals for those who are future oriented may be a useful nursing strategy.

Expenditure of time can be broken down into three components (Schwartz, 1982): (1) the amount of time it takes for one person to reach another for an interaction; (2) the amount of time a person who has arrived for the interaction must wait for another's presence; and (3) the time spent after the first two barriers are overcome. People with chronic conditions make many trips to clinics, physicians' offices, and treatment centers. Travel to and from, travel delays, interruptions and delays during an appointment (e.g., telephone calls, emergencies), and so forth, are variations on the three-part division of how time is spent.

In our society, people spend a great deal of time in obtaining medical care. In 1970, the head of a household averaged 45 minutes waiting at the doctor's office in addition to the time spent getting there. In one study, when waiting was held constant, impatience was significantly associated with race, but not income. Using a measure of impatience, Schwartz (1982) found that African-Americans exhibited less tolerance of delay than whites.

Health care professionals need to examine the amount of time family members must wait before being seen by health care providers. Can schedules be altered to lessen waiting time? Can necessary activities (e.g., filling out forms, participating in short educational programs) appropriately fill the waiting time?

Family systems manage time based on their general characteristics (Ausloos, 1986). Families represented by rigid transactions are those with closed, impermeable boundaries, rigid rules, and little or no change. In these families time is arrested. For example, parents may fail to recognize that their adolescent is no longer the toddler they remember. They block out new information that might make a difference in their functioning. Families with chaotic transactions are characterized by boundaries that are too open and permeable: Rules are generally absent, and there is constant, but not permanent change. To these families, time is in motion, and they have difficulty making plans and getting places on time, if at all. New information gets into the family, but it is not remembered and therefore of little use to them. In the middle of the continuum between rigid and chaotic transactions are families with flexible transactions. They have semipermeable boundaries, flexible and negotiable rules, and alternate between periods of change and stability.

Mead (1955) believed that the past was one's social structure, composed of habits that develop through interactions with others, and it influenced present behavior to a great extent. Present behavior is influenced, also, by the actual situation, and the future acts as a control on present behaviors. Hendricks (1982) talks about **lived time,** in that each action in the person's present experience is incorporated into a temporal framework, composed of personally meaningful events; it is modified as new events are experienced. Memory is essential to the construction of this framework.

Culture and Time

The possible cultural interpretations of the temporal focus of human life are the past, present, and future (Kluckhohn & Strodtbeck, 1961). Societies have to deal with all three elements but differ in their preferential ordering of the alternatives (rank-order emphases). It is possible to make predictions about a society or part of a society if one knows its rank-order preference. For example, Spanish-Americans place the present time in first-order position. They pay little attention to the past and regard the future as vague and unpredictable. They do not plan for the future or hope it will be better than the past or the present. The Chinese, however, prefer the past, believing that nothing new ever happens in the present or will happen in future; it all happened in some distant past. Modern European countries have strong leaning toward the past (traditions), whereas Americans tend to disregard the past. Americans place their emphasis on the future, which is expected to be bigger and better than past or present. However, even within American society, cultural differences influence emphasis on the present or future.

Time is the core of cultural, social, and personal life. Each culture has its own patterns of time. Hall (1983) points out that to function abroad we need to learn the language of time as well as the spoken language. The abstract concept of time duration, a characteristic of technological societies that measure costs in time and money, seems absent in many other cultures, suggesting that the value of time is learned and depends on one's cultural setting (Luce, 1971). To function within the health care system (culture), clients need to learn our idiosyncratic language, including our notions of time. It is equally important to understand clients' perception of time to help them function within the health care system.

Hall (1983) suggests two different types of time that can explain cultural differences: polychronic time (P-time) and monochronic time (M-time). Polychronic time refers to doing many things at once. It stresses the involvement of people and completion of transactions rather than adherence to preset schedules. In P-time, appointments are not taken seriously and are frequently broken. P-time is treated as less tangible than M-time, and time is rarely expressed as "wasted." Mediterranean and Middle Eastern people tend to use polychronic time. They are almost never alone; even at home, they interact with several people at once and are continually involved with one another. Tight scheduling consequently becomes difficult, if not impossible. In occupational situations, administrators identify all components of a person's job but leave the time schedule for accomplishing them to subordinates.

Monochronic time refers to doing one thing at a time. M-time cultures tend to make a fetish of management, though at times life in general is unpredictable. It is difficult to tell exactly how long a person or set of transactions will take; what may take an hour to accomplish today, may take only 10 minutes tomorrow. In the Western world, schedules dominate activities. Because M-time is thoroughly integrated into Western culture it is treated as the only logical way of organizing life. Yet, it is not inherent in a person's biological rhythms or creative drives, nor does it exist in nature. It is arbitrary, imposed, and learned. Schedules frequently can and do cut things short just when they are beginning to go well. M-time tends to seal off one or two people from the group and intensifies relationships with one or at most two or three other persons. In occupational situations, administrators schedule the activities of subordinates but leave the analysis of the activities involved in the job up to the individual.

American time is both polychronic and monochronic, although M-time dominates the official world of business, government, the professions, entertainment, and sports. Most people equate P-time with informal activities and multiple tasks and responsibilities such as go on in the home. Occupational roles in industrialized societies have many temporal qualities, including the importance attached to speed and efficiency, coordination and scheduling, frequency of payments, and so on. Of all the cultures, the present-day Western world is most frantically time conscious.

In a culture like ours, the group past becomes dim as it recedes and events of 20 years ago are "ancient history." The total effect leads to an impression of time speeding up; the more one has buried in the past, the faster the present will appear to move. Although great value is placed on the future in the United States, many cultures value the past (Mead, 1955). In cultures like the Near Eastern, the past is kept alive and nearly everything today is viewed as rooted in the past. Under conditions of social instability, one's perspective of time may be destroyed (Coser & Coser, 1983). When people can no longer maintain a meaningful sense of the connection between their current images and images of the future, they make little effort to bridge the past and the future in their present experiences. Temporal integration is facilitated by a stable social context that encourages the belief that present actions will have some measurable impact on future outcomes, that what will happen in the future is to some degree both predictable and controllable.

Social Class and Time

Differences can be seen between social classes and their perceptions of time: Studies of the role of American business executives suggest "the sense of the perpetually unattained," with one goal following on the heels of another. This role dominates middle-class experiences, shaping a life-style that puts a high premium on control and foresight rather than enjoyment and retrospection (Seely et al, 1956, p. 357). Upper- and middle-class people "occupy positions and pursue careers," they do not "work and have jobs." The career pattern is built on "timetable norms" with a future referent built into them. People's self-esteem depends upon comparison of their own rate of progress with that of coworkers. Chronic conditions in adults or children have the potential to disrupt the timetable and interfere with self-esteem. Parents of children with chronic conditions may also suffer a disruption in their career pursuits.

In contrast to the middle class, the occupation life of the "working class" is one that generally proceeds on a flat level. There are few differences in pay or responsibility from job to job, or year to year. Many believe there is little point to working hard to get somewhere because there are few places to go (Kahl, 1962, pp. 205–206). Manual labor in Ameri-can society rarely holds the possibility of upward movement.

A characteristic of the lower class is an inability to imagine the future or to sacrifice present for future satisfaction (Banfield, 1968). A trait peculiar to the subculture of poverty is strong orientation to the present with relatively little ability to defer gratification and plan for the future. In addition, there is a sense of resignation and fatalism. Recent studies have demonstrated the role of situational realities in determining the choices people make in such contexts. Impulses are likely to be deferred only when future rewards can be confidently predicted, and when people sense the goals they anticipate are under personal control at least to some degree. Since these conditions are rarely found among those who live in poverty, most are likely to develop a fatalistic outlook on their lives, if only to protect their self-esteem in the presence of repeated frustration. "If the facts of a person's past and present are extremely dismal, then about the best he can do is to show that he is not responsible for what has become of him" (Goffman, 1961, pp. 150–151).

Development of Sense of Time

Development of the ability to experience and estimate time occurs gradually as children mature (Schilder, 1981). There is general agreement that as egocentricity diminishes, sense of time increases. A sense of time duration is not developed until after age 5 or 6 years and continues to develop until the child is about 13 or 14. The notion of time is a highly abstract mental schema based on inner imagery, symbolic representations, and language. Synthesizing these elements into an adult's sophisticated temporal awareness and abstract conception of time is a high-level intellectual achievement.

Preschool children   Awareness of time is thought to develop slowly, along with the gradual establishment of coordinated motor activities, from repeated goal-oriented encounters with the world (Wessman & Gorman, 1977). Children become oriented to the notion of cyclic activities as they adapt to the regular pattern of everyday existence (Fraisse, 1963). Gradually, they master temporal relationships by organizing, into sequences, periods of time they have experienced. Until about 2 years of age, time is in the present and related to subjective experiences. To the young child, time is not clearly separated from notions of distance and velocity (Piaget, 1971). Because children lack the adult conception of clock time, their assessments of time are confused and disorganized. They use observed distances and speeds to assess the time of moving objects. Initially, children will say that something moves faster, and therefore it takes more time; later, they say it moves faster and consequently it takes less time. The first statement results from the object's actions—faster means farther and therefore more time.

According to Elkind (1971), the concept of time can be subcategorized as psychologic, clock, and calendar. The preschooler relies on psychologic time, in which intervals are based on events that occur, such as bedtime, mealtime, or a favorite television program. Time is not reversible, and it is difficult for the young preschooler to use the terms *before* and *after* correctly. When trying to explain future events to a preschooler, anchor these events with familiar events, such as "after lunch" or "when this television program is over."

Between 2 and 6 or 7 years, preoperational children deal with environment solely in terms of "before-the-eye" reality. They can draw inferences and anticipate further ramifications of present events. Gradually, they can bring images of future consequences to bear on present actions and delay gratification for short and specified periods of time.

Children learn to extend time into the past and future, but only within a limited time frame that is close to the present. Although an early concept they learn relates to speed (hurry, slow), their ability to predict time or to arrive somewhere on time is limited. They learn gross differentiations (daytime, nighttime) and somewhat finer distinctions (lunchtime, bedtime), but often these times are related to places, such as the dinner table for lunchtime or the bed for bedtime. Elkind (1971) suggests that one reason children dawdle may be associated with not believing it to be lunchtime until they are at the table or bedtime until they are in bed.

A child who is to wait for a promised future reward must not only be able to maintain a faithful image of that distant event, but must also be able to experience now and throughout the waiting period some of the satisfaction that will be experienced upon receiving the reward. Otherwise the child has no incentive for rejecting an alternative lesser reward available immediately. Telling children that taking medicine now will make them feel better is meaningless in early years.

Temporal language

In studying the temporal aspects of early language, Church (1966) noted that the first references to past and future are initially couched in the present tense, although past and future tense forms appear soon after. For example, toddlers appear to recall isolated past events and have a sense of future that is even less well articulated than the past. They are likely to anchor all temporally distant events, past or future, with a single term, such as *tonight*. Words referring to intervals of time (*hour, day, year*) or points in time (*last week, yesterday, tomorrow*) may be used but have no stable meanings. Toddlers can understand more complex temporal statements they can say.

In a study of nursery school children, Ames (1946) found that statements indicating present time came first, then statements indicating future, and finally statements about past time. From 18 to 30 months, the majority of time-related words used dealt with the present. Mastery of a particular time concept was acquired in successive levels. First, the child was able to respond appropriately to a temporal expression, then to use it in spontaneous conversation, and eventually to correctly answer questions related to the concept. For example, at 18 months the child might respond to the phrase "pretty soon" by waiting; at 24 months, he might use the phrase spontaneously; and at 42 months answer the question "When is mommy coming for you?" with, "She'll come pretty soon." The preschooler who is told that something will happen soon envisions the event taking place in the next few minutes; a teenager may interpret the same time frame, depending on circumstances, to mean hours or days; and an elderly person may think of weeks.

Fraisse (1963) summarized the ages by which the majority of children could understand and correctly use terms related to time. This summary is presented in Table 8–1.

School age children

Older children and adults think of time in relation to the constant, uniform movements of clocks and the regular, established durations of seconds, minutes, hours, days, and years. By 7 or 8 years, they grasp the notion that movement is an abstract concept independent of the movement of clocks, people, and growing things. By 8 or 9 years, most children can distinguish between the time spent traveling and the distance traveled, and thus they have the sense of a general uniform time separate from the events they observe. The mastery of clock time occurs in the early school years, when the child recognizes that time progresses in an orderly fashion and is unidirectional. After mastering clock time, the school age child begins to understand calendar time. The rigid schedule of the school day enables children to develop concepts of what they can accomplish in a given period of time. Although notions of historic time are still somewhat vague, children become fascinated with historical episodes and their place in time. People like pioneers, pilgrims, and astronauts take on a special fascination, especially if they have a distinctive style of dress.

Much research on topics such as estimating time spans and delay-of-gratification behavior shows that children generally make large gains between the ages of 5 and 10 years in mastering and extending temporal conceptions. This research also points out the role social and cultural influences play in such learning. As children grow during the early school years, they are generally able to endow future events with a sufficient sense of reality so they may prefer, or at least be able to wait for, delayed rewards.

School age children are unlikely to integrate distant anticipations of their adult years into their sense of identity or awareness of their life span as a whole. According to Piaget (1971), preadolescents have not yet attained intellectual capacities to comprehend the psychologically distant, the abstract, and the hypothetical. The preadolescent might fail to maintain a clear distinction between realistic expectations and conceptions that reflect unrealizable, wish-fulfilling fantasies. By the close of childhood the near future is well delineated, e.g., age-graded sequences yet to come in school; but adult years are likely to remain beyond reach, standing isolated and unconnected with actual future experiences. As such they remain available for the projection of wish-fulfilling fantasies, offering possibility of escape from the frustrations of current reality. When things are going well in the life of a child, the distant future seems to be of comparatively little interest. However, for those who feel acute frustrations in the present, the future offers a welcome haven.

Adolescents An adolescent's orientation toward the distant future will be substantially different from that of a child. By 14 or 15 years of age, anticipations of the future are largely restricted to realizable objectives and realistic expectations rather than wish-fulfilling fantasies. Gradually, adolescents begin reflecting on the long-range implications of current experience. Past failures or present feelings of pessimism foreshorten perspective on the future and tend to narrow and make defensive the present orientation. Thus, a youngster who has grown up with a chronic condition will come to see it in a new perspective as its implications for the future become apparent.

To the adolescent, the reality of adult years looms greater than when the "real" future was limited to concrete extensions of the present situation or to events already experienced. Integration of the distant future probably is made easier by an overarching conception that views time as an abstract continuum, encompassing all its separate movements in an irreversible succession. The adolescent now conceives of time abstractly. The future is that part of the continuum that is open to reasonable expectation and planning.

According to Erikson (1968), the unification of past, present, and future depends on a meaningful structure of personal time. The need for this synthesis is a central feature of the adolescent identity crisis. To formulate a coherent plan for adult life, the adolescent must examine and clarify what he or she is, and wishes to become. In Erikson's terms, an adolescent successfully achieving such integration has a sense of "temporal perspective," while one failing to do so experiences "time confusion." There are great differences in the degree to which individuals realistically plan their future and effectively utilize their time.

Youngsters who tend to view a future of almost

Table 8-1 Child Understanding and Correct Use of Terms Related to Time

Age (Years)	Time Concepts and Terms
4	Recognize special days of the week, e.g., Sunday
5	Tell whether it is morning or afternoon
6	Identify day of the week
7	Identify month
7–8	Identify season
8	Identify year
8–9	Identify day of the month

Source: Adapted from Fraisse, 1963, pp. 179–180.

unlimited possibilities are likely to have been socialized in families in which time was viewed as pointed to the future. Such a view is likely to be maintained only in a society of stable social institutions and by people who have relatively ready access to opportunities for personal advancement. Children who grow up in poverty tend to receive rather different messages about their prospects for the future.

Adults   Three social processes are related to timing in adult development (Kimmel, 1980). The first is the implicit notion that adults should follow a **timetable** of events closely related to age, e.g., marriage, parenthood, widowhood, first job, second job, and retirement. The second social process is the **social clock** that tells us if we are "off–time" or "on–time" (Neugarten, 1968) in achieving the events on our timetable. When events occur off time, that is either too early or too late according to social norms, they may precipitate a crisis. These first two processes involve events related to people in general, whereas the third process is related to individual **timing events.** These timing events are significant for adult development only if they affect the self in some way by bringing it to one's consciousness. For example, a previously active gentleman remarked following a stroke, "I guess I have to face the fact that I'm not young anymore."

During middle age, one's perspective of time changes. Neugarten (1968) examined time perspectives in middle age of high-status men and women. The subjects generally viewed themselves as being between generations, in relation to family and the wider contexts of work and community. Both sexes talked of a difference in the way time was perceived, in that one's life becomes "restructured in terms of time-left-to-live rather than 'time-since-birth'."

A controversy regarding the psychologic characteristics of older age stems from Cumming and Henry's (1961) formulation of **disengagement** as a general feature of aging. This theory postulates that the aging individual gradually withdraws from society. In the later years, the individual recognizes that one's personal future is limited and that time is insufficient to fulfill all hopes and plans. Anticipating death, the person constricts life plans and activities. Evaluations of disengagement theory (Kastenbaum, 1969; Kimmel, 1974; Neugarten, 1968) indicate that although patterns of increasing constriction characterize the later years of many individuals, for many individuals involvement in life continues to be high.

Life goals and development   Buhler (1968) described five phases of a person's life history that change as one develops an expanded concept of time. They are:

1. Birth to 15 years: the phase before the self-determination of life goals
2. Young adult years (15 to 25): tentatively determine life's goals. At this stage a person first grasps the idea that one's life belongs to oneself and represents a time unit with a beginning and end. Life goals are conceived, and the person sees herself or himself in a historical perspective.
3. Adult years (25 to 50): specify, determine definite goals, and implement them. According to Buhler, the healthy adult lives primarily in the present and sees the future tied to present life in meaningful continuity.
4. Climacteric years (45 to 65): time of assessing the foregoing life and its relative degree of fulfillment. It is a time of reorientation and self-assessment that includes taking stock of the past and revising plans for the future. There may be anticipatory thinking about the last years of life.
5. Later life after 65 years: the final phase of rest and retirement. This phase is characterized by great individuality. Some people show a great decline and marked restriction of activity while others enjoy feelings of essential fulfillment. Health and general life circumstances play an important part in how people respond during this phase.

Perception of Time

Time perception is a complex phenomenon that is not fully understood and is difficult to measure. Traditionally, time has been measured according to some external, culturally defined standard (Moore, 1982). Although such time measure is useful for understanding the duration of activities, it is not useful for examining a person's experience of time. "One cannot clearly distinguish between past and present time even though the present is more subjectively real and the past is more objectively real. The past is prior to, or in a different mode of being than the present, but it is not clearly distinguishable. Past, present, and future instants merge and fuse" (Watson, 1988, p. 60).

Time means different things to different people,

under differing circumstances and in different places. It does not have the same consistency for someone waiting in the physician's office, working on an interesting project, being on vacation, or being hospitalized. Temporal judgment differs even over very short periods of time for the same individual (Fraisse, 1963). People tend to judge time subjectively in relation to clock or objective time. They may underestimate, overestimate, or accurately estimate given time intervals. "Real" time for an individual cannot be equated with the clock time of minutes and seconds (Hall, 1959). For example, Tompkins (1980) found that time passes more slowly when movement is restricted and Scott (1980) found that for patients having a breast biopsy, the number of stimuli, vigilance, and feelings about being in control were related to time perception under noncritical circumstances.

Hoagland (1977) and Goldstone (1967) suggested that perceived time duration was a biologic function of metabolism, and Fraisse (1963) and Bentov (1977) hypothesized that the rate of perceived time duration was a function of individual consciousness. Ornstein (1969) suggested that perceived time duration was a combination of both the quantity and the complexity of information processing. If events are large and a person is emotionally absorbed in them, duration is perceived as short. Bentov's model of time was an index of consciousness that is a ratio of Subjective Time/Objective Time, and Newman (1979) developed a model of perceived duration as a ratio of Awareness/Content. The factors related to awareness include emotional state and attention to a task; those related to content are body movement, metabolism, and external events.

Piaget (1971) indicated that Time is equal to Power (Energy) divided by Work (Time = Power/Work). When one is doing a task, if power is increased, time seems to diminish. If the amount of work is increased, however, and the person's ability to do the task remains the same, time seems to increase. For example, a person's perception of the time it takes to walk on dry pavement would be shorter than the same person's perception of the time it takes to walk through heavy snow. Imagine the impact that crutches, canes, wheelchairs, and walkers might have on this formula. Distortions in time judgments by both children and adults are fairly common because the individual is never directly judging time but is labeling the end result of a subjective equation of time (Piaget, 1971; Voyat, 1977).

There are two opposing views of how we estimate time duration (Prisely, 1968). The first view suggests there is a linear and positive relationship among presented stimuli so that as stimuli become more complex, one's estimation of time duration increases. That is, duration is lengthened whenever a procedure results in an increase in the number of stimuli one perceives. When input is decreased, the duration experience is perceived as decreased. Thus, when someone listens to a lecture that is clear, concise, and easy to follow, time seems to pass more quickly than when one listens to something complex that is difficult to understand. The other view hypothesizes a negative association between the complexity of stimuli experienced in a given interval and how time duration is assessed. From this perspective, a shortened time period is experienced when there is increased stimulus complexity. For example, when a bedridden person has a good book to read or interesting friends to talk with, time is perceived as passing more rapidly than when the person is lying in bed staring at blank walls. Hogan (1978) reconciles the two views by hypothesizing that time perception is not a linear but rather a U-shaped function of both personality and stimulus complexity.

Subjective impressions of time based on intuition and biologic rhythms are not very reliable. Although it is possible to judge time of day by internal cues (e.g., hunger, thirst, sleep) or by external environmental cues (e.g., position of sun, moon), these judgments are crude because they may be affected by internal states. For example, someone who is well fed will perceive the time to eat differently than will someone who is ravenously hungry (Gorman & Wessman, 1977).

A reliable and orderly clock gives a sense of an ordered and reliable social and physical world. Although some people find comfort in such order, others feel frightened and constrained by time limitations (Gorman & Wessman, 1977). For some families having a scheduled routine for medication and treatment provides structure, whereas for others set times may interfere with a flexible schedule.

In general, individual perspectives on time are constructed as guideposts and markers for the person's own meaning system and are formed to serve the person's pattern of needs. Aspects of time perception are important as people lead day-to-day lives. All people must work out their own conception of time flow and deal with their own past, present, and future. These perceptions constantly change because people live within time. People's perception of the passage of time becomes a major determinant in shaping their perception of how they may have changed over time (Cottle, 1977). For example, the presence of a chronic condition in a family for several years may be reflected in the family members' perception that they have grown stronger through adversity.

When a crisis occurs and people are totally absorbed in present experiences or exhausted by excessive fatigue, "the future will largely disappear from consciousness and anticipatory images will lose their power to motivate present behavior" (Cottle & Klineberg, 1974, p. 20). Indeed, Osgood (1962) suggested that when one is emotionally driven, one's time span contracts to the present moment; and Maslow (1968) described the "peak experiences" of creative people as an intense absorption in the present, when a person is most free of both the past and the future, most "all there" in the experience itself. If the future thus gains no entry into a present of intense absorption, feelings of severe dejection or discouragement may also constrain the capacity to bridge the past and future. We rarely expect the worst from the future and when we do we tend to think about other things (Cottle & Klineberg, 1974). When people confront the probability of something unpleasant, they tend to stop thinking about the future and turn instead to the present or to the past, where events are nonthreatening if only because they have already occurred. It is at this time that people may say they are living a day at a time and taking each day as it comes.

Images of one's personal future may lead to pleasant or unpleasant emotional states that intrude on current experience and motivate present behavior. This link between emotion and image is what may enable some individuals to postpone present gratification for the sake of imagined future rewards. Others, however, tend to restrict their perspective to the relatively immediate present in order to avoid confronting the prospect of an undesirable or seemingly unavoidable future. Disturbing thoughts of future prospects are motivating only as long as the person believes it is possible to do something now that might preclude an undesirable outcome.

A relatively restricted present orientation can operate as a "defensive" strategy, protecting a person from the pain induced by unpleasant anticipation. Under these circumstances, the present may be limited to those relatively short-range events that one feels can be controlled. Alternatively, the time span may be restricted to those areas of life that

offer more promising prospects or perhaps to images of distant events, so far off that they remain safely detached from the disturbing reality of immediate experience. The process of temporal integration (linking images of the future with conceptions of the past and the present) may appear to vanish when future prospects are bleak and motivation to think about the future disappears. Personality differences and the social context in which one finds oneself are likely to affect one's images of time.

Time drags when the body clock and the wall clock are not synchronized. Time dragging becomes a synonym for not having a good time. The message that time is dragging can be used to alert individuals to find out what is making them feel that way. Time away from a loved one moves at a snail's pace, whereas a rendezvous is over before one knows it.

Concentration and time perception   The degree of concentration required to complete a task is related to the rate at which time is perceived as passing. The events that cause a person or group to concentrate so hard that all sense of time is lost can be attributed to multiple causes. Concentration of any sort obliterates time.

Expectation and perception   Expectancy is a situation that leads people to be more sensitive to stimuli and become more vigilant than usual (Ornstein, 1969). The more vigilant a person becomes, the longer the experience is perceived to last. The saying that "A watched pot never boils" exemplifies increased vigilance. Knowing you are about to undergo a painful procedure can make a 15-minute wait seem like an eternity, while waiting 15 minutes for a waiter to bring your entree may pass quickly if you are engaged in stimulating conversation, or slowly if you are very hungry. Patients may perceive a lengthened waiting time for a nurse or other health care professional because of heightened vigilance during the waiting. Significant others may perceive a prolonged expectancy while awaiting the return of a loved one from surgery.

Age and time perception   Age affects how people experience time: The years go faster as one gets older. To a child age 5 or 6 years, a year seems infinite, while to someone age 50 or 60, the years begin to blend and are frequently hard to separate because they race by so fast! If one has only lived 5 years, a year represents 20% of one's life, but at 50 it represents only 2%. A young child may perceive a 30-

minute treatment as taking "forever," while to the adult it may appear to pass quickly.

Variables that may influence perception of time in the elderly include age, emotional state, imminent death, activity level, environment, outlook on the future, and the values attached to time (Strumpf, 1987). There also appears to be a positive relationship between a future orientation, overall satisfaction, a sense of well being, and adjustment in the elderly.

Strumpf (1987) studied the concept of time with 86 elderly noninstitutionalized women. On the Time Metaphor Test the women perceived time as moving neither rapidly nor slowly, whereas on the Time Opinion Survey, the majority of the women (76%) considered time as passing fairly or extremely rapidly. Fifty-seven percent thought that time was passing more rapidly than 10 years ago, but 84% did not seem concerned about time running out. On the Time Reference Survey about one third (36%) felt the present dominated their thinking. The past was rated as the most important time of their lives by 57% of the subjects, and 47% received the most enjoyment from thinking about the past.

Temperature and time perception Time perception has been studied in relation to physiologic processes for many years. Based on a series of studies, Hoagland (1977) concluded that body temperature affects perception of time. Higher temperatures speed up the body clocks and lower ones slow the clocks down. Alcohol can work on two levels. Because of the sense of stimulation and festivity, time initially moves faster, but since alcohol is a depressant, the ultimate effect is for time to drag.

Anniversaries and time perception Anniversaries are a cyclic manifestation of time. Yet, because of the subtle and omnipresent nature of our own internal timing mechanisms, many of us react to anniversaries of which we are not even aware. By the time people reach age of 60, they have so many of these hidden anniversaries (of triumph, failure, or disappointment) that sometimes they do not know whether it is an immediate situation or something forgotten that causes them to feel cheerful or depressed, or is causing time to speed up or slow down.

Environment and time perception Space and time are functionally interrelated (DeLong, 1981). The perception of time is influenced by multiple factors, including the scale of the environment. For example, working in a smaller environment makes time appear to move faster.

Anxiety and time perception A survey of the empirical findings concerned with the relationship between anxiety and the orientation toward future events is confusing. At one extreme, the presence of anxiety presupposes an anticipation of the future, while its absence suggests a lack of concern with future events. People who remain only moderately anxious can still retain a feeling of at least partial control over the future; in fact the sense of the connection between present and future may be enhanced. Anxiety is likely to be a major motivation in one's efforts to bring anticipations of the future to bear on present actions; to take steps in the present that may provide some reassurance regarding prospects of the future. In the event that reassurance is not forthcoming, this sense of personal control diminishes and anxiety may become increasingly intolerable. The person's efforts will now be directed to ways of reducing that anxiety.

As anxiety rises, perceived duration is judged longer in retrospect. That is, a person may suffer severe pain for approximately an hour, but in retrospect believe it lasted for 2 hours.

The feelings aroused by images of the future may profoundly affect a person's present emotional state. A person who despairs, however, and feels relatively powerless to control the future, is likely to make unconscious use of antepression (the gradual adjustment to extreme agony). Another way is to fashion an idyllic image of a distant future detached from the implications of present reality. In either event, hopelessness may result, and one lives only in present. The person loses feeling for sequence of time, is unable to plan for future or give up immediate pleasure satisfactions for greater ones in the near future (Cottle & Klineberg, 1974). A person may restrict personal perspective to those relatively short-range future events over which there is some personal control, or to those limited areas of life that offer promising prospects, or perhaps to images of future events so remote that they remain safely detached from the present.

Chronic Conditions and Time

Chronic conditions are long term by nature (Strauss et al, 1984). As such, they require repeated interaction over months and years between patients and health workers. In contrast, crises are by their nature time limited, lasting anywhere from a few days to a few weeks (Moos, 1979). At various times patients with chronic conditions will experience crises that may or may not be related to their condition. Interventions during times of crisis differ from interventions on an ongoing basis.

Time Phases

Rolland (1987) identifies five time phases of illness, noting that each phase has its own psychosocial tasks to be mastered. These phases are prediagnosis, diagnosis, acute, chronic, terminal or survival. Chronic diseases with an acute onset (e.g., stroke) require affective and instrumental changes that must take place in a much shorter time period than when the onset is gradual (e.g., Parkinson disease, muscular dystrophy).

Lawrence and Lawrence (1979) proposed a model of adult adaptation to chronic illness consisting of three overlapping stages, each stage having a beginning but no end. Stage I is characterized by shock, disbelief, denial, and independent behavior; Stage II involves developing awareness, anger, and dependent behavior; Stage III constitutes resolution of the loss, identity and role transition, and dependent and independent behavior. The interaction of the three stages results in adaptation, characterized by self-dependent behavior, hope, and bargaining. These stages, similar to many other stage theories, are inadequate for understanding the social context in which chronic illness occurs. Coombs (1984) extended the work of Lawrence and Lawrence (1979) to home nursing in Australia. Using a grounded theory approach (Glaser & Strauss, 1967) she identified two central concepts for home nursing. The first concept, aloneness, referred to the nurse, care recipient (chronically ill individual), and care giver (family member or significant other). Aloneness fell along a continuum from loneliness/isolation at one end to autonomy/reflection on the other end. Nurses were alone in being dependent on their own resources. Clients were often alone because they were homebound or isolated from society and past activities. The family was alone in adjusting to the patient's needs and often had a decrease in personal time, had to curtail social activities, and suffered from financial stress and anxiety. The second central concept, interaction, was not developed in the article. Coombs

notes that aloneness was a concept central to home nursing, whereas interaction was central to nursing in any situation. The principal effect of the nursing role was to change the family's narrow focus and facilitate adjustment to loss of functional status.

Stewart and Sullivan (1982) note the long prediagnosis stressor period for patients eventually diagnosed with multiple sclerosis (MS). In their study of 60 men and women with MS, it took an average of 5½ years to make a correct diagnosis. They identified three phases that nearly everyone went through: *nonserious phase,* lasting an average of 3 years; *serious phase,* lasting nearly 2½ years; and the final one, *diagnosis phase,* lasting up to 6 months.

Levy (1976) suggested three phases, similar to the stages of the grieving process, that patients go through in their psychosocial adjustment to maintenance hemodialysis. In Phase I, the honeymoon phase, patients and their families are hopeful that treatment will result in cure. In Phase II, the disenchantment and discouragement phase, the patient and family begin to realize that cure will not occur. In Phase III, long-term adaptation, they have accepted that living with chronic renal disease is a way of life.

From her research with women who have cancer, Scott (1980) drew the following conclusion. The crisis of the diagnostic phase of care and changes in ability to regulate emotions and process information (e.g., informed consent and judgments about future modes of therapy) have implications for the waiting period, teaching-learning aspects of hospitalized patients, and patient adaptation following discharge. Although her study was limited to patients with cancer, it probably holds true for other patients and their families, as well as for nonhospitalized patients.

Trajectories

The concept of **trajectory,** or the way disease progression is perceived over time by those involved, includes the ideas of direction, movement, shape, and predictability. Trajectories occur over time and move in some direction at varying rates of speed. The shape of a trajectory is the mental image of the direction and movement or course of the illness. The course of an illness trajectory may be altered by advances in technology. For example, the rapid downward trajectory of AIDS is slowly changing with advances in therapy. The course of childhood leukemia in the 1950s was rapid and downward; now children have prolonged trajectories, often with an outcome of cure.

Each type of disease (arthritis, diabetes) has some general pattern for its course (Strauss et al, 1984; Rolland, 1987). Downward trajectories, which Rolland calls progressive, may be either slow or rapid, and the condition worsens over time (e.g., emphysema, muscular dystrophy, cystic fibrosis). These diseases are usually symptomatic and progress in severity, with few periods of relief. In other cases, the condition reaches a plateau and remains stable throughout life (e.g., sensory loss). With a constant course, the individual is left with a residual deficit or functional limitation. In other cases, the trajectory varies with slight ups and downs (exacerbations and remissions). This relapsing or episodic course (e.g., diabetes, asthma, ulcerative colitis) has variable periods of stability, with few or no symptoms, and flare-ups, when symptoms become manifest. This episodic course tends to create uncertainty for clients, who do not know when to expect relapses or how severe they may be.

Regimen and Time

The amount of time needed to manage a chronic condition varies widely for everyone who may be involved in the person's treatment regimen. These treatments often necessitate daily activities and schedules to get them done. The extent to which time needs to be reordered depends, of course on the nature of the treatments and the disruption they impose on life-style. Some treatments may take only a few minutes, but others may take hours each day. In addition, some regimens, such as postural drainage or range-of-motion exercises, may need to be done two or three times a day. Some take so much time (e.g., days on dialysis, going to radiation therapy) that they are virtually the center of the patient's life (Strauss et al, 1984). Some treatments must be carried out on schedule and timed in relation to peaking of symptoms rather than flexibly altered to fit time schedule.

For some people, a treatment such as taking pills may not be much of a problem. Others manage time during treatments by doing other activities, such as listening to music, thinking, or doing job-related work. Parents may help their children do homework during treatments.

When therapy also involves going to the health facility it includes travel time and waiting time, making it difficult for those with chronic conditions to plan their day. People who must travel to medical centers to receive care may have to drive 2 to 3 hours one way. Others will take trains or buses and travel time may take 6 to 7 hours a day. Senior citizens who take public transportation may have to schedule appointments around times they can receive reduced rates.

Strauss and colleagues (1984) point out that clients are often left on their own to figure out how to handle basic temporal problems of (1) having too much time, as when the person can no longer work; (2) having too little time to do things other than manage the disease; (3) scheduling their days; and (4) timing of activities, such as taking insulin in relation to eating.

Quint (1969), referring to the importance of time for children with diabetes, stated that the child "can *never forget about time.* In fact, time becomes the ruler of his life" (p. 63). The key to the medical management of diabetes is the management of time and the maintaining of a regular schedule. She also noted that age of onset of an illness was another important temporal dimension.

Chronic Conditions and Time Perception

Although knowledge of chronic conditions and time perception is currently limited, it is relevant, nevertheless, for nursing care. As mentioned earlier, time perception is individual and related to context. Chronic illness is one variable that may influence a person's perceptions of time. For example, Fizpatrick, Donovan, and Johnson (1980) found that people with cancer who knew their status was terminal reported a shorter future temporal perspective and more time pressure, although they had more free time, than those without cancer. In addition, patients with cancer reported increased curiosity about the time following their death. Neuringer and Harris (1974) found that terminally ill hospitalized patients reported a great amount of time pressure. They focused on the future as regards accomplishing things before they died and providing for the future of their survivors. Studies by Smith (1979) demonstrated that for bedridden patients, the more ambiguous the emotional context, the longer the perceived duration of time.

Hospitalization Hospitalization of a person disrupts the usual time structure followed in the home or community. When a child is hospitalized, disruption also extends to at least one parent who remains in the hospital, as well as to family members remaining at home. Although some disruption is inevitable, nurses need to consider ways to make it more tolerable for the patient and family. Sometimes providing an explanation of the daily schedule can help them understand and anticipate these disruptions. Knowledge of the person's usual temporal organization (through assessment) can facilitate planning for discharge and help the family arrange interventions at times that are appropriate at home.

Adaptation and Time

A person's characteristic way of adapting to new problems changes over time (White, 1974). The way the problem is met the first time differs from the way it is met the fifth or tenth time. Adaptation strategies are created over time, not in an instant. Information needed for adaptation changes over time as does the person's physical and physiological status.

Nursing and Time

Nursing is a dynamic process that takes place over time. Time is an important consideration in planning and providing nursing care based on individual needs. Knowing a person's time frame is especially important when one is interacting with different cultural groups or people for whom time is of no particular importance. Of relevance to nursing are the recent policies that have decreased the length of hospital stays, necessitating changes in the planning of nursing interventions. For patients in the hospital, the nursing care plan is a 24-hours-a-day, 7-days-a-week guideline for promoting continuity of care over time. Knowledge of illness trajectories can facilitate planning interventions for client and family. However, as Peterson (1987) points out, the care plan does not take into account rapid changes that are likely to occur in the needs and stressors of patients (e.g., insulin reaction).

Winnicott (1964) and Stephens (1979) discuss the relationship of time to nursing in hospital settings, noting that nurses are the only professionals available to patients on a 24-hours-a-day basis. La Monica (1979) recognizes it takes nurses time to develop a relationship with patients that involves a more person-oriented rather than task-oriented interaction. Peterson (1987) reports that one study supports La Monica's belief, but others suggest that nurses may not develop relationships with patients who remain hospitalized for long periods because they tend to dislike such patients who do not get well quickly. Note that little is known about the time needed to develop person-oriented nurse-patient relationships in clinics, physicians' offices, or the home. With primary nursing care, there is a change in nursing responsibility from one 8- to 12-hour shift to 24-hour responsibility.

Assessment

Assessment involves obtaining information about the past, present, and future dimensions of time. Assessment of the past includes the patient's past medical history and biography, and a history of the present illness. Historical questioning leads to understanding how the individual or family system is currently coping with past stressors (Rolland, 1987). Try to obtain the person's views of the future trajectory and outcome of the present illness.

Assessment of time also includes the person's perception of time and orientation to time (Scott, 1980). Nursing assessments are based on rates, patterns, and change (Metzger & Schultz, 1982). Therefore, assessment of the patient's time perception and orientation needs to take place periodically. One way to determine discrepancies in time perception is to ask the person to estimate the duration of one minute, and compare the result with clock time. Guidelines for assessing time and time management are in Table 8–2.

Several instruments have been used to measure the concept of time. The Time Metaphor Test (Knapp & Garbutt, 1958) consists of 25 poetic descriptions of the passage of time, such as a dashing waterfall, a burning candle, or a vast expanse of time. Subjects are asked to choose five that most closely resemble how time is passing for them. The Time Opinion Survey (Kuhlen & Monge, 1968) questions the subjects' attitude about the speed of time passage, feelings of time pressure, orientation, and achievement in reference to past, present, and future time. The Time Reference Inventory (Roos, 1964) consists of 30 statements about past, present, or future time orientation. For example, respondents are asked to indicate the most important time of their lives, the most unhappy time, and the busi-

Table 8–2 Assessment of Time and Time Management

Area	Useful Information
Past	Onset of illness
	Relevant past health history and experiences
	Development prior to illness
Present	Stage of illness
Future	Future goals and plans
Time	Daily routine
	Describe
	Recent changes in routine
	Causes (e.g., change in disease, treatments, finances, support)
	Treatments
	Schedule
	How often **able** to do treatments
	Interferes with usual schedule
Availability of help	Would client use help?
How labor is divided	For usual routine tasks
	For situational tasks
Passage of time	Usually slow or rapid
	When pressured (more slowly or rapidly)

Strengths	Needs

est time. Strumpf (1987) noted some difficulties in using these instruments. Because these instruments were developed decades ago, they may not reflect changing temporal horizons. The use of metaphors to describe time may be problematic for older persons. Since time is private, personal, and difficult to measure with instruments, guided interviews may better capture the complex nature of time.

Selected Nursing Interventions

Timing of intervention The timing of intervention needs to be considered in planning care. For example, the amount of information that a family can absorb immediately after hearing a diagnosis is limited. At this point, only the "must know" information is appropriate. Plans to provide information in small doses over several time periods will be more effec-

tive than telling everything in one session shortly after the news of the diagnosis. Timing of teaching is particularly difficult in these days of cost containment and early discharge. Knowing that patients are often discharged before there has been sufficient time to help them appropriately is frustrating. Alternative strategies that take time into account need to be thought about, such as greater use of telephone-call follow-up (Hagopian & Rubenstein, 1990); scheduling appointments at times that are convenient for clients; and using teaching materials such as videotapes, audiotapes, and computers.

Once adults perceive a need for information, they want it as soon as possible (Knowles, 1973). Therefore immediacy of timing is important. Also, they want what they learn to be applicable immediately to solving a current problem. Once the client's perceived needs are assessed, it is possible to tailor a program of intervention specifically to these needs.

If there are general guidelines for information to be incorporated into a teaching plan, these can be modified to accommodate the immediate needs and then expanded.

Using clocks and calendars   Clocks and calendars serve to help persons with chronic conditions structure their time while in hospital and at home. An easy to read clock can be placed in the room in a way that it can be seen but is not constantly in view from the bed. Calendars also help keep the person oriented to time and can be used to mark off days and record significant or future events.

Volz (1981) suggests "time structuring" with children during hospitalization to help them organize their days and have some feeling of control. The nurse, parents, and child together determine how the child's day will be spent. A clock and a calendar are placed in the room and the child's hourly and daily schedule is outlined.

Summary

This chapter provided an overview of the concept of time as it pertains to the Contingency Model of Long-Term Care. Time can be described objectively, according to clocks or calendars, and subjectively, related to one's cultural background, developmental stage, and emotional state. Concentration, expectations, age, temperature, anniversaries, environment, and anxiety influence time perception.

The gradual development of children's ability to experience and estimate time was described and the implications for communicating with children at different stages were noted. The restructuring of time during middle age as regards "time–left–to–live" rather than "time–since–birth" was also discussed.

Time was described in its connection with the observation of events, as a primary organizer for activities and means of handling priorities and categorizing experience, and as a feedback mechanism for how things are going. Time can be scheduled according to rigid sequential orders, fixed durations, standard durations of clock or calendar, or its uniform rates of occurrence.

The trajectories and phases of chronic conditions and the time needed to manage treatment regimens were discussed, along with the disruption in the usual time structure caused by hospitalization. Different perceptions of time held by family members and health care professionals were noted to interfere with understanding, care planning, and patient acceptance.

Nursing was presented as a dynamic process taking place over time. Aspects of the nurse's role in assessment and intervention related to chronic illness and time were discussed. Nursing assessment was said to involve obtaining information about the past, present, and future dimensions of time and the timing of intervention needs to be considered in planning care. The use of clocks and calendars in helping persons with chronic conditions structure their time was described.

References

Ames, L.B. (1946). The development of a sense of time in the young child. *J Gen Psychol, 68,* 97–125.

Ausloos, G. (1986). The march of time: Rigid or chaotic transactions, two different ways of living time. *Fam Process, 25,* 549–557.

Banfield, E.C. (1968). *The unheavenly city: The nature and future of our urban cities.* Boston: Little Brown.

Bentov, I. (1977). *Stalking the wild pendulum.* New York: Putnam.

Buhler, C. (1968). The course of life as a psychological problem. *Hum Dev, 11,* 184–200.

Church, J. (1966). *Language and the discovery of reality.* New York: Random House (Vintage).

Coombs, E.M. (1984). A conceptual framework for home nursing. *Journal of Advanced Nursing, 9,* 157–163.

Coser, L.A., & Coser, R.L. (1963). Time perspectives and social structure. In A.W. Gouldner & H.P. Gouldner (Eds.), *Modern sociology: An introduction to the study of human interaction* (pp. 638–647). New York: Harcourt, Brace, & World.

Cottle, T.J. (1977). The time of youth. In B.S. Gorman, & A.E. Wessman (Eds.), *The personal experience of time* (pp. 163–189). New York: Plenum.

Cottle, T.J., & Klineberg, S.L. (1974). *The present of things future: Exploring of time in human experience.* New York: MacMillan Free Press.

Cumming, E., & Henry, W.E. (1961). *Growing old: The process of disengagement.* New York: Basic Books.

DeLong, A. (1981, Aug. 7). Phenomenological space-time: Toward an experimental relativity. *Science, 213,* 4508, 681–683.

Elkind, D.S. (1971). *A sympathetic understanding of the child six to sixteen.* Boston: Allyn & Bacon.

Erikson, E. (1968). *Identity: Youth and crisis.* New York: Norton.

Fitzpatrick, J.J., Donovan, M.J., & Johnston, R.L. (1980). Experience of time during the crisis of cancer. *Cancer Nurs, 3*(3), 191–194.

Fraisse, S.P. (1963). *The psychology of time.* (J. Lieth, Trans.). New York: Harper & Row.

Goffman, I. (1961). *Asylums.* Chicago: Aldine.

Goldstone, S. (1967). The human clock: A framework for the study of health and deviant time perception. *Annals of the New York Academy of Sciences, 138,* 767–783.

Gorman, B.S., & Wessman, A. E. (Eds.). (1977). *The personal experience of time.* New York: Plenum.

Gorman, B.S., & Wessman, A. E. (1977). Images, values, and concepts of time in psychological research. In B.S. Gorman, & A.E. Wessman (Eds.), *The personal experience of time* (pp. 217–263). New York: Plenum.

Guralnik, D.B. (Ed.). (1984). *Webster's new world dictionary* (2nd ed.). New York: Simon and Schuster.

Hagopian, G.A., & Rubenstein, J.H. (1990). The effects of telephone call interventions on a patient's well being in a radiation oncology department. *Cancer Nurs, 13,* 339–344.

Hall, E.T. (1959). *The silent language,* Greenwich, CT: Fawcett.

Hall, E.T. (1983). *The dance of life: The other dimension of life.* Garden City, NY: Anchor Press/Doubleday.

Hendricks, J. (1982). Time and social science: History and potential. In E.H. Mizruchi, B. Glassner, & T. Pasorello (Eds.), *Time and aging: Conceptualization and application in sociological and gerontological research* (pp. 12–45). Bayside, NY: General Hall.

Hoagland, H. (1977). Brain evolution and the biology of belief. *Science, 33*(3).

Hogan, W.H. (1978). A theoretical reconciliation of competing views of time perception. *Am J Psychol, 94*(3), 417–428.

Kahl, J.A. (1962). *The American class structure.* New York: Holt, Rinehart & Winston.

Kastenbaum, R. (1969). The foreshortened life perspective. *Geriatrics, 24,* 126–133.

Kimmel, D.C. (1974). *Adulthood and aging.* New York: Wiley.

Kluckhohn, F.R., & Strodtbeck, F.L. (1961). *Variations in value orientations.* New York: Harper & Row.

Knapp, R., & Garbutt, J. (1958). Time imagery and the achievement motive. *J Pers, 26,* 426–434.

Knowles, M. (1973). *The adult learner: A neglected species.* Houston: Gulf Publishing.

Kuhlen, R., & Monge, R. (1968). Correlates of estimated time passage in the adult years. *J Gerontol, 23,* 427–433.

LaMonica, E.L. (1979). *The nursing process: A humanistic approach.* Reading, MA: F.A. Davis.

Lawrence, S.A., & Lawrence, R.M. (1979). A model of adaptation to the stress of chronic illness. *Nursing Forum, 18*(1), 33–42.

Leach, E.R. (1961). *Rethinking anthropology.* London: Athalone.

Levy, N.B. (1976). Coping with maintenance hemodialysis. In S.G. Massry & A.L. Seller (Eds.), *Clinical aspects of uremia and dialysis.* Springfield, IL: Charles C Thomas.

Luce, G.G. (1971). *Body time.* New York: Random House.

Maslow, A.H. (1968). *Toward a psychology of being* (2nd ed.). New York: Van Nostrand Reinhold.

Mead, M. (Ed.). (1955). *Cultural patterns and technical change.* New York: New American Library.

Metzger, B.L., & Schultz II, S. (1982). Time series analysis: An alternative for nursing. *Nurs Res, 31*(6), 375–378.

Moore, G. (1982). Duration experience: A useful theoretical construct for nursing theory and research. *Nurs Papers, 14*(2), 37–44.

Moos, R.H. (1979). Social-ecological perspectives on health. In G.C. Stone, F. Cohen, N.E. Adler (Eds.). *Health psychology—A handbook* (pp. 523–547). San Francisco: Jossey-Bass.

Neugarten, B.L. (Ed.). (1968). *Middle age and aging.* Chicago: University of Chicago Press.

Neuringer, C., & Harris, R. (1974). The perception of the passage of time among death-involved hospital patients. *Life Threat Behav, 4,* 240–254.

Newman, M.A. (1979). *Theory development in nursing.* Philadelphia: F.A. Davis.

Ornstein, R.E. (1969). *On the experience of time.* Middlesex, England: Penguin Books.

Osgood, C.E. (1962). *An alternative to war or surrender.* Urbana: University of Illinois Press.

Pastorello, T. (1982). Time as a tool for policy analysis in aging. In E.H. Mizruchi, B. Glassner, & T. Pasorello (Eds.), *Time and aging: Conceptualization and application in sociological and gerontological research* (pp. 46–61). Bayside, NY: General Hall.

Peterson, M. (1987). Time and nursing process. *Holistic Nurs Pract, 1*(3), 72–80.

Piaget, J. (1971). *The child's conception of time.* New York: Ballantine Books.

Prisely, J.B. (1968). *Man and time.* New York: Dell.

Quint, J.C. (1969). Some thoughts on a theory of chronicity. *Proceedings of the first nursing theory conference* (pp. 67). University of Kansas Medical Center Department of Nursing Education, March 20–29.

Riegel, K.F. (1977). Toward a dialectical interpretation of time and change. In B.S. Gorman, & A.E. Wessman (Eds.), *The personal experience of time* (pp. 59–108). New York: Plenum.

Rolland, J.S. (1987). Family systems and chronic illness: A typological model. *J Psychother Fam, 3*(3), 143–168.

Roos, P. (1964) Time Reference Inventory. Unpublished manuscript. (Available from author, National Association for Retarded Citizens, Arlington, TX 76011).

Schilder, E. (1981). On the structure of time with implications for nursing. *Nurs Papers, 13*(3), 17–23.

Schwartz, B. (1982). The friction of time: Access and delay in the context of medical care. In E.H. Mizruchi, B. Glassner, & T. Pasorello (Eds.), *Time and aging: Conceptualization and application in sociological and gerontological research* (pp. 75–111). Bayside, NY: General Hall.

Scott, D.W. (1980). A matter of time. *Cancer Nurs, 3*(4), 301–302.

Seely, J.R., Sim, R.A., Loosely, E.W. (1956). *Crestwood Heights: A study of the culture of suburban life.* New York: Basic Books.

Smith, M.J. (1979). Duration experience for bed confined subjects: A replication and refinement. *Nurs Res, 28,* 139–144.

Stephens, G.J. (1979). *Nursing theory: Analysis, application, evaluation.* Boston: Little Brown.

Stewart, D.C., & Sullivan, T.J. (1982). Illness behavior and the sick role in chronic illness: The case of multiple sclerosis. *Soc Sci Med, 16,* 1397–1404.

Strauss et al (Eds.). (1984). *Chronic illness and the quality of life* (2nd ed.). St. Louis: Mosby.

Strumpf, N.E. (1987). Probing the temporal world of the elderly. *Int J Nurs Stud, 24*(3), 201–214.

Tompkins, E. (1980). Effect of restricted mobility and dominance on perceived duration. *Nurs Res, 29,* 333–338.

Volz, D.D. (1981). Time structuring for hospitalized school-aged children. *Issues Compr Nurs, 5,* 205–210.

Voyat, G. (1977). Perception and the concept of time: A developmental perspective. In B.S. Gorman & A.E. Wessman (Eds.), *The personal experience of time* (pp. 135–160). New York: Plenum.

Watson, J. (1988). *Nursing: Human science and human care.* Publication # 15-2236. NY: National League for Nursing.

Wessman, A.E., & Gorman, B.S. (1977). The emergence of human awareness and concepts of time. In B.S. Gorman & A.E. Wessman (Eds.), *The personal experience of time* (pp. 3–58). New York: Plenum.

White, R. (1974). Strategies of adaptation: An attempt at systematic description. In G. Coelho, D. Hamburg, & J. Adams (Eds.), *Coping and adaptation* (pp. 47–68). New York: Basic Books.

Winnicott, D.W. (1964). *The child, the family and the outside world.* Hammondsworth, Middlesex, England: Pelican Books.

Zerubavel, E. (1982). Schedules and social control. In E.H. Mizruchi, B. Glassner, & T. Pasorello (Eds.), *Time and aging: Conceptualization and application in sociological and gerontological research* (pp. 129–152). Bayside, NY: General Hall.

9 Orientation to Life

Orientation to life refers to system values, attitudes, and beliefs such as those related to issues of health, illness, life, and nursing and health care. We assume behavior is based on values, attitudes, and beliefs; therefore, they are important mediators of coping with chronic conditions, and as noted by Mullen, Hersey, and Iverson (1987) can predict lifestyle behaviors. Although it is difficult to differentiate between values, attitudes, and beliefs, we believe there is value in trying to do so. These concepts have common characteristics and also unique qualities. Figure 9–1 illustrates the relation of orientation to life to other variables in the Contingency Model of Long-Term Care. Note that a system's orientation to life can be part of its identifying characteristics and can influence coping strategies which, in turn, influence strengths, needs, and level of functioning. Because coping strategies may involve modifying val-

117

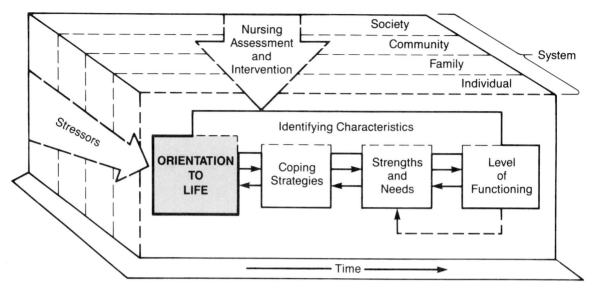

FIGURE 9–1 Relationship of Orientation to Life to Other Components of The Contingency Model of Long-Term Care

ues, attitudes, or beliefs, a broken line designates their potential role in changing these orientations. For example, believing that long-range planning is important in one's life may be altered to valuing "one day at a time" when a family member is diagnosed with cancer.

Values

Values can be viewed as standards or principles of worth that influence and shape behavior. According to Raths, Harmin, and Simon (1966), our values slowly evolve by a process of making choices, prizing them and acting in a consistent repeated way. Values are associated with a dimension of acceptability or unacceptability regarding the appropriateness of behavior and thoughts. Purtilo (1983) categorizes three sets of values: social, professional, and personal, noting that they overlap one another. Values are both unique to an individual and common to a family, group, or culture (Curtain, 1977):

Values are those assertions or statements the individual makes either through his/her behavior, words or actions which define what he/she thinks is important and for which they are willing to suffer, and even die—or perhaps to continue living. Each person is defined in terms of the value choices he/she has made, and even though it might not be ex-

picated, they do have a value system. In like manner, a civilization is defined in terms of the value choices made by those who constitute that civilization (pp. 35–36)

"Value orientations are complex but definitely patterned (rank-ordered) principles (Kluckhohn & Strodtbeck, 1961, p. 4)." They result from an interaction of cognitive, affective, and directive elements in the evaluative process that gives order and direction to human acts and thoughts as they relate to solving "common human" problems. Five value orientations are believed to relate to all human groups: (1) the character of human nature (human nature orientation), (2) the relation of man to nature (man-nature orientation), (3) the temporal focus of human life (time orientation), (4) the modality of human activity (activity orientation) (5) the modality of one human's relation to another (relational orientation).

Value orientations vary from culture to culture. The rate and degree to which an ethnic group becomes assimilated into a dominant culture depends in large part upon the "degree of goodness of fit of the group's own rank ordering of value orientations with that of the dominant culture" (Kluckhohn & Strodtbeck, 1961, p. 26). Dominant value orientations of the United States are individualism, future time, mastery-over-nature, doing, and a definition of evil-but-perfectible human nature (now changing).

Individual and Family

Every family has a unique culture, value structure, and history. Values are the means of interpreting events and passing information from generation to generation, but they are subject to changing interaction with the environment (Sedgewick, 1974). We have few data regarding how families learn to define health and illness and determine their health practices; who their sources of attitudes and opinions are; how beliefs, values, and attitudes are related to levels of education or concern about personal health; or what impact the beliefs, values, and attitudes of other social systems have on the family system.

Steele and Harmon say "a value is an affective disposition towards a person, object, or idea" (1979, p. 1). The major source of values is experience. Values represent something important and are those elements that indicate how a person has decided to use his or her life (Raths, Harmin, & Simon, 1966). When a chronic condition is diagnosed, values may be challenged and need to be replaced by new ones. For example, a family that values flexible mealtimes may have to alter these values to accommodate a member with newly diagnosed insulin-dependent diabetes who requires regularly scheduled mealtimes.

Children begin to form cultural and religious biases as young as 2 years of age (Raths et al, 1966). Customary ways of helping children acquire values are through moralizing, modeling, or assuming a laissez faire attitude (Wilberding, 1985). Moralizing is telling a child what is right or wrong, such as, "It's not right to make fun of somebody who is different." Modeling is setting a good example for others to follow, as in acknowledging the ability of a deaf person to communicate by addressing conversation to that individual. The laissez faire attitude assumes that children should do what they want in the belief that everything will turn out alright. These traditional approaches may be confusing, because children have many sources for obtaining values in addition to parents. As children grow, peers and religious teachings are increasingly influential (Kirschenbaum, 1977; Simon, Howe, & Kirschenbaum, 1972). For example, telling a child that it is not nice to stare at a person with cerebral palsy does not stop the curiosity and may make the child feel uncomfortable around handicapped people.

A nontraditional approach, values clarification, encourages the person to undergo the valuing process, in which critical thought is applied to affective matters (Raths et al. 1966). Raths and colleagues described the seven essential steps in the valuing process: (1) choosing freely, (2) choosing among alternatives, (3) choosing after thoughtful consideration of the consequences of each alternative, (4) prizing and cherishing, (5) affirming, (6) acting upon choices, and (7) repeating (Raths et al, 1966, pp. 28–29). The person must feel happy about and be willing to publicly affirm the choice. A true value will meet all seven criteria. One may infer that the person with chronic obstructive pulmonary disease (COPD) who smokes cigarettes, values smoking and its pleasure. The person has made a choice to smoke and acts on that choice. Value indicators are statements that, although not meeting all criteria, approach values. These include personal feelings, interests, worries, goals, and aspirations. Controversy exists about these criteria for the valuing process. To Kirschenbaum (1977), Rath's criteria are not operational. He believes the valuing process consists of thinking, feeling, choosing, communicating, and acting.

Assigning personal meaning to one's life experience and to pain and suffering appears to be the significant force that enables many to cope and grow under such circumstances (Taylor, 1983). For example, in a study of parents of children with cystic fibrosis, Burton (1975) noted that when parents were able to develop a positive outlook on their situation, their child's longevity increased. Venters (1981) found that parents of children with cystic fibrosis who could "endow the illness with meaning," that is could make sense philosophically out of what was happening to them, were able to cope better than those unable to do this. Examples of comments that express values about chronic conditions appear in Box 9–1.

Patient values should be incorporated in medical decision making (McNeil & Cravalho, 1982). Three basic value questions are of concern to the profession:

1. What is the relative importance to the patient of immediate versus long-term survival? That is, what is the patient's preference?
2. How do individuals value varying states of health?
3. How do preferences for survival at varying times interact with preferences for different health states?

For example, prospective parents must make decisions as to whether or not they will utilize prenatal

---

Box 9–1   *Value Statements about Chronic Conditions*

Parents of Chronically Ill Children

"God gave me this child for a reason."

"In the beginning you have to work with how upset you feel, but then after you accept the disease, you realize how relative it is . . . How bones are something you can deal with, how fortunate that the mental faculties are intact . . . "

Chronically Ill Adults

"Things are different now. People are more important to me."

"I never used to think I needed to contribute to charities, but since I had my heart attack, I give to the American Heart Association. It's important to support them."

"I knew God would help me."

"God doesn't give you any more than you can carry."

"It's made me more aware of life."

"If you don't have your health, you don't have anything."

---

diagnosis. Their decision will be based on the frequency of potential outcomes of a pregnancy and their values and attitudes toward these outcomes. The potential outcomes range from the birth of a normal child to the birth of an affected child, and include elective abortion or miscarriage resulting from prenatal diagnostic procedures.

Thus far, diagnoses analysis has considered mainly the economic costs of affected children, the cost of prenatal diagnosis, and disease frequency. Parents must weigh the short-term costs of the procedure versus the long-term costs of raising a chronically ill, handicapped, or retarded child. In addition, parents have to struggle with their values and beliefs about expected pregnancy outcomes if a problem should be identified. To date, the economic costs of high-tech procedures have received more attention than the psychologic concerns of families (Paucker, Paucker, & McNeil, 1982).

Another difficult decision is removal of life-support measures from a family member. Although the family and the critically ill individual may share common values, individuals cannot automatically make choices for others. They must weigh the potential outcomes of death or long-term, perhaps lifetime, dependency on machinery against the patient's beliefs about life-sustaining measures and desire to prolong life.

Community and Society

Values, attitudes, and beliefs of community members can lead to lack of understanding and resources. A community that does not value the needs of the handicapped will not support programs or resources (e.g., sheltered workshops, special olympics) or give generously to fund-raising campaigns.

Health Professionals

Values, attitudes, and beliefs of health care professionals are important determinants of the care they provide. Each professional group has its own value system in addition to its own technical language and techniques (Thomas, 1982). Since health professionals need to communicate with one another, these differing values and attitudes can be a barrier to their communication. However, as communication continues there is likely to be growth of shared values.

Robinson (1984) pointed out discrepant views of parents of hospitalized children and those of the health care professionals caring for them. She noted that the orientation of the health professionals is one of acute episodic illness and cure, whereas that of parents takes into account the long-term nature of the child's condition and its significance in family experiences. For the health care professional, a child's hospital admission tends to be an episodic event separate from the trajectory of the family's illness experience. Nurses caring for hospitalized adults also view hospitalization as an episodic event. In fact, the entire health care system, including financial reimbursement, tends to favor acute episodic care.

Davis (1988) notes that the current assessment of our society's values could affect health care policy in the future and that nursing needs to "acknowledge and clearly delineate its own values as a guide for influencing public policy, generally, and health care policy, specifically" (p. 289). She notes that dominant nursing values include respect for the individual's right to health care and responsibility for his or her own care, provision of health care by the best qualified practitioner, and holistic health care.

Nurses who value trust, respect, and individuality are likely to respond by listening, and questioning clients to determine what they value.

Attitudes

There are various definitions of the term *attitude,* but they all have a common characteristic: An attitude is a way of thinking and feeling that, in combination with situational and other dispositional variables, signifies a person's predisposition to behave in a particular manner (Rosser, 1971). Although attitudes are not directly observable, they can be inferred from verbal expressions and overt behavior.

Individual and Family

Attitudes toward chronically ill, disabled, or handicapped persons are a multidimensional phenomenon (Gottlieb & Switzky, 1982). They are affected by factors such as type of condition, its degree of severity, its length, and the time and place of contact one has with the person (Esposito & Reed, 1986).

Spread   There is a tendency to evaluate others on the basis of a single characteristic. This concept is called **spread** (Wright, 1960) (see Figure 9–2). When we perceive one physical imperfection about a person, we develop other perceptions from assumptions, either positive or negative, based on our first impression. This can be seen in everyday behavior when one assumes a blind person cannot hear and talks louder to that person. A person who cannot walk is assumed to be intellectually and affectively disabled as well. Also, it is often assumed that people who have been noncompliant in the past will always be noncompliant. Serious errors are made when it is assumed, for example, that the person with diabetes who is compliant about taking insulin is also compliant about exercise and diet.

People tend to attribute disease characteristics to the whole person, as evidenced when the person is referred to as the cystic, hemophiliac, asthmatic, or arthritic. The concept of spread should caution health care workers to be aware of their own perceptions. This "spread" to characteristics unrelated to the person's condition leads the healthy, ablebodied, nondisabled person to have little contact with the disabled. Negative spread is likely to occur when someone knows little about the person other than the presence of the disability (Wright, 1983).

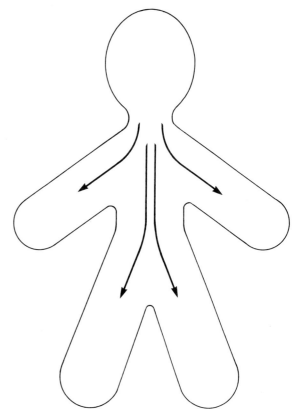

FIGURE 9–2   Illustration of the Concept of Spread

A similar concept is that of "identity spread" (Strauss & Glaser, 1975). Identity spread occurs when a chronic illness is obtrusive and others make assumptions that the ill person cannot work, act, or be like themselves.

Stigma   Stigma was defined by Goffman (1963) as an incongruence between an ideal social identity and the real social identity. Stigma tends to dominate social interactions unless the stigmatized person tries to normalize relationships by trying to hide the intrusive symptom. Not all persons with a particular chronic condition perceive their stigma to the same degree. For example, perceptions of stigma in people with epilepsy were found to vary with severity of seizures, age, gender, educational level, and perceived limitations and job discrimination (Ryan, Kempner, & Emlem, 1980).

Stimulus properties of the stigma determine how an observer will respond to the stigmatized person (Katz, 1981). The degree of stigma depends on such factors as the body part affected and whether or not the problem is physical or emotional, curable or incurable. Visibility of the condition refers to the degree of evidence of the stigma, such as a missing limb, and whether the observer knows about it. For example, an individual may have diabetes but her coworkers may not know about the condition. A person with crutches, however, cannot hide them. The extent to which the person creates discomfort or embarrassment in others is another variable influencing the degree of stigma.

A stigmatized person may be a threat to the healthy person and arouse apprehension. Conditions that are fairly well understood, such as heart disease, may cause less threat than those that are less well understood and relatively uncontrollable, such as cancer or AIDS. The degree of sympathy or pity aroused by the person with a chronic condition may influence observer response. Young, physically disabled children may arouse sympathy, whereas adults with a similar condition may not. Finally, the extent to which the disabled person is held responsible for an illness will influence others' response. A young woman commented to her uncle, recently diagnosed with lung cancer, that "I have absolutely no sympathy for you. You smoked all your life. You make me so angry."

Many groups in the United States, including those who have chronic illnesses or disabilities, are considered stigmatized, deviant, or of marginal social status (Katz, 1981). However, Goffman (1963) cautions that the social context is important because what may be discrediting in one setting may not be in another. For example, a group of people playing baseball may believe a person in a wheelchair does not belong in the group, whereas the person may easily be accepted in an office or with a group of wheelchair athletes.

American values of youth, physical attractiveness, and personal accomplishment contribute to perceptions of chronic conditions as deviant. People with these conditions may have physical deformities and be unable to do some things expected of "normal people" (those without the deviant characteristic). Affected people may have artifacts such as wigs, wheelchairs, and oxygen tubes, and life-styles that further set them apart from the rest of the population. A stigmatized person may be disqualified from full social acceptance.

Responses of "normal" individuals to deviancy may be either hostile and rejecting or friendly, sympathetic, and helpful. In addition, they may devalue, stereotype, or label the stigmatized person. State-

ments such as "He's just like all those others who can't see" or "Don't play with her, she's got CP [cerebral palsy]" are examples of such devaluation. On the other hand, making modifications to enable a disabled person to participate in an activity is an example of a friendly or helpful response. A youngster was observed changing the rules of a game of catch to enable a playmate in a cast to participate.

Stigmatized people may respond to the stares, cruel remarks, and exclusion from activities in various ways. Responses depend on factors such as personality characteristics (e.g., temperament), previous experiences, and the social context. They may choose to ignore the incident or deal with it directly. Other approaches include passing for normal, attempting to normalize life, or laughing it off ("These crutches are such a pain in the neck."). To pass for normal a person may choose not to reveal the presence of a disease on a job application or, if hearing impaired, refuse to wear a hearing aid. Others may try to cover up the defect, such as wearing a turban over a balding head, or wearing a long skirt or pants, or a long-sleeved blouse, to conceal leg or arm scars. Another response is to isolate oneself from situations that may be stigmatizing, such as avoiding swimming in order to avoid stares at a badly scarred body.

Critics suggest that although Goffman's theory may have been appropriate for the disabled when it was developed in the 1950s, it may not be true in the 1990s (Fine & Asch, 1988; Frank, 1988). Many social changes have occurred for the disabled in both legal status and empowerment. Frank (1988) pointed out that some disabled persons tend to be active rather than reactive in combatting stigma. That is, they insist on being visible as people with disabilities, thus making it open to society to deal with and increasing their self-empowerment.

Fine and Asch (1988) suggest that most social problems of disabled individuals can be understood within a minority-group framework. They challenge the following assumptions, and suggest looking beyond them: (1) Disability is solely a biological phenomenon and therefore uncritically treated as an independent variable. (2) Impairments are assumed to cause problems faced by the disabled. (3) The disabled person is a victim. (4) "Disability is central to the disabled person's self-concept, self-definition, social comparisons, and reference groups" (p. 11). (5) Being disabled is synonymous with needing help and social support.

Courtesy stigma refers to the spread of the disability to those affiliated with the stigmatized person and are regarded by others as having a spoiled identity (Goffman, 1963). People may react to the courtesy stigma by appearing normal without any effort, not attempting to appear normal, or trying to eliminate all information about their affiliation with the stigmatized person (Birenbaum, 1970).

Ambiguity   The concept of **ambiguity** (Preston, 1979) is closely related to stigma. Ambiguity refers to elements falling outside the specified range of normal variations and for which there is no alternative characteristic to account for the variation. The incongruence causes ambiguity. Both Goffman and Preston state that stigma is most severe when situations border on normal but are not normal. This situation is related to the concept of marginality discussed in Chapter 7.

Labeling   Labeling refers to the designation of a term or title for a particular condition. Conflicting conclusions exist about the effects of labeling handicapped individuals (Fiedler & Simpson, 1987). Several investigators report no effects from labeling, although others argue that such a practice is detrimental to the person. Labeling is thought to create barriers to understanding because it encourages defining people by a single dimension (the handicap) that then spreads to the person's character. On the other hand, others say there may be benefits from labeling because it reduces the discrepancy between expected and actual behavior, thus increasing peer acceptance. In addition, labeling may facilitate the process of obtaining needed services, available only to persons with a designated (labeled) condition.

Community and Society

Community and societal attitudes can help or hinder the implementation and improvement of services to persons with chronic conditions. Societal attitudes are a critical variable in removing psychologic and social barriers affecting the chronically ill and disabled. Unfortunately, many people still have negative attitudes towards those with chronic conditions.

Gething (1985) cites problems of disabled persons identified by Hastings (1980) that focus on reactions and attitudes of members of society. These problems include (1) exclusion and segregation from society, including deprivation of opportunities; (2) negative beliefs about disabled persons (e.g.,

they are frightening, incompetent, and lacking in confidence); and (3) poverty because of limited job opportunities and government assistance. Other barriers are architectural inaccessibility and a general lack of acceptance by society. As a result, many disabled individuals feel powerless (especially those living in institutions) and frustrated.

As with values, attitudes are thought to be learned through social experiences, mostly in childhood, and prejudice against the physically handicapped appears by 6 years of age (Richardson, 1970). People having close contact with the ill person are said to have an **insider** view of the disabled person. They accept the limitations but are also aware of the person's strengths and abilities. They believe it possible for the disabled person to have meaningful aspirations and achievements (Gething, 1985). Illness is seen as just one aspect of a multifaceted person with limitations due as much to environmental as personal characteristics. The **outsider,** who does not know the disabled person, tends to view the disability as tragic and to overestimate limitations and underestimate capabilities (Wright, 1983). Disability is viewed as permeating every area of functioning (difficulties, restrictions, frustrations).

Gething (1985) conducted a study of people with cerebral palsy (CP), their close relatives (insiders), and able-bodied people (outsiders) who did not know the people with CP. Insiders perceived fewer problems for the person with CP, except for public transportation, than did the outsiders. Close relatives identified more problems in areas concerning survival, daily care, mobility, and the future than did the disabled or the able-bodied. Relatives also assigned higher levels of problem severity to issues like communication, activities of daily living, people's staring, and the discomfort of the able-bodied. They also placed more emphasis on psychologic problems, attitudes of the able-bodied, and personal interaction.

Beliefs

Beliefs are personally formed notions and meaning that an individual has about the environment (Lazarus & Folkman, 1984). They are filters through which a person interprets stimuli. Beliefs and commitment influence how people cognitively appraise their situation. **Commitment** defines what is meaningful or important for a person and serves as a motive for behavior.

Families may have certain beliefs about health and illness. For example, they may believe that cancer is equated with death or a hysterectomy with the eradication of a woman's role (Williams, 1976). They may believe that illness is incapacitating and then have difficulty accepting gains in independence and self-care skills as the child or adult adjusts to the illness. Others may believe that illness is punishment for a sin or evidence of guilt (Safilios-Rothschild, 1970).

Kleinman (1980) distinguishes explanatory models from generalized beliefs about sickness and health care. General beliefs exist independently of, and prior to, any given episode of sickness. Explanatory models (EMs) are beliefs and perceptions that individuals hold about a specific disease. Even though EMs draw upon general belief systems, they are constructed in response to particular illness episodes and specific health problems. Explanations are related to etiology, onset of symptoms, pathophysiology, course of illness, and treatment (Kleinman, 1980). The degree of congruence between the patient's and health provider's EMs can affect the way the patient responds and follows a recommended treatment plan. EMs are powerful motivators of behavior regardless of how well thought out or rational they are. Each person has a different understanding and expectation of health care encounters, which when dissonant, are likely to increase stress for all involved. Anderson (1981) notes that although patients and staff may use the same language, they have different ideas about the meaning of these words. Using the same language may therefore intensify discrepancies because no one is aware of them.

Health Beliefs

To some extent, state of health and decisions to seek health care depend upon personal beliefs, attitudes, and values about health. For example, persons with positive attitudes toward cancer prior to receiving a diagnosis of cancer were found to have a more positive adjustment post-diagnosis (Edlund & Sneed, 1989).

Describing the differing cultural beliefs about health is beyond the scope of ths book, but it is essential that nurses become aware of the beliefs of the people with whom they are working. Beliefs influence the person's understanding of the chronic condition, as well as decisions regarding health care and following through with recommended regimens.

In addition, the beliefs influence how explanations need to be given to patients and families, as well as the possible course of therapy. For example, African-Americans tend to classify illness into natural and unnatural categories (Flaskerud & Rush, 1989). Natural illnesses occur because of God's will, as punishment for sin, or an encounter with the forces of nature without adequate protection. Natural illnesses are predictable and can therefore be prevented. They occur because of exposure to cold, dirt, and impurities in the air, food, or water that can enter the body: Going out in the cold or rain can lead to the flu, pneumonia, or tuberculosis. Laxatives, a good diet, rest, and prayer are believed to keep one healthy. Lack of moderation (e.g., eat or drink too much, stay out too late), improper diet, and stress are other causes of these illnesses. Natural illnesses are believed to be punishment for sin, God's will, or a test of one's faith. They can be helped through prayer or through a person whom God has blessed.

Unnatural illnesses are those caused by witchcraft and are the result of evil influences. Treatment for these illnesses comes from religion, magic, visible protection (e.g., charms, prayer cards), massage, and natural foods, herbs, or medicines. Flaskerud and Rush (1989) examined these beliefs as they related to AIDS and found that the same categories of beliefs about healing were present for this illness.

Several models attempt to explain why people seek health care services. They include Mechanic's Model (1978), the Health Belief Model by Rosenstock (1974) and Becker (1974), and the Chatterton Model. An understanding of these models, may help nurses assist patients having encounters with the health care system. Mechanic identified 10 variables that play a part in seeking help. These variables are listed in Table 9–1.

The Health Belief Model explains behaviors directed at prevention, decisions to seek health care, and compliance with medical regimes (Becker, 1974; Rosenstock, 1974). "Health behavior is any activity undertaken by a person believing himself to be healthy for the purpose of preventing disease or detecting it in an asymptomatic state" (Kasl & Cobb, 1966, p. 246). The model predicts increased likelihood of health care service use if the person perceives personal susceptibility to the disease, perceives the disease as harmful, and believes treatment is beneficial, with benefits of treatment outweighing the disease risk. These beliefs plus a cue to action (an emotional reaction to internal or external stim-

Table 9–1 Variables Influencing the Ill to Seek Help

Variable	Measure Pursued
Salience of symptoms	The more severe and visible the symptom, the more likely one will seek help
Perceived seriousness	The more serious the symptom, the more likely one will seek help
Disruption of activities	If symptoms interfere with normal activities, the more likely one will seek help
Frequency and persistence of symptoms	The more frequent the symptom, the more likely one will seek help
Tolerance threshold	When tolerance level has been reached, a person will seek help
Basis of appraisal	One's knowledge, attitudes, and values influence what one identifies as illness
Needs for denial	Amount of denial depends on amount of anxiety present, degree of aberrancy of problem, and amount of guilt associated with the problem
Competing needs	Other important roles and tasks may compete with help seeking behaviors
Alternative interpretations	A person may attempt to explain aberrant behavior within a range of normalcy
Accessibility of treatment	Barriers such as embarrassment, stigma, distance, time, economic constraints may interfere with seeking help

Source: Mechanic, 1978.

uli) influence a person's willingness to undertake health-related actions.

Using data from the Health Belief Model, Rosenstock and Becker report that prevention and detection services are most often used by younger or middle-aged persons, more often females, those who are better educated and have a higher income, and those of the white race. The same is true of diagnostic and treatment services.

The Chatterton Model (Rankin & Duffy, 1983), based on the Health Belief Model, examines the decision-making process used at each step from prediagnosis to consumption of health services. It helps health care professionals identify and provide the appropriate educational information needed at each step so that patients can make informed decisions. The decisions made are

1. Disease/no disease present
2. Perceived illness/no perceived illness
3. Perceived need for health services/no perceived need for health services
4. Decision to seek health care services/decision not to seek health care services
5. Consumption of health care services/no consumption of health care services

Most of these models are based on patient perceptions and not the perceptions of the health care professionals. The models assume that people perceive illness as an undesirable state and would prefer to be free of illness. Although this assumption is true for the majority of people, some have secondary gains from illness, such as freedom from responsibility, attention, and exemption from obligation.

Family Myths and Rules

Families have myths, rules, and themes that differentiate them from other family systems. These myths, rules, and themes are actually beliefs that have developed within the family that influence certain behaviors of the family members. Family myths are usually unchallenged beliefs about each family member and each one's position in family life (Ferreira, 1966). These myths may be challenged when a chronic condition is diagnosed and the family member believed to be the only person who can carry out a certain function (e.g., discipline the children) can no longer do so. Family rules provide order and direct how the system operates. These rules, which may be overt or covert, determine how information flows within the family and how much information is allowed into the family.

Children's views of health Natapoff (1978) studied 264 school children and found that children saw health as a positive attribute. Being healthy meant feeling good and doing the things they wanted to do, whereas being sick meant being unable to do the things they wanted. Most said they could tell whether others were healthy or sick by relying on perceptual data from use of their five senses. This study suggests that children's views of health differ from the traditional definition proposed by health professionals: the absence of disease or symptoms.

Folk beliefs   Some people believe that disease is caused by the supernatural intervention of witches, sorcerers, mediums or departed ancestors. It is not unusual for people to believe that environmental forces such as the wind, moon, and night air may play a part in the development of disease (McKenzie & Chrisman, 1977).

Many cultures use home remedies that include herbs, spices, teas, massage, sleep, and exercise, either alone or in combination with conventional medical therapy. Nurses must assess the presence of folk beliefs and combine the folk remedies into traditional regimes when possible.

Religious Beliefs

"Religious beliefs express the character of the social totality. . ." (Giddens, 1978, p. 88). Rituals are important in sustaining one's religious beliefs. Religious beliefs and symbols are kept separate from ordinary daily life.

> All religious beliefs presuppose a polar division of reality into two opposed classes of objects; those which are 'sacred' on the one hand, and those that are 'profane' on the other. Sacred things are the subject of attitudes of awe and veneration and thus are kept completely separate from life in the profane world (Giddens, 1978, p. 91).

Religion can be defined as a unified system of beliefs and practices related to sacred things. These practices unite into a "single moral community called a church all those who adhere to them" (Giddens, 1978, p. 92). There are two essential ideational components of religion. One is the provision of moral ideals and moral regulation; the other is the creation of a cognitive framework for understanding the world conceptually (Giddens, 1978). Every religion consists of practices, or rituals and ceremonials, in addition to beliefs. Each religion involves the existence of a church (i.e., a regularized social organization of believers) in which the social practices associated with it take place.

Wyszynski (1986) notes that problems exist in distinguishing between psychiatric symptoms and religious and cultural beliefs. Some cultures cultivate spiritualism, a belief that the dead survive as spirits and can cause harm to the living. Belief in spirits can be found in segments of the Hispanic population and in African-American communities.

Espiritismo, the Spanish term for belief in spirits, includes *mal puerto* (evil put on) and *mal ojo* (evil eye). Among some African-Americans *rootwork* refers to the working of evil upon someone. Patients believing in spiritualism may first go to a healer instead of seeking medical care, allowing their health problem to go undetected or untreated for a long time.

Miller (1985) compared loneliness and spiritual well-being in 64 chronically ill adults with rheumatoid arthritis and in healthy adults. Using the 20-item Spiritual Well-Being Scale, with two subscales measuring religious and existential well-being, she found that the ill subjects had higher spiritual and religious well-being than did healthy adults. It is possible that chronic illness may stimulate a person's valuing religion, having faith in God, and having a relationship with God.

Silber and Reilly (1985) studied spiritual concerns of 114 hospitalized adolescents. Using the Spiritual and Religious Concerns questionnaire, an 18-item Likert-type scale, the more seriously ill subjects had higher scores. Although belief in God and participation in religious activity seemed an inherent part of one's background and identity, spiritual and religious experience becomes more important in direct relationship to the severity of an adolescent's condition. Studies using different instruments conducted by Brandt (1987) and Hymovich and Baker (1985) support the strong role that religion plays in the lives of adults with cancer and parents of children with various chronic conditions and that prayer and belief in God are important coping mechanisms.

Spiritual Orientation to Life

The spiritual dimension is a unifying force that integrates physical, mental, emotional, and social dimensions and plays a vital role in determining one's well-being. The spiritual dimension is the central core, a grounding source for all other dimensions. The spiritual dimension concerns what the person identifies as purposeful or meaningful in life. What one selects as meaningful serves as an inner drive for one's accomplishments in life. The spiritual dimension transcends the individual and has the capacity to be a common bond between people. It consists of a sense of selflessness, a feeling for others, and a set of principles that govern conduct. The bond accounts for sharing warmth, love and compassion with others and could be perceived as a "caring center" (Banks, 1980).

According to Stoll (1989), spirituality is "the core of one's being; a sense of personhood; what one is and is becoming" (p. 6). It brings purpose and meaning to one's existence. Spiritual well-being is a satisfaction in a relationship with God, a perception of life as having meaning, and a satisfaction with one's life.

Spiritual distress is "distress of the human spirit . . . a disruption in the life principle which pervades a person's entire being and which integrates and transcends one's biological and psychosocial nature" (Kim, McFarland & McLane, 1987, p. 314). Spiritual distress can be characterized in ways such as questioning the meaning of suffering, the meaning of one's existence, or the moral and ethical implications of the therapeutic regimen. It can include verbalization of inner conflict about beliefs or concerns about one's relationship with a deity. It may be manifested in anger towards God or religious representatives. Sometimes spiritual distress can cause nightmares and sleep disturbances or alterations in behavior and mood as evidenced by crying, anger, withdrawal, anxiety, hostility, or apathy.

Assessment and Intervention

Assessment

Assessing orientation to life is a nursing responsibility, because values, attitudes, and beliefs influence what is important to families and how acceptable planned nursing interventions will be. For example, while some handicapped individuals may choose to spend time and energy dressing or feeding themselves, others may prefer to spend time doing something else, such as reading or socializing (Zola, 1982). Because one has the ability to do something does not necessarily mean it is the best thing to do or is something the person values. For example, Karen Killilea, an adolescent with cerebral palsy, spent years learning to walk with crutches and braces but eventually decided she had greater mobility in a wheelchair. She gave up walking for more efficient use of her time and energy by using the wheelchair (Killilea, 1963).

Some people may find it difficult to discuss their beliefs, and it is important to acknowledge and respect their wish in this matter. It is helpful, however, to distinguish whether a family belief system is based on the premise of internal or external (powerful other, chance) locus of control. Of special relevance to nursing is the issue of health locus of control. Two instruments may be useful: the Health Locus of Control Scale (HLC) (Wallston et al, 1976) and the Health-Specific Locus of Control Beliefs Questionnaire (Lau & Ware, 1981). The HLC in an 11-item scale with a 6-point Likert format, an alpha reliability of 0.72, and test-retest reliability of 0.71 over an 8-week interval (Cohen, 1988). The Health-Specific Locus of Control Beliefs Questionnaire is a 28-item instrument measuring "beliefs about self-control over health, provider control over health, chance health outcomes and general health threat, health care attitudes, health status perceptions, and value placed on health" (Cohen, 1988, p. 283).

Spirituality   Assessment of a person's spirituality involves both observation and interviews (Carson, 1989). The spiritual portion of most nursing histories only identifies religious affiliation. The health professional can ascertain spiritual needs by specific questions geared to the four areas of spiritual concerns (Stoll, 1989). These include questions related to the person's (1) concept of God, (2) source of strength and hope, (3) importance of specific religious practices, and (4) perception of the relationship between one's spiritual beliefs and state of health. Guidelines for areas to explore in assessing a person's orientation to life and spirituality are included in Table 9–2. Some people may find it difficult to discuss spirituality and it is important to acknowledge and respect each person's right to his own values and beliefs.

Questions to determine spirituality include:

"Is religion or God significant to you?"

"Is prayer helpful to you?"

"Does a God or deity function in your daily life?"

"What is your source of strength and hope?"

"Do you feel your faith is helpful?"

"Do you ever ask why is this happening to me?" (Stoll, 1989, p. 154).

Table 9–2   Guidelines for Assessing Orientation to Life*

Topic	Useful Information
Health	Values placed on health
	Beliefs about health, illness, death, hospitalization
Treatment	Expectation about type of treatment needed
Expectations	Expectations of treatment outcome
Religious beliefs	Religion
	Importance of religion or God
	Importance of prayer
	Amount of reliance on religion at times of stress
Spirituality	Source of strength and hope
	If ever asks why this is happening
	If a God or deity functions in daily life
Health system beliefs	Satisfaction with past experiences with health system (doctors, nurses, hospitals)
Strengths	**Needs**

*The following questionnaires may be useful: Health Locus of Control Scale (HLC) (Wallston et al, 1976), Health-Specific Locus of Control Beliefs Questionnaire (Lau & Ware, 1981).

Selected Interventions

Modify Attitudes

Negative attitudes often interfere with a person's ability to function with a chronic condition. Altering these attitudes is essential if changes in public policy are to occur and be effective. Nurses can play an important role in modifying negative attitudes by providing for close relationships between the handicapped and others, providing factual information through educational programs, changing the individual's attitudinal environment, and legislating against discrimination.

"The preferred strategy for changing attitudes is to create cognitive dissonance by increasing awareness of conflicts among knowledge, feelings, and behavior" (Henderson et al, 1979, p. 153). Many social scientists believe attitude theory has limited application in changing attitudes because attitudinal changes follow changes in behavior. They recommend focusing on behavioral change rather than on altering opinions and attitudes (Janis, 1975). When legislation against various forms of discrimination is enacted, it often takes a long time before it is actually implemented, primarily because of the attitudes of the public.

Interactions between disabled and nondisabled are often strained and accompanied by uncertainty, anxiety, and discomfort (Kleck, Ono, & Hastorf, 1966). One way to reduce tension is to acknowledge the disability. Disabled people need a repertoire of social skills to facilitate social encounters (Resnick, 1984). However, since physical appearance is also important in relationships, these social skills may be inadequate to encourage or sustain relationships because able-bodied people have a tendency to stay away.

While attempts to modify patients' attitudes continue, there is no impressive evidence that such interventions have been effective, especially for persons with serious impairments. Mechanic (1986) suggests that it is probably more effective to try to achieve change indirectly than directly through psychotherapy.

Provide close contact between handicapped and others   One approach to modifying attitudes is the "contact model," whereby contact with handicapped people is expected to lead to improved attitudes of the nonhandicapped. Results of this approach are equivocal: Some researchers find no change in attitudes, others find increased positive attitudes, and still others find increased negative attitudes following contact (Esposito & Reed, 1986). In addition, there is little evidence that positive changes, when they do occur, can be maintained over time.

On the other hand, frequent close contact between the handicapped and nonhandicapped is expected to lead to gradual but deep change. The underlying premise is that familiarity diminishes fear of the unknown, especially since such fears are often unfounded or based on ignorance. Integration should begin in the preschool years. Increased interaction could provide both groups with an improved perspective on the values, standards, and aspirations of one another.

A recent approach to helping children understand disabled youngsters is the use of a troupe of puppets with and without disabilities (Meehan, 1981). Called The Kids on the Block, the puppets were designed to teach children in kindergarten through sixth grade about disabilities and the feelings associated with them. Among these puppets' problems are obesity, deafness, cerebral palsy, leukemia, epilepsy, and diabetes. Puppets express the feelings of both normal and disabled children and show how each can communicate with the other. However, they do not deal with problems of the able-bodied or teach them how to interact with the disabled. The disabled puppets have good self-concepts and help the able-bodied puppets and the audience feel at ease with them. This depiction tends to present an ideal situation rather than a real-life situation, where disabled children may have low self-esteem and lack ability to put others at ease. Children in the audience have an opportunity to ask questions of the puppets. Complete kits of puppets can be purchased, along with a guide covering puppetry, handicaps, and mainstreaming, including scripts, classroom activities, and resources.

Rosenbaum et al (1986) compared three types of interventions to modify attitudes of children age 9 to 13 years toward disabled peers. Group I was a buddy program in which the children had direct contact with disabled youngsters, group II children saw the Kids on the Block (KOB) program, group III combined the buddy and KOB programs, and group IV was a control group. The KOB program had no greater effect on the children's attitudes than did the control group. Only 11% of the children in the combined KOB and buddy program showed improved attitudes, while 67% of those in the Buddies alone group showed significant changes. This study points out the value of direct contact in changing attitudes. Although direct contact is effective for changing attitudes, it cannot always be provided. Effective alternatives must be sought.

Direct educational programs Approaches to modifying attitudes with at least short-term effectiveness for college students have included a panel of disabled people speaking with the students in class or students viewing a videotape of the panel speaking (Donaldson & Martinson, 1977). Another approach used with children (Cleary, 1976) and adults (Stauffer, 1974) is simulation of various disabilities, such as deafness, hemiplegia, and blindness. Simulations can include equipment such as wheelchairs, crutches, and ostomy bags.

Increasing numbers of books about children with disabilities (Engel, 1980) and chronic illness are available for helping children learn about others different from themselves. Books encourage the growth of positive attitudes on the part of normal children. Meeting the disabled child through a nonthreatening story may reduce anxiety and fear that might have been felt if first meeting the disabled person face to face. Through vicarious experience, the able-bodied can identify with the problems and aspirations of the disabled child (Baskin & Harris, 1977). Criteria for evaluating such books are listed in Box 9–2.

Fiedler and Simpson (1987) described two curricular approaches to modifying the attitudes of nonhandicapped high school students toward handicapped peers. Two types of curricula were used. In the categorical approach students received information about the definitions, causes, and characteristics of disabling conditions. This approach has proven effective in imparting cognitive information but has the danger of labeling and perhaps stereotyping the handicapped person. The noncategorical curriculum focused on generic concepts, such as values, conformity, individual differences, labeling effects, and normalization. Results showed that both approaches were effective in modifying attitudes, but the categorical approach consistently resulted in more-positive attitudes than did the noncategorical curriculum. Females were found to hold significantly more favorable attitudes toward handicapped persons than did male counterparts.

Change attitudinal environment

Box 9–2   *Criteria for Evaluating Children's Books to Modify Attitudes Toward Disabled Persons*

1. Are the text and illustrations appropriate for the child's developmental level?
2. Is the book centered on people? Is it contemporary realistic fiction or is it unrealistic?
   Is the disabled protagonist a child?
3. Does the book have good literary quality?
   Are the characterizations strong?
   Is the disabled character a real person with basic needs, aspirations, strengths, and weaknesses?
   Is the plot well developed?
   Is the conclusion plausible?
   Is the setting clear and believable?
4. Do text and illustrations give accurate information about the disability?
   Is the nomenclature accurate?
   Is the description of the handicapping condition consistent with medical and psychologic practice?
   Are the accoutrements and paraphernalia associated with the disability correctly described and utilized?
   Are the social, psychological, and emotional ramifications of exceptionality developed in a credible manner?
   Are the genesis, current conditions, and prognoses harmonious with reasonable expectations?
   "Is the resolution of the story (not) dependent on improbable events or illogical behavior on the part of the characters?" (Baskin & Harris, 1977, p. 50).
5. Does the book generally reflect positive attitudes toward disability and the disabled? (Engel, 1980, pp. 28–29).

Source: Baskin & Harris, 1977.

Advocacy

Social change is inconvenient and sometimes painful. An independent movement of consumers (e.g., parents, people with disabilities) and their allies have developed organized ways to monitor and change human service agencies. Health care professionals need to learn how to be advocates for this population as well as for the individuals and families with whom they work. The techniques they use are listed in Box 9–3.

Values clarification   Clarifying values helps one develop a set of beliefs that result in consistently successful actions toward ourselves and others. Values clarification can help the nurse personally as well as professionally with patients. It can be used personally for growth and ethical reflection. Our own values direct our commitments to helping, healing, and combatting pain and illness. Engaging patients in the valuing process may help them gain understanding of their own lives and clarify what is impor-

Box 9–3   Advocacy Strategies

Demonstrations
  marches
  sit-ins
  vigils
  picketing
Making demands
  bill of rights
  list of grievances
Letter writing
Fact-finding forums
  town meetings
  investigation panels
Education
  speeches
  posters
  newspapers
Model programs
Demystify technical aspects of situation
  translate research findings, diagnostic terms, etc., into terminology patients and other nonhealth-care individuals can understand

Nurses can assist school personnel with curricula to modify attitudes or, if programs do not exist, could help identify the need for them, plan curricula and also participate in the programs. Although exact curricula are yet to be determined, available findings offer guidelines.

tant for them. The nurse can then use this information to focus intervention on those areas valued by the person. Values clarification may help improve compliance in some patients.

The aim of values clarification is patient reflection on a situation to determine what is important. This technique is called the clarifying response (Raths et al, 1966). The nurse has the patient focus on an issue and then asks questions to determine what is prized. The patient is encouraged to think about the possible choices and the alternatives and consequences of his or her behavior. The patient should have time to think about the situation, without expectation of immediate answers. When exploring values, the nurse must be nonjudgmental and realize that the individual is ultimately responsible for his or her own care. In certain matters, however, the professional code of ethics must be kept in mind.

Supporting spirituality Dewey (1976) suggests it can be supportive to provide opportunities for people to express their feelings and concerns with a religious person. Sometimes, she notes, just being with a patient can be meaningful. She believes that people who are dying may just want someone to be with them so that they are not alone. Conveying a sense of worth, dignity, and respect for the values of every individual is another way to support a person's spirituality.

Summary

System values, attitudes, and beliefs, components of orientation to life, are powerful forces that influence response to health and illness. Knowledge of one's own as well as others' orientation is essential to meaningful and effective interactions. Values are standards or principles of worth that influence and shape behavior. Attitudes are hypothetical constructs predisposing one to respond in a particular way to some aspect of the environment. Various attitudes toward those with chronic conditions are explored from the perspectives of deviance, stigma, labeling, spread, and ambiguity. Beliefs are personally formed notions and meanings that an individual has about the environment. Although not directly observable, values, attitudes, and beliefs can be inferred from verbal expressions or overt behavior. Spirituality reflects the totality of values, attitudes, and beliefs.

The nurse's role in assessing client's values, attitudes, beliefs, and spirituality was explored, as were selected nursing interventions. The primary focus of the intervention section was on strategies to modify negative values, attitudes, and beliefs related to chronic illness. These approaches included providing close contacts between the handicapped and others, providing factual information through educational programs and the use of books, changing the individual's attitudinal environment, and legislating against discrimination.

References

Anderson, J. (1981). An interpretive approach to clinical nursing research. *Nurs Papers, 13,* 6–12.

Banks, R. (1980). Health and the spiritual dimension: Relationships and implications for professional preparation programs. *J Sch Health, 50,* 195–202.

Baskin, B.H., Harris, K.H. (1977). *Notes from a different drummer.* New York: R.R. Bowker.

Becker, M.H. (1974). The health belief model and personal health behavior. *Health Educ Monogr, 2,* 324–473.

Birenbaum, A. (1970). On managing a courtesy stigma. *J Health Soc Behav.* 11(Sept), 196–206.

Brandt, B.P. (1987). The relationship between hopelessness and selected variables in women receiving chemotherapy for breast cancer. *Oncol Nurs Forum, 14*(2), 35–39.

Burton, L. (1975). *The family life of sick children: A study of families coping with chronic childhood disease.* London: Routledge and Kegan Paul.

Carson, V.B. (1989). *Spiritual dimensions of nursing practice.* Philadelphia: W.B. Saunders.

Cohen, R.F. (1988). Measuring attitudes toward chronic illness. In M. Frank-Stromborg (Ed.), *Instruments for clinical nursing research* (pp. 269–295). Norwalk, CT: Appleton & Lange.

Cleary, M.E. (1976). Helping children understand the child with special needs. *Child Today,* 5(4), 6–10.

Curtain, L. (1977). Human values in nursing. *J NY State Nurses Asoc,* 8(4), 31–40.

Davis, G.C. (1988). Nursing values and health care policy. *Nurs Outlook, 36*(6), 289–292.

Dewey, D. (1976). Function of religion in clinical practice. In B.H. Peterson & C.J. Kellog (Eds.), *Current perspectives in oncologic nursing* (pp. 151–153). St. Louis: Mosby.

Donaldson, J., & Martinson, M.C. (1977). Modifying attitudes toward physically disabled persons. *Except Child, 44,* 337–341.

Edlund, B., & Sneed, N.V. (1989). Emotional responses to the diagnosis of cancer: Age-related comparisons. *Oncol Nurs Forum, 16*(5), 691–697.

Engel, R. (1980). Understanding the handicapped through literature. *Young Child, 35*(5), 27–32.

Esposito, B.G., & Reed II, T.M. (1986). The effects of contact with handicapped persons on young children's attitudes. *Except Child, 53*(3), 224–229.

Ferreira, A.J. (1966). Family myths. *Psychiatr Res Rep 20,* 86–87.

Fiedler, C.R., & Simpson, R.L. (1987). Modifying the attitudes of nonhandicapped high school students toward handicapped peers. *Except Child, 53*(4), 342–349.

Fine, M., & Asch, A. (1988). Disability beyond stigma: Social interaction, discrimination, and activism. *J Soc Issues, 44*(1), 3–21.

Flaskerud, J.H., & Rush, C.E. (1989). AIDS and traditional health beliefs and practices of black women. *Nurs Res, 38*(4), 210–215.

Frank, G. (1988). Beyond stigma: Visibility and self-empowerment of persons with congenital limb deficiencies. *J Soc Issues, 44*(1), 95–115.

Gething, L. (1985). Perceptions of disability of persons with cerebral palsy, their close relatives and able bodied persons. *Soc Sci Med. 20*(6), 561–568.

Giddens, A. (1978). *Emile Durkheim.* New York: Penguin Books.

Goffman, I. (1963). *Stigma: Notes on the management of spoiled identity.* Englewood Cliffs, NJ: Prentice Hall.

Gottlieb, J., & Switzky, H.N. (1982). Development of school-aged children's stereotypic attitudes toward mentally retarded children. *Am J Ment Def, 86,* 596–600.

Hastings, E. (1980). Be grateful and shut up: Some personal experiences. *Breakthrough.* National Bulletin of the International Year of Disabled Persons, Camberra, No. 3. (cited in Gething, [1985.])

Henderson, J.B., Hall, S.M., & Lipton, H.L. (1979). Changing self-destructive behaviors. In G.C. Stone, F. Cohen, N.E. Adler (Eds.). *Health psychology—A handbook* (pp. 141–160). San Francisco: Jossey-Bass.

Hymovich, D.P., & Baker, C. (1985). The needs, concerns and coping of parents of children with cystic fibrosis. *Fam Relat, 34,* 91–97.

Janis, I.L. (1958). *Psychological stress: Psychoanalytic and behavioral studies of surgical patients.* New York: Wiley.

Kasl, S.V., & Cobb, S. (1966). Health behavior and sick role behavior. *Arch Environ Health I, 12,* 246–266 and II, *12,* 534–541.

Katz, I. (1981). *Stigma: A social psychological analysis.* Hillside, NJ: Lawrence Erlbaum Associates, Publishers.

Killilea, M. (1963). *With love from Karen.* New York: Dell.

Kim, M.J., McFarland, G.K., & McLane, A.M. (1987). *Pocket guide to nursing diagnosis.* 2nd ed. St. Louis: Mosby.

Kirschenbaum, H. (1977). *Advanced value clarification.* LaJolla, CA: University Associates.

Kleck, R., Ono, H., & Hastorf, A. (1966). The effects of physical deviance upon face-to-face interactions. *Hum Relat, 19,* 425–435.

Kleinman, A.M. (1980). *Patients and healers in the context of culture.* Los Angeles: University of California Press.

Kluckhohn, F.R., & Strodtbeck, F.L. (1961). *Variations in value orientations.* Evanston, IL: Row, Peterson.

Lau, R.R., & Ware, J.F. (1981). Refinements in the measurement of health-specific locus-of-control beliefs. *Med Care, 19*(11), 1147.

Lazarus, R.S., & Folkman, S. (1984). *Stress, appraisal, and coping.* New York: Springer.

McKenzie, J.L., & Chrisman, N.J. (1977). Healing herbs, gods, and magic. *Nurs Outlook, 25*(5), 326–329.

McNeil, B.J., & Cravalho, E.G. (Eds.). (1982). *Critical issues in medical technology.* Boston: Auburn House.

Mechanic, D. (1986). *From advocacy to allocation: The evolving American health care system.* New York: Macmillan.

Mechanic, D. (1978). *Medical sociology.* 2nd ed. New York: Free Press.

Meehan, T. (1981). Puppets are people disabled but different . . . *Biomed Commun, 9*(8), 18–19.

Miller, J.F. (1985). Assessment of loneliness and spiritual well-being in chronically ill and healthy adults. *Journal of Professional Nursing, 1*(2), 79–85.

Mullen, P.D., Hersey, J.C., & Iverson, D.C. (1987). Health behavior models compared. *Soc Sci Med, 24*(11), 973–981.

Natapoff, J.N. (1978). Children's views of health: A developmental study. *Am J Pub Health, 68*(10), 995–999.

Paucker, S.G., Paucker, S.P., & McNeil, B.J. (1982). Implications of parents' attitudes on alternative policies for prenatal diagnosis. In B.J. McNeil & E.B. Cravalho (Eds.), *Critical issues in medical technology* (pp. 343–357). Boston: Auburn House.

Pellegrino, E. (1976). Lecture delivered to the International Institute of Health Care, Ethics, and Human Values, Mt. St. Joseph College, Mt. St. Joseph, Ohio, July. Cited in L. Curtain, (1977). Human values in nursing. *J NY State Nurses Asoc, 8*(4), 31–40.

Preston, R.P. (1979). *The dilemmas of care: Social and nursing adaptations to the deformed, the disabled and the aged.* New York: Elsevier.

Purtilo, R.B. (1983). Ethics in allied health education: State of the art. *J Allied Health, 12,* 210.

Rankin, S.H., & Duffy, K.L. (1983). *Patient education: Issues, principles, and guidelines.* Philadelphia: Lippincott.

Raths, L.E., Harmin, M., & Simon, S.B. (1966). *Values and teaching: Working with values in the classroom.* Columbus, Ohio: Charles E. Merrill.

Resnick (1984). In R. Blum (Ed.), *Chronic illness and disabilities in childhood and adolescence.* San Diego: Grune & Stratton.

Richardson, S.A. (1970). Age and sex differences in values toward physical handicaps. *J Health Soc Behav, 11,* 207–214.

Robinson, C.A. (1984). When hospitalization becomes an 'everything'. *Issues Compr Pediatr Nurs, 7,* 363–370.

Rosenbaum, P.L., Armstrong, R.W., & King, S.M. (1986). Improving attitudes toward the disabled: A randomized controlled trial of direct contact versus kid-on-the-block. *Dev Behav Pediatr, 7*(5), 302–307.

Rosenstock, I.M. (1974). Historical origins of the health belief model. *Health Educ Monogr, 2,* 328–335.

Rosser, J.M. (1971). Values and health. *J Sch Health, 41,* 386–390.

Ryan, R., Kempner, K., & Emlem, A. (1980). The stigma of epilepsy as a self-concept. *Epilepsia, 21,* 433–444.

Safilios-Rothschild, C. (1970). *The sociology and social psychology of disability and rehabilitation.* New York: Random House.

Sedgewick, R. (1974). The family as a system: A network of relationships. *J Psychiatr Nurs, 12,* 17.

Silber, T.J. & Reilly, Sr. M. (1985). Spiritual and religious concerns of the hospitalized adolescent. *Adolescence, 20,* 217–224.

Simon, S.B., Howe, L.W., & Kirschenbaum, H. (1972). *Values clarification: A handbook of strategies for teachers and students.* NY: Hart Publishing.

Stallwood, J., & Stoll, R. (1975). Spiritual dimension of nursing practice. In I.L. Beland & J.Y. Passos (Eds.). *Clinical Nursing.* 3rd ed. New York: MacMillan.

Stauffer, D.T. (1974). Disability simulation. *Phys Ther, 54*(10), 1084–1085.

Steele, S.M., & Harmon, V.M. (1979). *Values clarification in nursing.* New York: Appleton-Century-Crofts.

Stoll, R. (1989). The essence of spirituality. In V.B. Carson *Spiritual dimensions of nursing practice* (pp. 4–23). Philadelphia: Saunders.

Strauss, A.L., & Glaser, B.G. (1975). *Chronic illness and the quality of life.* St. Louis: Mosby.

Taylor S.E. (1983). Adjustment to threatening events: A theory of cognitive adaptation. *Am Psychol, 38,* 1161–1173.

Thomas, D. (1982). *The experience of handicap.* London: Methuen.

Venters, M. (1981). Familial coping with chronic and severe childhood illness: The case of cystic fibrosis. *Soc Sci Med, 15A,* 287–297.

Wallston, B.S., et al. (1976). Development and validation on the health locus of control (HLC) scale. *J Consult Clin Psychol, 44*(4), 580.

Wilberding, J.Z. (1985). Values clarification. In G.M. Bulechek & J.C. McCloskey (Eds.), *Nursing interventions: Treatments for nursing diagnoses* (pp. 173–184). Philadelphia: Saunders.

Williams, M.A. (1976). Easier convalescence from hysterectomy. *Am J Nurs, 76,* 438–440.

Wright, B.A. (1960). *Physical disability, a psychosocial approach.* New York: Harper & Row.

Wright, B. (1983). *Physical disability—A psychological approach* (2nd ed.). New York: Harper & Row.

Wyszynski, A.A. (1986). The impact of spiritualism on the cancer patient. *Journal of Psychosocial Oncology, 4*(3), 93–98.

Zola, I.K. (1982). Denial of emotional needs in people with handicaps. *Arch Phys Med Rehabil, 63,* 63–67.

SECTION IV
Contingency Variables: Stressors and Coping Strategies

This section contains three chapters relevant to the stressor and coping strategy contingency variables. Chapter 10 presents an overview of the stressor concept and its definitions and conceptualizations. This chapter also discusses selected developmental and situational stressors associated with chronic conditions. Four major categories of stressors associated with chronic conditions are related to (1) the illness and its management, (2) external and internal resources, (3) relationships, and (4) life-style adjustment.

Chapter 11 presents a similar overview of coping concepts, definitions, and conceptualizations. Four sets of coping categories are discussed in detail: (1) managing the condition; (2) coping with feelings; (3) communicating thoughts and feelings; and (4) accepting, refusing, and giving support.

Chapter 12 provides guidelines for assessment of individual and family stressors and coping strategies. It also suggests instruments to use when further in-depth assessment is needed in certain areas. Specific strategies for preparing people for stressful events, reducing stressors, and enhancing coping abilities also appear.

10　Stressors and Potential Stressors

Stressors are contingency variables that represent major concern and difficulty for all systems. Various definitions and conceptualizations of stressors are discussed in this chapter. They are followed by selected developmental and situational stressors that may be associated with chronic conditions.

Figure 10–1 illustrates the relationship of stressors to the Contingency Model of Long-Term

137

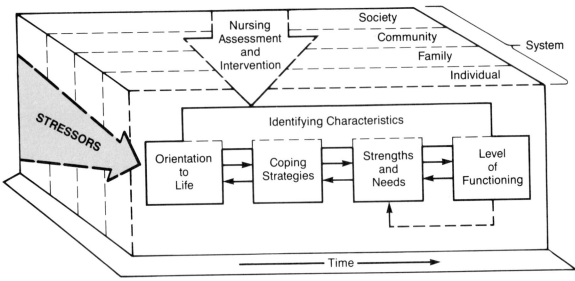

FIGURE 10–1   Relationship of Stressors to Hymovich's Contingency Model of Long-Term Care. Stressors are major contingency variables that may challenge the system's orientation to life, necessitating new or modified coping strategies, influencing strengths and needs and ultimately the system's level of functioning.

Care. Stressors are major contingency variables that may challenge the system's orientation to life, necessitating new or modified coping strategies, and influencing the needs and strengths and, ultimately, the system's level of functioning.

Definitions

Stress and **stressors** are difficult terms to define and are sometimes used interchangeably to refer to an environmental event, condition, or characteristic. Attempts to develop precise definitions have failed because they do not distinguish all stressful events from all nonstressful events. Because precise definition is difficult, it is important to know how events are perceived in a given situation. For example, in research literature, definitions of stress and stressors differ with the needs of each study. Studies examining physiologic aspects of stress may operationally define stress in terms of pulse, blood pressure, and respiratory changes, whereas a study of psychologic aspects may define it as a high score on Spielberger's State-Trait Anxiety Scale (1983).

Stress can be viewed as a transaction between a person and the environment that is cognitively appraised by the person as taxing or exceeding personal resources for coping with it (Lazarus & Folkman, 1984). Gatchel and Baum (1983) describe stress as a process "unfolding in a sequence of events and feelings and involving a number of factors that by themselves can be quite complex. Stress involves environmental and psychological events, interpretations of them, and behavioral and physiological responses" (p. 41).

Gatchel and Baum (1983) define **stressors** as the environmental or psychologic events to which the person responds. McCubbin and McCubbin (1987) define stressors as part of their T-Double ABCX model of family adjustment and adaptation as life events or transitions "impacting upon or within the family unit" that produce, or may potentially produce, change in the family social system (pp. 4–5).

Several nursing models, such as those of Neumann (1980) and Clarke (1984a, 1984b) are based on the concept of stress. According to Clarke (1984b), stress arises from a mismatch between demands on the person and the person's ability to cope. *Demand* denotes "an internal or external stimulus which is perceived by the individual as requiring an adaptive response" (Clarke, 1984a, p. 6). From our perspective, the difficulty with these models is that they are not sufficiently comprehensive for the broad field of chronicity.

Panel members of the Institute of Medicine (IOM), recognizing that there is no single satisfactory definition of the term, define stressors as "any events or conditions that elicit physical or psychosocial reactions" (Elliott & Eisdorfer, 1982, p. 8). Building on this definition, Elliott and Eisdorfer suggest that stressors are those internal (individual) or external (environmental) events or conditions that change (activate) the individual's present state and produce significant physical or psychologic reactions (consequences). Consequences, or outcomes, may be short term, prolonged, or cumulative and can be physiologic, emotional, or social. Events or conditions may be potential stressors, based on their probability of becoming stressors for a particular person under a given set of circumstances.

As used in the Contingency Model of Long-Term Care, **stressors** are any stimuli, or the absence of stimuli, in the environment or internal to the system, that can tax or exceed the system's resources for adapting and for accomplishing tasks, and that elicit a response from the system. Stressors may be actual (elicit a response) or potential (could elicit a response). **Potential stressors** are events or conditions known to be stressors that, for some individuals under certain circumstances, have a probability of becoming stressors. The absence of an event, such as an unmet expectation, can also be a stressor or potential stressor. Stressors can be described by their intensity, quantity, and temporal pattern. For example, a family may indicate having serious (intensity) financial, child care, and equipment difficulties (quantity equals three difficulties). Although the child care and equipment stressors occur periodically, the financial problems have been long standing (temporal pattern).

Stressors may be developmental or situational. **Developmental stressors** are stressful events that occur during the course of one's normal growth and development and can strain or surpass the system's ability to cope. The birth of an infant, a child beginning school, or a person retiring from a job are examples of developmental stressors.

Situational stressors are stressful events that arise as the result of a stressful event and can strain or surpass the system's ability to cope. They are superimposed on developmental stressors and tasks and are due to events such as accidents, illness, or death. Operationally, stressors are defined as any areas that individuals or family systems indicate are problematic, or potentially problematic, for themselves or for members of the family.

Concept of Stressors

Stress is a complex phenomenon consisting of many variables and processes. Historically, interest in stress came from its potential role in causing illness. Cannon (1929, 1935), among the first to use the term *stress*, suggested it contained both physiologic and psychologic components that could disrupt an organism's homeostasis. Selye's work on stress as a syndrome of response to noxious agents is well known (Tache & Selye, 1985). Lazarus and colleagues (Lazarus & Cohen, 1977; Lazarus & Folkman, 1984) added a psychologic dimension to the concept that will be discussed later in this chapter.

There are many conceptualizations of stress. In psychology these conceptualizations come from the psychodynamic and the behaviorist approaches. The psychodynamic approach is based on Freud's contributions. Stress is considered mainly an intrapsychic conflict leading to defensive operations (e.g., denial, projection, repression) aimed at reducing drive tension (anxiety). In contrast, the behaviorist model assumes behavior is determined to a large extent by external events in the social environment. Initially, this approach centered around stimulus-response (S-R) psychology (See Chapter 4). From this perspective, stress is either an external stimulus impinging on the person **or** an internal stimulus (e.g., hunger, thirst) to which the person reacts in some way.

One widely accepted approach to stress is the transactional approach of Lazarus and his colleagues, which has influenced development of the Contingency Model of Long-Term Care. Lazarus and Folkman (1984) argue that any approach to stress, either as a stimulus or a response, is circular in nature. Stress stimuli within the environment may be (1) major, often catastrophic changes such as natural disasters or war that affect large numbers of people; (2) major changes such as chronic illness or death that affect only one or a few persons; or (3) daily hassles, the little things that happen to a person, such as being stopped in a traffic jam or running out of an ingredient for a recipe (Lazarus & Cohen, 1977). Positive events or the absence of change, such as chronic boredom or loneliness, have the potential to be stressful (Lazarus & Folkman, 1984). Daily hassles are other potentially stressful events that are likely to occur in the presence of chronic illness. As one woman said, "It's all the little things that keep happening that seem so bad, not that he's in the hospital."

Early research focused on the biologic and nonspecific responses associated with various stimuli, whereas more recent research and theory development focus on the person's appraisal and contextual cues that evoke stress responses. Lazarus (1966) emphasized the role of perception and cognitive appraisal in the stress response and argued that an event only becomes a stressor if it is appraised as threatening.

A socioecologic approach to stress emphasizes the impact that other individuals, or the sociocultural environment, have in mediating (producing or reducing) stress. For example, expectations and demands may produce stress while social support may serve to reduce it (Moos & Schaefer, 1986). Stress results from environmental, social, and physical demands as well as constraints and resources within the environment. Stress is the person's reaction to the event or challenging environment.

Lazarus (1971) suggested that the definition of stress include the entire phenomenon of stimulus, response, and intervening variables. The Institute of Medicine (IOM) takes the conceptualization a step further and includes the consequences of the phenomenon. A framework developed by the IOM, encompasses all definitions of stress: stressors, reactions to stressors, consequences of stressors, mediators, and the relationships between these variables (Elliott & Eisdorfer, 1982). Within this context, stressors are conceived of as stimuli; reactions (the biologic and social responses) to the stimuli; and consequences or outcomes (the physical or psychosocial results of the reactions). Mediators are modifiers or filters that define the context in which the sequence (stressor—reaction—consequence) takes place. Within the Contingency Model of Long-Term Care, stressors are conceived of as stimuli requiring action, although it is recognized that these stimuli are often the result of other stimuli.

Stressors and Health

The relationship of stress and health has appeared in the literature for many years. Biologic components of stress were initially studied in relation to adrenal hormones. Since then, hormones such as insulin, growth hormone, prolactin, and luteinizing hormone were found responsive to stress. Hormonal responses vary from person to person, situation to situation, and time to time. They are controlled by the brain and can be affected by various genetic, biologic, environmental, and psychosocial mediators (Hamburg, 1982).

Selye (1975) proposed that people subjected to noxious stimuli develop a General Adaptation Syndrome (GAS) consisting of three stages: (1) alarm reaction (prior to adaptation), (2) resistance (optimal adaptation), and (3) exhaustion (loss of adaptation). Selye's early definition of stress as a synonym for stimulus changed to a more specific response to physical and emotional stimuli called stressors. His research supported the belief that social and psychologic factors are important in health and illness, and has influenced research in neurobiology, medicine, and psychosomatic medicine (Elliott & Eisdorfer, 1982).

People experiencing any of a wide variety of stressful events or situations are at increased risk for developing physical and mental disorders (Hamburg, 1982). This does not mean the stressful event is the only or even the primary cause of the disorder, but it may be the decisive factor or "straw that breaks the camel's back." Combinations of recent stressful events such as death of a loved one, birth of a child, loss of one's job, or divorce, increase the risk of becoming physically or mentally ill (Elliott & Eisdorfer, 1982). On the other hand, stressful marital relationships may result in divorce, followed by diminished stress. However, our understanding of these relationships is limited because of conceptual and methodologic problems in assessing these variables. Age, sex, social networks, social environment, family history, and available coping modes have been linked to increased prevalence of different types of illness.

Research has shown a "small, but reliable, association" between childhood stress experiences and a variety of child health outcomes. Citing several studies, Boyce (1985) notes that more children are exposed to psychologic stresses now than in the past. For example, children experience stressors before, during, and following parental divorce. A decade ago it was estimated that by 1990 one third of all children in the United States would have experienced divorce in their families (Select Panel, 1981). While data with chronically ill or disabled children are needed, it can be anticipated that these children will be subjected to the same stressful events as their healthy peers; and superimposed on these events will be additional stressors associated with the chronic condition.

Most early definitions equated stressors with adverse events and stress with negative outcomes, excluding the possibility of positive outcomes. It is now evident that not everyone exposed to a stressor will have adverse health effects. The way stress may enhance growth and development under some circumstances is of increasing interest. It has been suggested that people exposed to a severe life stressor may have increased self-esteem and be able to perform better in similar situations at a later time. Children can master threatening events and achieve personal growth by using their ego resources and drawing on social supports (Murphy, 1962). In addition, they learn empathy and may be able to take advantage of new situations. Other positive outcomes of stress might include increased physical stamina, improved coping styles, and strengthened social ties (Elliott & Eisdorfer, 1982). Whether stressful events lead to growth, temporary difficulty, or trauma probably depends on (1) their pervasiveness and persistence, (2) timing in the life course, (3) available personal resources for reacting to them, (4) availability of opportunities to act on the environment, (5) meaning given to the experience (Benner et al., 1980; Elliott & Eisdorfer, 1982), and (6) previous experience coping with stress (Hill 1949; McCubbin & Thompson, 1987).

Stressors and Life Events

The importance of stimuli as sources of stress led to the study of stressful life events (Dohrewend & Dohrewend, 1974). Life events are stressors that require change in a person's ongoing life pattern (Holmes & Rahe, 1967). Stress is the physiologic and psychologic response to these stressors, especially when an imbalance between environmental demands (life change) and the individual's ability to meet these demands is perceived. Life events such as getting accepted into a university or receiving a promotion are usually pleasant, but others, like being diagnosed with a chronic condition, are negative or unpleasant. Positive and negative life events may have different physiologic and psychologic consequences for the person, including different hormonal responses. Negative events are stronger predictors of disease outcomes than are positive ones (Elliott & Eisdorfer, 1982).

A common method of assessing the impact of stress on health is to measure major life changes. However, life events inventories, such as Holmes and Rahe's Social Readjustment Rating Scale (Holmes & Rahe, 1967), often fail to distinguish between antecedents and consequences. The scale is based on the assumption that all events, even positive ones, cause stress. The relationship between these life events and health outcomes is weak and does not predict the likelihood of future illness (DeLongis et al, 1982). Because life-events scales view life events as stimuli, there is no way to take into account the reciprocal nature of stressors and coping strategies. For example, events such as sexual difficulties or divorce may be the result of some underlying problem rather than the risk factor for it. The issue is whether the stressful event was the cause of the current situation or the consequence of something else. As Engel (1962) noted, "The judgement as to whether or not [a particular situation] constitutes a stress for an individual cannot be made from the nature of the external event alone, but requires knowledge of the response as well. A separation may constitute a welcome release as well as a loss . . ." (p. 264).

Coddington (1972a; Heisel et al, 1973) extended life-stress research to children. He developed a series of life-event questionnaires for children at the preschool, elementary, junior high, and senior high school levels. Research indicates an increase in life change units with age (Coddington, 1972b) and a positive correlation between life events (especially undesirable ones) and measures of psychologic impairment in children.

Hassles and uplifts   Daily hassles are repeated or chronic strains of everyday life (DeLongis et al, 1982). Seemingly minor stressors (hassles) in daily life may be more powerful predictors of health outcomes than are major life events (Kanner et al, 1981; Pearlin & Schooler, 1978). Major life events are considered distal measures of stress, whereas hassles are proximal measures, that is, immediate perceptions of social environment. Distal environmental events may not be experienced as stressors, while proximal measures represent stressors here and now as appraised by the individual. In recent studies, hassle scores were found to be more strongly associated with somatic health than were life-events scores. The frequency of various daily hassles over a period of 9 months was significantly related to psychologic symptomatology (Kanner et al, 1981).

Stressors and Time

The IOM proposed four broad categories of stressors, differentiated primarily by their duration: (1) acute time-limited stressors, like waiting for surgery; (2) stressor sequences, a series of events that take place over time but result from a single event, like visits to the health care provider for a chronic illness; (3) chronic intermittent stressors that may occur daily, weekly, or monthly, such as daily radiation therapy or medications; and (4) chronic stressors that persist a long time but may result from a single incident, such as chronic illness or permanent disability (Elliott & Eisdorfer, 1982). Reactions may occur over an extended time with stressor sequences and chronic stressors.

When stressors occur "on-time" (the time customarily expected) the outcome may be quite different than when they occur "off-time" (Neugarten, 1979). For example, if a mother with a chronic condition dies before her 30-year-old son who takes care of her, the stressor would occur on time. However, the son's dying before his mother would be atypical and considered off time. In this instance, consequences of the son's death would produce a different outcome and necessitate finding alternative care arrangements for his mother. An elderly woman at the funeral of her son said, "This isn't right, I'm not supposed to bury my son, he's supposed to bury me."

Focal Stressor Events

A **focal stressor event** is a circumstance or event that causes the individual or family system to evaluate its situation and determine the presence of a need. It can be any developmental or situational stressor, or potential stressor, creating a need within the individual or family system for assistance, either from someone within the system or someone outside of it. Any event that has the potential to precipitate a crisis may be a focal stressor event, such as diagnosis of a chronic condition, exacerbation of the condition, admission to the hospital, or need for a new piece of equipment. The meaning of a focal stressor event depends on how the event is perceived by the person and the outcome that results from it. Some focal stressors may be growth promoting, others may be growth inhibiting, and others may have no effect on growth. While the consequences (outcome) can be evaluated as good (desirable) or bad (undesirable), the focal stressor itself cannot be evaluated in that way (Elliott & Eisdorfer, 1982).

Crisis Events

Crisis theory is based on the concept of homeostasis (Caplan, 1964). Emotional balance is maintained by learned coping techniques used to resolve common daily-life stressors. When these stressors become overwhelming, a crisis develops and the system can no longer use its previous coping strategies effectively to solve its problems. Periods of disorganization and upset occur during which the system makes unsuccessful attempts to solve the problem. For the Contingency Model of Long-Term Care the concept of **crisis** is redefined as a state precipitated by a focal stressor event for which the system's current coping strategies are ineffective. Crises are not pathologic experiences, tend to be self-limiting, generally lasting from 4 to 6 weeks, and lead to some eventual level of adjustment (Caplan, 1964).

Crisis has been defined in various ways (see Table 10–1) and used interchangeably with *stress*. Erikson (1965) classified crises as either developmental (maturational) or situational. Developmental crises are normal or expected occurrences in the

Table 10–1   Definitions of Crisis

Definition	Source
"any sharp or decisive change from which old patterns are inadequate"	Hill, 1949, p. 51
"provoked when a person faces an obstacle to important life goals that is, for a time, insurmountable through the utilization of customary methods of problem-solving. A period of disorganization ensues during which many abortive attempts to solution are made"	Caplan, 1961, p. 18
"the experiencing of an acute situation where one's repertoire of coping responses is inadequate in effecting a resolution of the stress"	Miller & Iscoe, 1963, p. 196
"an upset in a steady state"	Caplan, 1964, p. 40
"an event in which the individual's normal coping abilities are inadequate to meet the demands of the situation"	Fink, 1967, p. 592
Developmental crisis: ". . . a turning point, a crucial period of increased vulnerability and heightened potential. . ."	Erikson, 1968, p. 96

process of psychosocial development. They occur at various points in the developmental life cycle and, to some degree, can be prepared for and predicted (e.g., a child beginning school). Situational crises are external events (e.g., diagnosis of a chronic condition) beyond the control of the system and generally cannot be prepared for or predicted.

Crises present both danger to the system and opportunity for growth. The danger lies in the potential of crisis to overwhelm the system. At the same time it provides opportunity for growth because individuals are more receptive to therapeutic interventions during times of crisis. Intervention could lead to a higher level of functioning on the part of the individual or family system in crisis.

Aquilera and Messick (1982) suggest that three balancing forces must be present when a significant stressor is encountered: (1) realistic perception of the event, (2) adequate situational support, and (3) adequate coping strategies. When one force is missing, a crisis will occur. People with a support network have a buffer against the negative psychosocial effects of crisis and are aided in adapting to crisis situations.

Most crises, whether developmental or situational, occur within a family context and may be superimposed on one other. For example, a father may be newly diagnosed with cancer at the time his infant daughter is born, or a mother may be hospitalized the week her child begins school. In both situations, a maturational crisis (birth, school entry) is associated with a situational crisis (diagnosis, hospitalization).

Family crises.

Hill's (1949) theory of stress evolved from a study of separation and reunion in families during World War II. He described the ABC-X family crisis model. The stressor event (A) interacts with the family's crisis-meeting resources (B) and the family's definition of the event (C) to produce the crisis (X). Hill identified the family's definition of the event (C), that is, the extent to which the family believes it can handle the stressor, as an important determinant of the severity of the crisis. No stressor event has a uniform interpretation for all families; some families may interpret the event as stressful, but others may not. Stressful events may occur outside the family (e.g., war, floods, political or religious persecution) or within the family (e.g., suicide, divorce, nonsupport). Burr (1973) refined the definition to suggest that a crisis creates change in the family system.

Families may emerge from a crisis either stronger, weaker, or at about the same level as before the event. Time is important in understanding family vulnerability to stress and its regenerative power. Family resources are identified as role structure, flexibility, and previous experience with crisis.

Two models (MacVicar & Archibald, 1976; McCubbin & Patterson, 1983) were developed based on Hill's (1949) ABC-X crisis model. In the MacVicar and Archibald model, nurses examine the characteristics of the event, its perceived threat to the family, resources available to the family, and the family's past experience with a similar situation.

McCubbin and colleagues' (McCubbin & Patterson, 1983; McCubbin & Thompson, 1987) expansion of Hill's model, Double ABCX, takes into account the postcrisis impact of an event on the family in addition to the precrisis variables. They recognized that additional emerging events can become new stressors. Thus, the second A refers to a "pile-up" of events. In addition, it emphasizes the significance of past events in determining perceptions of current events. The Double ABCX model has been expanded to "incorporate the role of family types as a critical family strength which will help explain the family's adaptation to both normative and situational stressor events over time and to highlight additional clinically relevant variables for study" (McCubbin & Huang, 1989, p. 437). A series of assessment instruments and considerable research have been based on this model.

Variables Affecting How Events Are Appraised

Whether a person perceives an event as a stressor or a crisis is determined by many factors, including length, frequency of occurrence, controllability, time of occurrence (on-time or off-time) in the life cycle, the extent to which it is anticipated, and the expected consequence (Elliott & Eisdorfer, 1982). Other variables influencing perception of the event are personal resources, effectiveness of the coping strategies used, age of the person, and the amount of social support available.

Since family members are likely to be affected differently by any given stressor event, both individual and family resources need to be considered. Family resources differ from individual resources in that they represent the interdependence among family members (Walker, 1985). The way one member responds to stress has the potential to create stress for other family members. In addition, when family members agree on the nature of a stressor and work together toward a common goal, it is more likely to be reached than if there is disagreement.

Stressors Associated with Chronic Conditions

The types of stressors encountered by any system vary from individual to individual, family to family, and time to time. The extent to which any event is perceived as a stressor is contingent on system identifying characteristics, orientation to life, time of occurrence, strengths, needs, and level of functioning. While it can be expected that families will experience stressors, many are resilient and can cope with most of them. As indicated previously, a stressor for one is not necessarily a stressor for another. For example, loneliness may be a stressor for someone with many friends and a large family, but not for a person who has lived alone for a long period and learned to live in an independent, self-sufficient manner (Gurklis & Menke, 1988).

While we do not want to paint a completely negative image of people with chronic conditions, we do want the nurse to be familiar with the **potential** stressors they may encounter. Nursing assessment and intervention involve identifying potential stressors, assisting family coping with stressors encountered, and preventing those that can be prevented, while at the same time supporting individual and family strengths. Nursing assessment and intervention related to these stressors are discussed in Chapter 12.

The following section describes common stressors and potential stressors for chronically ill individuals and family members. The major categories of stressors are (1) condition and management stressors, (2) external- and internal-resource stressors, (3) relationship stressors, and (4) life-style–adjustment stressors. These stressors and potential stressors are listed in Table 10–2. Specific stressors for children and adults with chronic conditions as well as those for spouse, parent, sibling, and care giver are described in this chapter. Although these categories represent potential stressors, they also represent potential strengths for the patient and family. What may initially be a stressor may become a strength over time and vice versa.

Table 10–2 Stressors and Potential Stressors

Condition and Management Stressors	Relationship Stressors
Nature of the condition	Within the family
Knowledge and information	Communication
Technology	Marital
Time	Parent-child
Nutrition	Sibling
Hospitalization	Outside the family
	Extended family
Resource Stressors	Friends
External Resources	Support system
Health care	
Educational	**Life-style Adjustment Stressors**
Vocational	Roles and responsibilities
Financial	Independence/Dependence
Housing	Social isolation
Child care	
Internal Resources	
Health	
Energy	
Self-concept, Self-esteem	
Feelings	

Box 10–1   *Statements About Managing Condition Stressors*

"Couldn't see any definite results. I didn't feel the treatment was necessary." (Parent)

"It's hard to know exactly what you should do." (Parent)

"I don't know how I could've managed without my husband. He's been great. He comes with me to all of my appointments and asks all of the questions." (Patient)

"By the time I finish with breakfast, the dressing, bath, irrigating the catheter, and getting him out of bed and back again, it's time to start all over again." (Spouse)

"If I could only get rid of the pain." (Spouse)

"It's a real pain to do." (Child)

Condition and Management Stressors

Multiple stressors are involved in managing chronic conditions. These stressors pertain to the nature of the condition, knowledge and information, technology, time, nutrition, and hospitalization. Comments made by patients and family members about these stressors are in Box 10–1.

Nature of the condition   Stressors vary depending upon the type of condition, including its symptoms, treatments, and trajectory. Thus, pain and limitation of movement are likely stressors for patients with arthritis, whereas respiratory distress is a potential stressor for patients with asthma or cystic fibrosis. The manifestations and ultimate outcome of many conditions are often difficult to predict; a chronic condition may become multiple diseases; many are degenerative over time and involve other organ systems. Further, they may increase susceptibility to other illnesses, necessitating additional care for prevention or treatment. Some chronic conditions require powerful chemotherapy and major surgery, thus adding additional iatrogenic disability. As diseases progress, the length of time between exacerbations may decrease and become more difficult to reverse. Prognosis may lead to feelings of hopelessness and powerlessness in patient and family, thus

increasing the stressors associated with management.

Knowledge and information   Three general types of stressors are related to knowledge and information: (1) adequacy of information, (2) timing of information, and (3) dissemination of information to others, such as health care professionals, friends, and the general public. Examples of statements made by chronically ill children, adults, and their families regarding knowledge and information stressors are in Box 10–2.

Children.

Potential stressors for children in relation to knowledge and information are threefold: receiving inadequate information, misunderstanding what they hear or are told, and not being updated as their cognitive capabilities change. These stressors are likely to occur for the child who has the chronic con-

---

Box 10–2   *Statements About Knowledge and Information Stressors*

"I'm overwhelmed with all there is to learn." (Patient)

"Doctors don't tell me nothing." (Child)

"That pediatrician really blew it when he didn't pick it up." (Parent)

"He had a really bad coughing spell, and someone said they'd call the paramedics." (Spouse)

"Neither of us knew enough about cystic fibrosis—other than that it was a fatal disease. They didn't tell us much." (Parent)

"She (another parent) came and told us everything about what happened to her girls, what I was going to have to do, what was necessary to buy, and the expense and the work, which would be very hard on me. It was just too much. It was like an avalanche." (Parent)

"I don't think I have any questions. The doctor told me what to expect, and I read the booklet." (Patient)

"We were just so uninformed. We didn't know anything when I was diagnosed." (Patient)

dition, the child's siblings, and children of chronically ill parents. Health care professionals need to understand the thinking of young children and how their concepts of illness change over time. Chapter 4 describes children's perceptions of illness at Piaget's stages of preoperational, concrete operational, and formal operational thinking. A small study of children with cystic fibrosis (CF) and their siblings revealed that both groups indicated lack of knowledge about the disease and that their parents rarely spoke about it to them (Hymovich, 1981). They were also concerned because peers, neighbors, and others did not know about the condition.

Adults.

Patients and families frequently mention problems they have in obtaining information about the chronic condition and its management. Knowledge may be lacking concerning the basic physiology, course, and treatment of the condition, as well as the complications that may occur and the ways to prevent them. There may be lack of knowledge about the health care system and resources available to help the families. Clients often have little information about the emotional and social responses caused by the condition and management of them. In addition, they may lack information about problem solving, decision making, and action taking needed for self-care (Armstrong, 1987).

Parents.

In addition to stressors related to their child's chronic condition and the health care system, parents are concerned about lack of information pertaining to child and family developmental needs and tasks. Parents have expressed concerns about having inadequate knowledge, the amount and timing of the information, and the overload of information (Hymovich, 1981). Parents want information about the physical, emotional, intellectual, and social development of their chronically ill child and the child's siblings (Hymovich & Baker, 1985), discipline and limit setting (Singer & Farkas, 1989), and the disease and its management (Hodges & Parker, 1987). McKeever (1981) found the majority of fathers of chronically ill children were dissatisfied with the factual knowledge they received about the progression of their child's condition.

One third of 161 parents of children with cystic fibrosis expressed worry about the responsibility of caring for their child and whether they were giving proper care (Hymovich and Baker, 1985). Three

fourths of the parents expressed concern specifically about their ability to manage the chronic condition. With older children, parents were concerned about whether their child was performing treatments and eating properly when away from home.

Community Members.

Patients and their care givers express concern about the knowledge gap of community members regarding chronic conditions, disabilities in general, and their particular condition. Community members such as primary and secondary school teachers who had children with diabetes in their classrooms indicated lack of knowledge about the disease (Bradbury & Smith, 1983) and did not feel they had received sufficient information. School nurses were information sources for less than a fourth of the teachers, and medical staff provided even less information. The most common source of information was the children and their parents, who may also be inadequately informed. Teachers felt printed materials would be the best medium for providing information they needed.

Technology

More stressors are likely as clients are expected to manage ever more complex technology. It is not unusual to see high-tech equipment such as respirators, oxygen tanks, ventilators, and intravenous lines in the home that previously were used only in the hospital.

Home Care.

Home care of children and adults with complex medical problems is on the rise. Although the purpose of home care is to enable care givers to provide as normal a life as possible within the limits imposed by the condition, it also presents stressors for the family. Families are required to manage equipment, usually with numerous other people who come to the home to ensure its proper functioning. They may have nurses or home health aides in their home most or all of the day. In addition, there are problems when the personnel fail to show up, are late, or are inconsiderate of the family. Privacy is lost, and parents may lose some control over their child rearing. Taking care of someone in the home requires support beyond the usual health care.

Time

While time is a mediator of stressors, it can also be a stressor. Managing some conditions may involve many hours each day. Time may be spent in dressing, eating, personal hygiene, elimination programs, taking medications, doing treatments, preparing special meals, filling out insurance forms, traveling to doctors, and making arrangements for health services as well as other condition-related tasks.

Time may be a focal stressor during the diagnostic phase because both individual and family are dealing with the unknown. They hope for the best while having to prepare for a feared diagnosis. Worse yet, the diagnostic period may last for years before a definitive diagnosis is reached (Mailick, 1984). In a study of patients with multiple sclerosis, the prediagnosis phase was reported to average 5½ years. Time is also a focal stressor during countless waiting periods throughout the course of the illness: there is waiting for the results of tests and the effectiveness of medications or therapy, and waiting to have surgery, and waiting for someone to return from surgery.

Nutrition Many chronic conditions such as diabetes, hypertension, and heart disease require special diets. These dietary restrictions may be stressors for the entire family as well as the patient. Those involved in buying and preparing food need to know which foods are allowed and which are not. Some treatments (e.g., radiation therapy, chemotherapy) may necessitate special diets or cause symptoms that interfere with good nutrition, adding another stressor for the family. Infants and young children who are irritable or listless present special difficulties for parents when it comes to feeding. Loss of appetite at any age generally creates stress among family members.

Hospitalization Hospitalization may occur for various reasons. Emergency admission may be related to a chronic condition, such as insulin shock or an asthmatic attack, or an unrelated event such as an accident or appendicitis. The affected person may require short-term admission for an elective procedure or repeated or prolonged hospitalization because of the chronic condition (bleeding episodes, pneumonia) or its treatment (chemotherapy, bone marrow transplant, orthopedic surgery). Hospitalization is likely to add new family stressors, but it may also give the family some relief.

When repeated hospitalizations are required, patients and families need to adjust and readjust to hospital and home, each with different life-styles, rules, and expectations of behavior. As Massie (1981) so aptly put it, they are "constantly passing between the two worlds of 'hospital' and 'normal' life, observing in doing so how little the two worlds seemed to know of, or care about, the other" (p. 16). Hospital personnel change, and the patient and family have to become accustomed to new care givers. Personnel, too, must become acquainted with or review the person's history and obtain updated information. For clients who have told their story (given their history) many times, repeating it can be disturbing.

People entering the hospital can be viewed as guests entering a microsociety composed of a physical structure and a social structure (Hymovich, 1977). Because of the hospital's formal structure, routines and schedules are considered essential and often lead to depersonalization of the patient. People lose their privacy, are displaced from their social environment, and are not consulted regarding many decisions made about them (e.g., scheduling of tests) (Fuchs, 1987). Loss of identity occurs as they wear hospital clothing and face many bodily intrusions (injections, intravenous therapy, examinations, weighing, collecting specimens). Time schedules and routines are different in the hospital than they are at home.

Each position (patient, family member, nurse, physician) within the hospital has an associated set of norms or expectations that specify behaviors. Patients and family members are expected to behave in ways that may be foreign to their usual patterns. They generally become dependent on the members of the institution for many activities they could control at home, such as diet, medications, and exercise. The role of the hospitalized patient needs to be viewed within the context of other roles the person already occupies: A child patient may also be a son or daughter, sibling, chronically ill child, and student. An adult patient may be a mother or father, spouse, breadwinner, bowler, and school board member. It is often not possible for the patient to continue fulfilling these roles while hospitalized, yet the roles influence responses to the hospital situation.

Patients and families must adapt to five phases of the hospital experience: (1) prehospitalization, (2) transition from home to hospital (admission), (3) hospitalization, (4) transition from hospital to home (discharge), and (5) posthospitalization (Hymovich, 1977). The hospitalization phase can be divided into a number of subphases (e.g., preoperative, operative, postoperative, diagnostic, treatment, convalescent), depending upon what will happen to the patient.

As patients and family members encounter each phase, their roles are altered. Three stages of role performance are associated with the phases of hospitalization. The first stage, role preparation, occurs during prehospitalization as the family prepares for admission. At this time they try to determine potential expectations and how they will manage the situation. Once the patient is hospitalized (transition to hospital and hospitalization), role enactment occurs, whereby the family behaves according to its perceptions of expectations. For example, parents of chronically ill children may consider themselves experts in their child's care, yet their expertise is often neglected once the child is in the hospital. They must now share the responsibility for their child's care with nurses and other health care personnel (Burke, Costello, & Handley-Derry, 1989; Knox & Hayes, 1983). Likewise, a daughter who has determined the most appropriate medication schedule to keep her elderly mother pain free is forced to abdicate this role as the hospital medication schedule takes precedence.

The length of time one is hospitalized mediates adjustment. Parents of hospitalized youngsters found that as they became more familiar with the routine, they could predict what was going to happen, thus reducing some of their uncertainty (Knox & Hayes, 1983). The final stage, role resolution, begins during discharge and continues post-hospitalization. During this stage family members work through the hospital experience and become readjusted to their roles at home.

The multiple stressors associated with the hospital experience can be classified as environmental or personal. **Environmental stressors** include those related to the physical environment, such as strange equipment, sights, sounds, and smells. Within the social environment are unfamiliar care givers, values, routines, communication patterns, rotation of personnel, separation from friends and family, and an unfamiliar emotional climate. In addition, the death of other patients, emergency procedures, and even the discharge of new acquaintances who are supportive can be stressful. **Personal stressors** impinge on the personal self and include the condition itself, threats to bodily integrity, and threats to personal identity.

Repeated hospitalizations cause disruption in normal family functioning, including established roles. Changes in these roles can be a source of stress for those who are hospitalized, their care givers, and those who remain at home. When treatment

protocols during intermittent hospitalizations fail to take into account previous and subsequent home management, continued family adaptation may be threatened. The family is an untapped resource during hospitalization (Strauss et al, 1984). Despite the fact that the family is virtually ignored, especially with adult patients, Strauss identified the work families must do while a member is hospitalized. This work, superimposed on other roles and responsibilities, involves sentimental or psychologic work to help the patient endure the situation, legal administrative work, and making crucial decisions.

Children.

The predominant concerns of young children hospitalized for acute illnesses are separation from parents, loss of family environment and experience, body intrusion, bodily integrity and punishment (Douglas, 1975; Ritchie, Caty, & Ellerton, 1984). Although single hospital admissions of a week or less are not associated with behavior difficulties, prolonged or repeated hospitalizations in early childhood are associated with increased educational and behavioral disturbances in adolescence (Douglas, 1975; Quinton & Rutter, 1975; Thompson, 1986). Whether the hospitalizations cause these disturbances is unknown because additional factors (e.g., chronic family stress in disadvantaged homes) are also associated with repeated hospitalizations. When repeated hospitalizations occur because of a chronic condition, Rubenstein (1984) believes it is the hospital admission, not the illness, that is responsible for later disturbance.

Although many children are cared for at home, others (e.g., those who are ventilator dependent, children with AIDS who have been abandoned) may be hospitalized for long periods, often months or even years. For others, there may be frequent repeated hospitalizations, which interfere with family relationships and functioning. In addition, parents have to cope with frequent rotations of residents and nurses, each with differing child-rearing beliefs (Scharer & Dixon, 1989).

Few studies focus on children's reactions to long-term or repeated hospitalization. A series of play interviews was used to assess the concerns of hospitalized children ages 2 to 4 years (Ritchie et al, 1984). The results of this study with four groups of children (healthy [$n = 20$], short-stay acute illness [$n = 20$], short-stay chronic illness [$n = 32$], long-stay chronic illness [$n = 10$]) suggest more similarities than differences between the groups. Major concerns of children in all groups were exploration and autonomy. Body intrusion was of concern to the chronically ill children. Interestingly, the percentage of play behaviors related to separation was low for all groups of children, probably because unlimited visiting was permitted. These patterns of behavior did not vary over time. Although there are methodological limitations to this study, it is an important step for trying to discriminate the similarities and differences among healthy, acutely ill, and chronically ill children.

Most research has focused on the adverse effects of hospitalization, while few studies have looked at its beneficial effects. The ability to master anxiety and develop competence in handling new situations is important for fostering growth.

Adults.

When symptoms of the chronic condition become out of control, hospitalization may be necessary, usually creating many stressors for patient and family. Patients, usually in charge of their own care, have to relinquish control and become dependent on the health care team. Their knowledge and experience unrecognized, they are expected to be cooperative and to comply with the hospital routines. Hospitalization forces many intrusions on patients, often confronting them with the necessity for a change in their previous life-style (Gull, 1987). They are separated from family and friends and forced to adapt to strangers. Patients may react to hospitalization with depression and grief.

Discharge and Posthospitalization Returning home from the hospital can also be difficult. Family role stability, altered as family roles shift when a member is hospitalized, necessitates reorganization again when the member is discharged. Table 10–3 compares the stressors of being admitted to the hospital to being discharged to home.

Patients may feel many, often conflicting emotions. While in the hospital attention was focused on them; at home they may no longer be the focus. They may still be worried or misunderstand what happened in the hospital. If children were hospitalized for corrective procedures, they may feel frustrated when they are not instantly better after hospitalization. Parents or care givers of adults may feel apprehensive about their ability to provide care without the assistance of hospital staff. The patient may be apprehensive, especially if there were prob-

Table 10–3 Hospital Admission and Discharge Stressors

Stressor	Admission	Discharge
Control	Lost	Reassume some or all
Physical strengths	May decrease	May increase or decrease
Role	Many are lost	Some or all regained
Values	May change	May change
Life-style	Altered	May be modified
Self-esteem	Altered	Altered, may improve
Uncertainty	Increased	May be initially increased, then decreased

lems that occurred following a previous hospitalization.

Children's behavior following hospitalization is likely to change (Droske, 1978). Changes include demand for increased attention from the mother, increased intensity of reaction to temporary brief separation from the mother, and disturbances in sleep behavior, such as resistance to going to bed, waking during the night, restlessness, increased response to noise, and night terrors.

Resources

Resource stressors are of two kinds: those internal to the individual or family and those that are external. Again, depending upon the situation, resources may be stressors, strengths, or needs.

External Resources External resources are related to health care, education, occupation, finances, housing, and child care. Chapters 6 and 7 discuss the impact of chronic condition on community resources and the stressors they impose on the patient and family. Box 10–3 contains statements of patients and their family members about these external resources.

Health Care.

A number of external resource stressors are related to the health care system, including inaccessibility, long waits, and lack of services, especially in communities where the full range of services is not

Box 10–3   *Statements Reflecting External-Resource Stressors*

Health Care System

"Every time we go in we have a different doctor and he's got to read her record." (Parent)

"I need to see the doctor soon because I've got another appointment upstairs at 1:00 and I don't want to be late." (Patient)

Education

"I had to drop out of school. I just couldn't keep up, and I didn't want to fail." (Child)

"I know he's behind the other kids in school. But what can you expect? He's got leukemia." (Parent)

Occupation

"My boss has been real good. He lets me come in late and leave early. But I am expected to work through my lunch time, and I don't take big breaks." (Patient)

"I have to keep working, even if it kills me. Some days I think it will." (Patient)

Finances

"If I don't work, I don't know how I'll pay the mortgage." (Patient)

"I just don't know what to do. How am I going to pay?" (Spouse)

Housing

"We really need to put in a wheelchair ramp. He's getting heavy now, and I can't carry him up the stairs anymore." (Parent)

"I'm sure glad we own our house free and clear. I don't think we could have managed if we had to pay rent or mortgage payments." (Patient)

Child Care

"I can't find someone to come in for a few hours in the afternoon so I can run errands and get caught up." (Parent)

"Nobody wants to take care of her. They're afraid that something might happen." (Parent)

Transportation

"It takes three buses to get here. I start at 6:00." (Patient)

"I need to get a ride to get here. I don't drive and I live all alone. My son works, so he can't bring me." (Patient)

available. Coordination between autonomous providers and continuity of care within even a single agency are cited as difficulties. The impersonal nature and strange environment often give the patient and family the feeling of "being a number" and fear that they may get lost in the system. Although we talk about the importance of their being part of the health care team, they are often left out of deliberations affecting care.

Trying to deal with the errors of computerized billing systems can be frustrating, intimidating, and often futile. Often patients lack the energy or knowledge to deal with these frustrations. They spend hours trying to rectify errors, being shuffled from one nameless person to another, no one willing to assume accountability.

Educational.

Educational resources are potential stressors for chronically ill children and adolescents, and parents. Specific stressors include finding schools near home willing to admit the child; having the child take medications in school; and obtaining services such as occupational, speech, or physical therapy. Other problems include restrictions in school activities because of complications, restricted parking privileges, forced enrollment in adaptive physical education classes, curtailing of class schedules; and exclusion from activities such as field trips, physical education, and recreation. Returning to school after diagnosis, surgery, prolonged hospitalization, or therapy can be difficult for children. Children may have difficulty getting around the building (e.g., consequence of amputation) and have to deal with overprotective teachers and peer teasing. School phobia involves about 10% of children with cancer.

Occupational.

Temporary or permanent loss of employment creates numerous stressors: emotional stress due to loss of self-esteem, financial stress from loss of income, worry about other people's reactions to obvious disability, telling the boss, threat of loss of insurance or job. People may be unable to function as before, which can be upsetting because they want life to go on as it did in the past. They may have a physical problem, such as loss of strength or mobility, that interferes with performance. Change of appearance because of disease or treatments can be an additional stressor, especially if appearance is important to the position.

During adolescence, youngsters may find they

have limited choices because of their condition or others' prejudice. In general, youngsters with chronic conditions are less likely to have permanent employment and tend to have manual jobs (Blum, 1983). It is difficult to know whether marital and vocational status is reflective of the individual's abilities or the attitudes and prejudices of society.

Financial.

Chronic conditions are expensive and may require sophisticated, expensive medical care. Even without these expensive services, the costs of routine monitoring, intervention during crises, long-term drug therapy, and services for multiple health professionals lead to financial stress. For example, expenses of caring for a child with spina bifida include braces, catheters, other disposable medical supplies, physical therapy, orthopedic or special shoes, wheelchairs, special educational services or home tutors (McCormick, Charney, & Stemmler, 1986). For the insured, many costs are at least partially reimbursable. Financial impact not only includes the direct cost of the condition but also indirect costs such as time lost from work, additional income needed, and decrease in number of hours worked. Children of chronically ill parents and siblings of chronically ill children also mention financial strain as a stressor (Harder & Bowditch, 1982).

Out-of-pocket costs.

Out of pocket long-term care can be more expensive than acute care and hospital care. With acute or hospital care, bills are usually covered by health insurance. For example, several years ago an elderly couple reported out-of-pocket expenses of $1,000 a year when they were not really sick, but much less the year they were sick and hospitalized. McNaull (1981) noted annual costs during treatment often exceeded annual income during the initial period of diagnosis and treatment. In 1981, the average monthly out-of-pocket nonmedical costs for parents of children with cancer were reported to be $129, or $1538 a year (Cairns et al, 1981). Expenses included transportation, parking, food, gifts for child and siblings, telephone calls to relatives, and lost salary income. Out-of-pocket expenses are primarily for medications and insurance premiums.

Third-party benefits.

Third-party coverage for chronic conditions mainly emphasizes institutional care and acute health care. Benefits under different settlements are confusing, complex, and difficult to understand. One third of over 150 parents of children with cystic fibrosis expressed concern about having adequate insurance to meet their child's medical expenses (Hymovich & Baker, 1985). For those with chronic conditions, insurance coverage can be problematic. Policies generally do not cover preexisting illness. Changing jobs may mean lack of coverage for an ongoing condition, at least for a time. In addition, the ceiling on coverage often precludes continued financial assistance throughout the person's lifetime.

Housing.

For some families, housing can be a stressor. The presence of chronic illness or disability may influence where a family chooses to live. In some cases, families living close to a medical center may refuse to move, even for job-related opportunities (McKeever, 1981). In other cases, the home may have to be adapted to meet the special needs of the affected family member. When the house is located far from medical care facilities, rather than travel long distances, families may choose to move closer. Unfortunately, moving can create additional financial and psychologic stressors.

Child care.

Obtaining adequate child care can be problematic for parents of youngsters with chronic conditions. For example, 55% of the mothers of children with long-term tracheostomies reported difficulty in finding adequate child care (Singer & Farkas, 1989). Child care may be a source of stress because of decreased family financial status or the complex needs of child. People may be unwilling to care for the child, or parents may be afraid to trust others with the care of their child. For parents with chronic conditions, the problem may be finding someone quickly in an emergency, or finding someone for extended periods while the parent is temporarily unable to care for the child.

Internal resources Internal, or personal, resource stressors are related to the health status, energy, self-esteem, and feelings of family members. Box 10–4 includes statements of family members related to their personal resources.

Health.

Persons with chronic conditions

Chronic conditions have the potential to interfere with growth and nutrition, although interference does not occur in any consistent pattern. Altered physical development may result from the condition itself, physical discomfort, medications, or treatments. Susceptibility to infections may be increased because of the condition or the medications and treatments received. Nutritional status and weight may be affected by poor appetite, allergies, or inability to exercise or feed oneself. Physical discomfort may inhibit eating patterns, making eating an effort and thus interfering with nutritional intake. Other health-related stressors unconnected to the chronic condition may include acne in adolescence, headaches, insomnia, and anxiety; worries about health, height, or weight; and menstrual (dysmenorrhea, irregular bleeding) or menopausal concerns.

Family members.

Care givers of chronically ill children and adults are likely to neglect their own health while caring for the ill member. For example, in Hymovich's studies of parents of chronically ill children, nearly half the parents rated their own health as fair or poor, and about a third rated the child's siblings' health as fair or poor (Hymovich, 1982; Hymovich & Baker, 1985).

Siblings of chronically ill children may become preoccupied with their own health. Health changes have been reported for these youngsters, including sleep disturbances, enuresis, appetite problems, headaches, muscle or stomach pain, and recurrent abdominal pain (Daniels, Miller, Billings, & Moos, 1986; Lavigne & Ryan, 1979; McKeever, 1983). Siblings of children with rheumatoid arthritis report having more allergies and asthma than siblings of healthy children and are at risk for developing heightened medical consciousness (Daniels et al, 1986).

Energy.

Family members may run out of physical and psychologic energy, due to the overall nature of care and level of involvement (Lipsky, 1985). For example, fatigue is a problem for mothers of children with long-term tracheostomies (Singer & Farkas, 1989). Poor sleep or awakening several times during the night was reported by wives of men with chronic obstructive lung disease (Sexton & Munro, 1985).

Self-concept, self-esteem, and body image.

Children and adults with chronic conditions face potential stressors related to changes in self-concept, self-esteem, and body image. When chronic illness or disability occurs, "confidence and hopes are undermined, the experience is usually difficult to account for, no end is in sight, and self-perception—the sense of identity—is assaulted by changes in the body and its functional performance" (WHO, 1980, p. 24). Self-concept and self-esteem are affected by developmental level, visibility of body changes, personal meaning of changes and illness, and attitudes and responses of others.

Self-concept.

Self-concept is defined as "the beliefs and feelings that one holds about oneself at a given time" (Andrews & Roy, 1985, 124). Self-concept affects various aspects of daily life, including one's mood state and interpersonal relationships (Blum, 1984). It develops as an internalized concept in relation to the perceptions of significant people in one's environment. In childhood, the major determinant of self-concept development is behavior of others toward the child (Greenspan, 1979). Of prime importance are parental perceptions of the condition and the children themselves. Stereotyped attitudes, especially negative ones, influence social expectations and the self-image of disabled people. Rejection by those who are not chronically ill can lead to feelings of self-consciousness, fear, maladjustment, and withdrawal (Gething, 1985). Any change in self-concept may negatively affect relationships with friends, colleagues, and peers.

A newly acquired chronic condition may lead to confusion about role identity (Gething, 1985), especially if it affects major aspects of one's life. According to Weinberg and Williams (1978), people born with a visible chronic condition are more likely to "accept" it and incorporate it into their body image and self-concept than are those who acquire it later. They are less likely to view it as a tragedy but see it as a fact of life or an inconvenience. People with invisible disabilities, such as epilepsy, often face conflicts when they disclose their disability to others (Falvo, Allen, & Maki, 1982). Zola (1982), himself disabled, argues that many disabled people live in an unrealistic emotional world because they are taught that they should not feel angry, frustrated, or vulnerable. In addition, nondisabled people are less apt to express their full range of emotions. Instead, they try to hide their reactions in front of those who are disabled.

Harvey and Greenway (1982) developed a measure of parental adjustment to a child's handicap that they called "primary mood." They found that when both parents had a similar primary mood, children's self-concepts were higher than when parents were dissimilar in their measures of primary mood. The mother's primary mood measure had a greater influence on the child's self-concept than did the father's mood.

Disabled youngsters often have a prolonged adolescence (Strax & Wolfson, 1984), especially when they have been overprotected and sheltered. Most of their psychologic growth occurs within the nuclear and extended family because experiences with peers have been limited. Their identity crisis is even more profound than that in able-bodied peers because they lack role models. This has implications for peer relationships because self-acceptance must be achieved before the disabled can be accepted by others.

Adolescents have a heightened sensitivity to physical appearance and functioning. At this age being just like one's peers is very important, and being different is synonymous with being imperfect. Adolescents have to adapt to an altered body image and prolonged dependence on others, at least for certain aspects of their medical-care needs. Questions of reproductive competence occur with chronic conditions such as myelomeningocele, and of longevity and long-term productivity for others (e.g., cystic fibrosis).

Self-esteem.

Self-esteem, a major component of self-concept (Beck, Rawlings, & Williams, 1984), is defined as an evaluation of one's worth in relation to one's ideal and the performance of others (Meisenhelder, 1985). Self-esteem may be important in successful adolescent coping with chronic conditions. For example, it has been associated with improved medication compliance in teenagers with chronic diseases such as diabetes (Jacobson, Houser, & Wolfsdorf, 1987) and renal failure (Korsch, Fine, & Negrete, 1978). Unexpected or undesirable side effects of medications such as hirsutism, facial disfigurement, or weight gain may also contribute to noncompliance (Dolgin et al, 1986; Korsch et al, 1978). Children are likely to have difficulty when there is parental concern for bodily functions (e.g., stools [CF] or urine [diabetes].

Lower self-concept and lower self-worth than those of healthy children have been reported for children with chronic conditions (Ferrari, 1987; Hayden, Davenport, & Campbell, 1979; Harvey & Greenway, 1984; Patton, Ventura, & Savedra, 1986; Savedra, 1977). Physically handicapped children (spina bifida, cerebral palsy), whether attending regular or special school, were found to have a lower sense of self-worth, greater anxiety, and a less integrated view of self than did their healthy siblings and a control group of healthy children (Harvey & Greenway, 1984). Siblings of children with diabetes had lower self-concepts with regard to intellectual and school status, and happiness and life satisfaction (Ferrari, 1987).

Adolescents who perceived their chronic illness as having a significant impact on themselves had a lower self-concept than those perceiving minimal impact (Zeltzer et al, 1980). Some studies found lower self-concept scores in children and adolescents with chronic conditions than in their healthy peers (McAnarny et al, 1974; Moen, Wilcox, & Burns, 1977; Swift, Seidman, & Stein, 1976), but other studies found no significant differences between self-concept scores in these two groups (Adams & Weaver, 1986; Burns & Zweig, 1975; Jamison, Lewis, & Burish, 1986).

Societal values toward chronic disorders tend to be negative, so children and adults are likely to incorporate these negative values into their own self-concept, with consequent low self-esteem. Although some physically handicapped people may regard themselves negatively, this is not always the case. Dixon (1981) found that visibly handicapped persons (amputation, spinal cord injury, stroke) tended to identify with others in similar circumstances, whereas those with less visible conditions (arthritis, emotional disturbance) tended to separate themselves from similar groups.

Reactions of professionals to the ambiguity of chronic conditions can affect one's identity, because health care professionals generally treat the person as one who is ill (Patton, Ventura, & Savedra, 1986). For example, a woman with newly diagnosed cancer of the breast is labeled a "patient," referred to or treated as sick, and required to undergo treatment that often interrupts her life-style, including job, roles, and responsibilities. Although she considers herself the same competent person as before diagnosis, she begins to wonder whether her identity has changed. Consciously or unconsciously, she may question who she is, what roles are appropriate for her now, and what she can expect to be able to do.

Body image.

The presence of a chronic condition can have a significant impact on body image. **Body image** is defined by Schilder (1964) as "the picture of our own body which we form in our mind, that is to say the way in which the body appears to ourselves" (p. 11). Body image is a part of self-concept and consists of one's idea about the size, shape, and functioning of the body and its parts. It goes beyond the physical body and includes clothes, jewelry, and hairstyle. In the chronically ill, body image can incorporate objects and equipment such as tubes, drains, canes, wheelchairs, and ventilators. Body image can also spread into space and incorporate the bed or even the room of the chronically ill. Body image is a learned phenomenon made up of physiologic, psychologic, and social components.

Body image changes continually from infancy to adulthood as we grow, develop, and respond to our internal and external environment (Selekman, 1983). In physiologic terms, body image develops as neurological and sensorimotor development progresses and infants begin to see themselves as separate from the environment. Psychosocial development of body image begins around 9 months as self-recognition and object permanence develop. Psychosocial factors such as attachment to a care-provider, classical conditioning, toilet training, cognitive development, and sexual awareness contribute to body-image development.

As children leave the protection of their home environment during the preschool and school years, new social contacts begin to influence body-image development. Fairy tales, childhood folklore, dressing up, and conforming to peer-group norms contribute significantly to developing body image. Physiologic maturation, obsession with body weight, clothes, and body appearance are body-image–forming factors during adolescence.

Changes to body image are difficult to accept, and threats to it are often met with anxiety. Changes in physical status necessitate adaptation to maintain a positive self-concept (Roy, 1984). General appearance may be affected by the disease or therapy, and undesirable cosmetic changes may affect one's body image and self-concept. These may include loss of hair; weight gain or loss; scars; being too thin, too fat, or too short; disfigurement from radical surgery; loss of hair; mastectomy; or amputation. Sometimes changes are insidious, such as gradual wasting of the body or clubbing of the fingers, yet they can be just as devastating to one's image. In addition, the disabled person may be denied fashionable clothing or attractive hairstyles.

How visibility influences self-concept is equivocal. Evidence from studies of children with juvenile rheumatoid arthritis, hemophilia, partial sightedness, and partial deafness suggests that with a mild or moderate degree of disability, children are more vulnerable psychologically than if the condition is severe. On the other hand, degree of disability may be less crucial than how the child feels about the condition. Heightened conflicts and increased ambiguity tend to occur with mild disabilities. These children could be considered marginal; that is, they need to deal with a conflict in identity associated with a duality of self. They relate to others either as "normal" or "deviant." There is a pull between needing, acting, and wanting to be normal on the one hand and the presence of disability that prevents doing everything others can do. The mildly or moderately affected child does not evoke support and sympathy as does the more severely disabled child. The fact of being ill (taking medication, special diets, limited activity) is the primary cause of maladjustment rather than specific conditions (Eiser, 1980).

For people of any age, touch is an important intervention. It can help one develop a more accurate picture of body parts, but more importantly, it signifies acceptance of one's body.

Feelings.

Feelings of adequacy in performing treatments, preventing complications, and meeting daily needs are important components of one's ability to care for oneself or for a chronically ill family member. Examples of statements made by family members regarding their feelings are in Box 10–5.

Chronic sorrow.

The concept of chronic sorrow, suggested by Olshansky in 1962, was based on clinical observations of parents of mentally retarded youngsters. She noted the mourning of these parents did not have the same characteristics of time-bound grief that ended in acceptance. Instead, the parents experienced a prolonged sadness persisting throughout the child's life. This prolonged sadness was called **chronic sorrow.** It means continuously living with the knowledge and grief of the condition. Intensity of sorrow was determined by parental perceptions of the severity of their child's limitations, and parents' characteristics, e.g., personality, religious beliefs, social class, and ethnic background. Although chronic sorrow pervades the parental thinking, it does not inhibit experiencing joy from their retarded child.

Chronic sorrow remains a poorly understood concept and is a fruitful area for research. Few formal studies of chronic sorrow have been reported since Olshansky originally described the concept. A descriptive study was conducted by mailing a questionnaire to parents and social workers (Wickler, Wasco, & Hatfield, 1981). Over two thirds of the 32 parents who responded indicated experiencing chronic sorrow. Four periods were particularly stressful for these parents: the child's walking, entry to school, 21st birthday, and siblings' surpassing the affected child's development. The parents indicated that chronic sorrow was a periodic rather than continuous phenomenon that resurfaced when developmental milestones were missed. Damrosch and Perry (1989) reported that almost all mothers ($n = $ 21 of 22) and fathers ($n = $ 17 of 18) of children with Down syndrome indicate the presence of chronic sorrow. Although there was no significant difference for the total sample, there was a significant difference in mother-father pairs, with mothers experiencing significantly more chronic sorrow than did their husbands.

Often, persons with chronic conditions and family members are told to forget about it, put it behind them, or get on with their lives and not think about it. These clients may then feel they are abnormal for having deeply pervasive thoughts and are likely to conceal these feelings. One parent, after hearing the concept for the first time said,

> "I believe it's really true. For years after my child was diagnosed, I would worry that he would bleed. It was always on my mind. I was told I was crazy and had to forget about it. But I can't forget. How can I ever forget? I feel so much better just knowing I'm not the only person who feels that way."

The notion of chronic sorrow has been expanded to include all serious chronic conditions of childhood (Lawson, 1977; Tenbrink & Brewer, 1976; Young, 1977). It has not appeared in the adult

---

Box 10–5   *Examples of Statements Reflecting Feelings*

"It just never goes away." (Parent)

"I don't know, all of a sudden it comes back with a vengeance. I could be in the middle of something wonderful, and then I remember I may not be around next spring." (Patient)

"I don't seem to have any control. Things just happen. Just when I think I've got a handle on it, some new problem pops up. It's awful." (Patient)

"Nobody ever asks me what I think about it" (Child)

"Sometimes I get really really mad. . ." (Sibling)

"It's a time-consuming hassle." (Patient)

"It's no burden—she has such a mild case of it." (Parent)

"I thought it would be nice if they could both go to school, and I could have 2, 2½ hours for me. . .very selfish. . ." (Parent)

"Any time you realize that she has CF, you're just all empty inside." (Parent)

Table 10–4   Clinical Examples of Uncertainty

Ambiguous and unpredictable symptoms
Probable results of treatment
Fluctuating course of symptom remissions, exacerbations
Incomplete diagnosis
Unclear explanations
Lack of information
Unclear feedback concerning progress toward health

Source: Mishel, 1981.

literature, although we believe it can be expanded to include all age groups. Investigation of concept characteristics to differentiate normal from pathological aspects of chronic sorrow is needed. Other unknowns are whether the concept applies to all chronic conditions and to chronically ill adults. Despite need for further research to understand the concept, it can be useful clinically.

Uncertainty.
"Uncertainty is the inability to determine the meaning of events and occurs in a situation where the decision-maker is unable to assign definite values to objects and events and/or is unable to accurately predict outcomes" (Mishel & Braden, 1988). Perceived uncertainty is a judgment about a situation that cannot be adequately categorized or structured because sufficient cues are missing. An event judged to be uncertain consists of one or more of the following characteristics: (1) vagueness, (2) lack of clarity, (3) ambiguity, (4) lack of predictability, (5) inconsistency, (6) probability, (7) multiple meaning, or (8) lack of information (Mishel, 1981, p. 259). Clinical examples of uncertainty appear in Table 10–4. There are four forms of uncertainty related to the illness situation: ambiguity about the condition, complexity of treatment and the health care system, inadequate information about the diagnosis and seriousness of the condition, and expected course of the disease and prognosis.

Perception of uncertainty may be due to the objective nature of the stimulus or a deficiency in the person's perceptual skills (Mishel, 1981). Uncertainty limits a person's appraisal of an event to one of threat. It implies unanswered questions, while certainty implies an understanding of the situation. When sufficient cues are lacking, the situation can not be structured or categorized and is then judged as uncertain (Molleman et al, 1984).

The feeling of uncertainty can be a dominant stressor for families when a chronic condition is present. Jessop and Stein (1985) suggested it may be related to psychologic and social correlates of child and family functioning. Their research indicated that children whose conditions were not visible suffered from increased ambiguity, and thus uncertainty. They hypothesized that lack of visibility may lead to disagreement among parents and providers about the course of action, and disagreement in the family's perception of the child.

Like adults, children may feel uncertain. For example, children who do not know what to expect when they visit the clinic or undergo x-ray may experience uncertainty. Adolescents with diabetes talk of their uncertain future regarding marriage, having children, and complications of diabetes such as blindness (Meldman, 1987).

Gathering information can reduce uncertainty, but sometimes the process may increase anxiety. For example, learning about side effects of chemotherapy may reduce uncertainty about treatment but increase anxiety about hair loss or nausea. It may even add additional uncertainty about how one will handle side effects.

Lack of self-efficacy.
People with chronic conditions, because of the uncertain nature and accompanying losses, are prone to feelings of hopelessness and powerlessness (Miller, 1983). Helplessness, hopelessness, and powerlessness appear to be manifestations or outcomes of lack of control. Control is "the **real** or **perceived** ability to determine outcomes of an event" (Gatchel & Baum, 1983, p. 80). White (1959) referred to a desire for control as "effectance motivation" and the sense of control over the environment as the achievement of "efficacy." Bandura (1977) later described self-efficacy as the belief that one can do what is needed in order to get desired outcomes. However, control may be a motivator of behavior only in situations where it will actually make a difference in outcome (Rodin, Rennert, & Solomon, 1980). The mistaken belief that one actually determines an outcome, when in reality it is determined by chance or other factors, is termed "illusion of control" (Langner, 1975). This illusion provides one with a sense of perceived control when objective control does not exist. Studies suggest people tend to overestimate the amount of control they actually

have, and that this perceived control reduces stress even when actual control is absent (Gatchel & Baum, 1983; Langner, 1975). Real or perceived control appears to be an effective mediator of stressful situations (Rodin, Rennert, & Solomon, 1980).

Averill (1973) described three dimensions of personal control: behavioral, cognitive, and decisional. Kobassa (1979) also specified three types of control: (1) cognitive control, which involves appraising and interpreting the meaning of stressful events and incorporating them into an ongoing life plan; (2) decisional control, or the choice among various courses of action to handle stress; and (3) coping skills, which are suitable responses to stress. Kobassa's coping skills are similar to the behavioral-control dimension noted by Averill.

Helplessness.

Lack of control over stress can induce a form of helplessness that suppresses performance. Seligman (1975) proposed a theory of learned helplessness in which he suggested that people learn to be helpless. Learned helplessness results when there is a **noncontingent** relationship between response and behavior, that is, the chances of something happening are independent of what the person does. Helplessness typically occurs following repeated exposure to uncontrollable events. The person who perceives traumatic events to be uncontrollable recognizes that response and outcome are independent of each other.

Evidence from laboratory studies, as well as studies in the natural environment, shows that repeated exposure to uncontrollable situations leads to loss of motivation to initiate voluntary responses that control other events, emotional disturbance such as anxiety and despair, and cognitive impairment that interferes with subsequent learning (Gatchel & Baum, 1983). For example, a woman hospitalized with complications of her chronic condition expressed helplessness by saying, "What's the use? No matter what I do, it still gets worse. Nothing I do ever works." Once lack of control is experienced, people have difficulty realizing that their responses in the past have been successful. Trauma produces heightened emotional responses, often manifested in fear, anxiety, and depression. Seligman suggests that helplessness and depression may be associated and that perhaps helplessness is a cause of depression. He notes that both are characterized by passive behavior, negative expectations (as in the previous example), and hopelessness. However, more re-

search is needed to determine these relationships. In instances such as loss of a significant other or loss of status, death has been attributed to helplessness.

Helplessness may be mediated by expectations for control (Wortman & Brehm, 1975). Initial exposure to uncontrollable events arouses **reactance** (purposive, control-seeking responses) as long as the person expects to be able to control outcomes. Initially, people resist loss of control and become helpless only when they have depleted their ability to regain control. Gatchel & Baum (1983) suggest loss of control may be a stressor under some circumstances, and helplessness may be the result of that stressor. The extent to which people perceive lack of control as personal, that is, due to one's own failure or lack of skill, or as universal, that is, caused by external factors, is it thought to contribute to helplessness (Abramson, Seligman, & Teasdale, 1978). Abramson and colleagues distinguished between personal and universal helplessness, global (across a wide range of situations) and specific (narrow range) helplessness, and stable (recurrent) versus unstable (short-lived or intermittent) helplessness.

Hopelessness.

Related to the theory of helplessness is the work of Engel (1968, 1971) on hopelessness. Hopelessness occurs when a person believes that nothing can be done to change a situation, does not feel worthy of help, and has feelings of giving up. If the cycle is not broken, depression and hopelessness occur. Engel identified characteristics of the "giving-up-given-up" complex as (1) a feeling of giving up, feeling helpless or hopeless; (2) low self-esteem; (3) loss of gratification from roles in life; (4) disruption of a sense of continuity between past, present, and future; and (5) reactivation of memories of previous periods of giving up.

Schmale and Iker (1975) examined the effects of hopelessness and loss on physical illness. They studied 40 women with abnormal Papanicolaou smears and were able to predict the outcome of a biopsy in 31 cases. The women diagnosed as having cancer had experienced a significant sense of loss, accompanied by feelings of hopelessness, 6 months earlier.

Powerlessness.

Powerlessness is another concept that includes the notions of helplessness, hopelessness, and loss of control. Powerlessness can be defined as a feeling that one's actions will not affect an outcome (Miller,

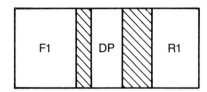

FIGURE 10–2   Relationship Between Dying Person (DP), Friend (F1), and Relative (R1). The diagonal lines represent emotional investment.
Source: Modified from Aldrich, 1963.

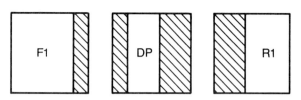

FIGURE 10–3   Loss Anticipated by Friend (F1), Dying Person (DP), and Relative (R1) at Death. The diagonal lines represent loss.
Source: Modified from Aldrich, 1963.

1983) or that one lacks personal control over certain events or situations (Carpenito, 1989). Characteristics of powerlessness include (1) passivity; (2) nonparticipation in care and decision making; (3) dependence on others that may lead to anger, resentment, or guilt; and (4) verbal expression of loss of control over situations or outcomes. Stapleton (1983) noted these manifestations of powerlessness in patients with chronic renal failure (CRF). In addition, she identified the following characteristics: (1) lack of information-seeking behaviors, (2) failure to disclose relevant health information, (3) expressions of loss of hope, and (4) crying and expressions of depression.

Death.
Aldrich (1963) suggested the dying patient's anticipation of loss of all human relationships is of greater concern than the threat of death. Relationships of the dying person are represented in Figure 10–2. The squares represent the dying person (DP), relatives (R), and friends (F). The diagonal lines inside the squares represent the limits of major emotional investment that overlap in proportion to the extent of interpersonal involvement. The area of overlap between the dying person (DP) and a casual friend (F1) is small in comparison to the larger overlap between the dying person and his close relative (R1). This means that the relationship between the dying person and his relative is more significant to both than the relationship between the patient and friend.

At the time of death, the friend and relative suffer a loss in proportion to the quantity of the relationships with the dying person. See Figure 10–3. They experience grief in order to fill the gap left by the dying person. For both the living and the dying, this grief can be anticipatory and may begin at diagnosis or when it is recognized that death is imminent.

Theoretically, the dying person, who is losing a friend as well as a relative, has anticipatory losses equal to the sum of the losses of all of his friends and relatives. This is shown in Figure 10–4. Aldrich believed that the more friends, relatives, and close relationships a dying person has, the more grief and suffering he will experience. As the dying process continues, the dying person becomes more concerned with himself and less concerned with others, and the significance of relationships with others is reduced, as well as the anticipated loss.

Patients with cancer are often preoccupied with thoughts of dying during the first months after diagnosis (Weisman & Worden, 1979). Patients with high "emotional distress" were found to have more disease symptoms and greater feelings of vulnerability and distress than those with low emotional distress (Worden & Sobel, 1978).

Death anxiety (Waechter, 1971) has been shown through death imagery (any association, description, or reference to death or death-related topics, funerals, separation, in response to an ambiguous pic-

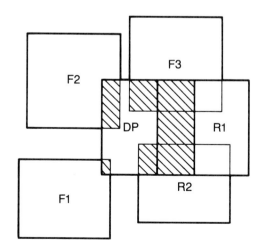

FIGURE 10–4   Dying Person's Relationships and Total Anticipated Losses at Death. The diagonal lines represent loss; F = friend; R = relative; DP = dying person.
Source: Modified from Aldrich, 1963.

ture). The findings suggest that intrusive procedures used to treat chronic conditions may be traumatic enough to produce death anxiety in children. A developmental progression in death imagery was noted, with older children undergoing intensive procedures having increased projection, and younger children using an "all or nothing" approach. That is, the younger either use imagery throughout the story or do not refer to it at all.

Relationships and Communication

Within the family The presence of a chronic condition changes the immediate social structure of the family. Roles may be altered if, for example, the breadwinner can no longer work or a parent must reduce participation in the children's activities. Role alteration is likely to create an identity crisis for the previous breadwinner and perhaps for the spouse who must now take on new roles, or for the parent who had not been working but must now remain at home to care for the sick child. See Box 10–6 for statements of family members about relationship and communication stressors within the family.

Communication.

Communication patterns within the family are likely to change when someone is diagnosed as having a chronic condition (Carandang et al, 1979; Spinetta & Deasy-Spinetta, 1981; Versluys, 1980). The patient may be excluded from discussions to protect him or her, or because the person no longer can participate fully in role responsibilities. Family members may not include the disabled person because of hostility toward the person and the changes he or she has caused in the family. Youngsters of chronically ill or dying parents, or siblings of chronically ill children, may be sent away or excluded from discussions. Conversations may stop abruptly when the child enters the room or take place in whispers out of the child's hearing. Healthy children feel isolated and excluded from a major family problem (Spinetta & Deasy-Spinetta, 1981).

Turk (1964) noted the pattern of diminished communication spreads to other aspects of family life, producing a generalized "web of silence." Parents are likely to feel uncomfortable when discussing the condition. In addition, parents report they "do not want to worry" the child, or they fear losing control in front of the child. When parents are upset and irritable themselves, they find it difficult to be patient with their children. In addition, some parents

---

Box 10–6 *Statements Reflecting Relationship Stressors*

". . . felt he [husband] was nagging at me and it was all my responsibility and why didn't he do it himself sometimes." (Parent)

"I think for a while it [marital relationship] was perhaps, strained, because we didn't understand. . ." (Spouse)

"I think it's hard to be close physically. . .if you don't feel emotionally like making love, you know, you don't just do it for the physical aspects of it." (Spouse)

"If it hadn't been for me, she would have had the abortion and we wouldn't have all this misery and heartaches. . .she was right. I think that made a wedge between us about it. . .we're just not as close as we were before." (Parent)

"I just don't know what to do. He won't eat. He won't go out. He just sits around all day and cries." (Spouse)

"I feel so guilty. My daughters are so busy and it's so hard for them to help me. They come, but I know they don't have time. And I can tell they resent it." (Patient)

"If you're not around 'cause you're sick, people forget who you are and then you have to take time to explain why you were gone." (Peters-Golden, 1982). (Patient)

"When I cough it sounds like I'm choking. The other kids are afraid to be around me. I don't have a lot of friends." (Child)

"Dealing with friends was hard. . .[when you] face other people, you relive it." (Parent)

"People would comment on how thin she was." (Parent)

---

may be unable to put the information into language that their children can understand, or they do not know how much to tell the children.

Children with chronically ill parents or siblings often feel isolated because they are not interacting with others in the family. They feel left out and uninvolved in both the family and the ill person's care, despite their deep interest, and deprived of parental time and attention. The time parents spent with the chronically ill child was reported as the most frequently perceived unresolved problem, even though children recognized the ill child's need. Children also felt slighted as regards physical care, recreational experiences, and material items. Life-style for siblings changed as their number of chores increased and the ill child could get away with misbehavior (Harder & Bowditch, 1982). When anxiety is prolonged and not openly discussed within the family, siblings may feel guilty and have unnecessary fantasies that they caused the condition (Fife, Huhman, & Keck, 1986).

Adults.

Patients may be reluctant to express anger to family or health care providers for fear of alienating the people on whom they depend. This reluctance may lead to anger, frustration, and despair. On the other hand, the patient may become controlling and demanding and try to manipulate family members. These communication problems can be especially problematic for patients with certain conditions. For example, the respiratory problems of patients with chronic obstructive pulmonary disease (COPD) may be aggravated by strong emotional states, so the patients learn to control their emotions to avoid acute episodes of their disease. They live with emotional restraint and may be viewed by others as apathetic and withdrawn (Shekelton, 1987).

Psychosocial functioning of spinal cord injured (SCI) individuals was found to be strongly associated with maintaining the marital relationship, and marital status was a powerful predictor of independent living outcomes (DeJong et al, 1984).

Spouse.

Chronic conditions can upset the balance of reciprocal marital interactions (Evans et al, 1987; Parmelee, 1983), creating unique sources of strain (Miller, 1990). Discrepancies can be noted in patients' and spouses' responses to openness and frequency of communication. Similar differences are noted for parents of chronically ill children. Spouses may not share concerns or fears about the future with each other. Husbands and wives may differ in their views of the support they receive and give (Antonucci, 1985), and increasing helplessness of one partner may eventually lead to dissolution of the marital dyad if the care giver receives inadequate support (Miller, 1990). Parents of chronically ill children may differ in their perception of the child's needs as well as their own and may not be able to support each other (Stein, 1989). There are also reports of parents who believe their child's condition

has brought them closer together and strengthened their relationship (Darling, 1979; Friedman, 1987; Korn et al, 1978).

Roles and responsibilities.

When illness occurs, family members' role responsibilities are likely to shift. These role changes can produce significant stressors for chronically ill children (Shapiro, 1983; Singer & Farkas, 1989) and adults (Evans et al, 1987). They are also stressors for parents and siblings of chronically ill children (Bernheimer, Young, & Winton, 1983), for care givers of adults (Horowitz, 1985), and for children of chronically ill parents (Greer, 1985). Among potential stressors likely to interfere with role performance are hospitalization, preoccupation of other family members, schedule changes, the emotional and physical condition of the family members, and child care by other than those usually responsible. Children may be required to take on household chores for which they are not physically and emotionally ready (Kerr & Bowen, 1988). An example of shifting responsibilities can be seen in a study of women with breast cancer (Green, 1986). Mothers decreased family responsibilities for about 6 to 12 months and then returned to their prediagnostic patterns. Differences in shifting responsibilities to family or friends were noted between partnered and nonpartnered families.

Marital relationships.

Although the divorce rate does not appear to be increased in families with chronically ill children, marital distress increases (Sabbeth & Leventhal, 1984). Divorce estimates for families in which one spouse has a spinal cord injury (SCI) are somewhat higher than in the general population (Baxter, 1981; Urey & Henggeler, 1987).

Among adults, colon cancer, colostomies, and genitourinary or gynecological cancers may interfere with relationships. Partners may be reluctant to be intimate with each other and may even make separate sleeping arrangements. Sometimes reluctance is based on misconceptions (fear of catching cancer), but factors such as fear of hurting a spouse or odor may play a role. Concerns expressed by patients and family members or significant others may also be related to sexual dysfunction (Comarr & Vigue, 1978; Stam, Bultz, & Pittman, 1986; Urey & Henggeler, 1987).

Stressors noted for spouses of persons with COPD include fear of exacerbating symptoms, resulting in little or no interest in marital relations; loss of freedom resulting in diminished recreation and social activities for the spouse; worries when away from spouse, leading to timed shopping trips; and decrease in family income that necessitates taking a job or working longer than originally planned.

Parent-child.

An infant's chronic condition may disrupt development of attachment between infant and parents. Infant irritability or listlessness, difficulty in feeding, and social unresponsiveness because of sensory or neurological deficits limit positive feedback to parents. In addition, frequent or prolonged hospitalizations may disrupt parenting and family development.

Learning skills of interpersonal relationships may be hindered by the emotional climate in home. Parents may become indulgent, rejecting, neglectful, or let up on discipline. The home environment may also restrict the child's repertoire of coping skills. Social isolation can mean inadequate social stimulation and is likely to occur when the youngster is dependent on parents. Daily routines are likely to be deviant because of the nature of the condition or treatments and, at times, because of hospitalization.

Prolonged dependency can hinder development of autonomy. A youngster may be physically independent of parents but may remain emotionally dependent on them. Adolescents who have moved out of their parents' homes may have to move back in because of their condition. When this happens, the youths, while grateful for the assistance, become angry at their parents because returning represents loss of control.

Siblings.

Siblings report the following stressors when they have a chronically ill brother or sister: being left alone (Iles, 1979), feeling anxious (Cairns et al, 1979; Lavigne & Ryan, 1979), isolation from family and peers (Cairns et al, 1979; Taylor, 1980), negative body image (Cairns et al, 1979), feelings of inferiority (Taylor, 1980), inadequate knowledge (poorly informed) (Taylor, 1980), deprivation (Taylor, 1980), and adjustment and behavior problems (Lavigne & Ryan, 1979; Tew & Lawrence, 1979). Siblings may fear the patient's or their own death and contracting a similar condition, and they may feel envy and anger toward the ill child (Koch-Hattem, 1986). Most studies of siblings of children found feelings of guilt for the condition (Iles, 1979; Koch-Hattem,

1986; Kramer, 1981; Sourkes, 1980), although one earlier study did not find guilt to be present (Gogan, 1977).

Outside the family

Relationships with friends.

Chronically ill individuals, and often other family members, report changes in relationships with extended family and friends. A study by Peters-Golden (1982) found that over half of a sample of women with breast cancer reported people feared or avoided them, and 72% felt others misunderstood them. Peer relationships for school children may suffer because of the stigma of disease or because of frequent or prolonged school absences. Parents speak of the difficulty they have in telling their parents, friends, and neighbors about their child's diagnosis.

Relationships with health care professionals.

Another major relationship stressor has to do with relationships between the individual and family system and the health care system. Actions of health professionals can be stressors at various times throughout the course of the illness trajectory. Potential stressors include poor communication (failing to answer questions honestly or directly, providing false reassurances); insensitivity; lack of respect and trust; rudeness; difficulties resolving conflicts; and staff incompetence (Chesler & Barbarin, 1987). Other stressors for parents include exclusion from consoling their child during treatments or procedures. The mother of a child with osteogenesis imperfecta said, "They wouldn't let me in when she was x-rayed. I could hear her screaming. I know how to hold her right. They were wrong. I finally got the doctor to write me a letter saying I could go in any time I wanted." In a study of 17 adolescents with cystic fibrosis, Patton, Ventura, & Savedra (1986) found that professionals, including school personnel, failed to communicate at the adolescent's level.

Cassileth et al (1980) suggested there may be lack of sustained professional interest in patient symptoms, on-going communication, and concern for the patient as a person. This was supported in a retrospective study of 158 taped communications from cancer patients (Thorne, 1989). Patients perceived 61.5% of the information and 90.5% of the advice offered by nurses and physicians as **not** helpful. Most of the unhelpful instances were associated with communication style (lack of concern). One woman, who suspected she had cancer, requested a thorough examination and was called "a crazy hypochondriac." Shortly after the incident, her cancer was diagnosed.

Support system.

Close relationships can create potential for conflict, and some may inhibit independence and personal growth, placing the person at risk in later-life situations that require independent problem solving. On the other hand, people who avoid personal relationships may show no apparent negative effects from lack of a support system. Some people may be hard to get along with and be less likely to have many confiding relationships. Life events that carry stigma, such as the diagnosis of epilepsy or AIDS, may lead to rejection rather than support from neighbors and the community.

Evidence suggests that having a social support system can buffer the effects of stress and crisis (Boyce, 1985; Friedland & McColl, 1987; Gatchel & Baum, 1983), but support systems can be a potential stressor to the individual and family. First, the presence of a support system does not always mean that support is available to the person. Second, different types of supports may serve different functions. Third, families with conflicts, critical attitudes, or strong emotional reactions may aggravate rather than alleviate the stressful situation. Grandparents who cannot come to terms with their grandchild's chronic condition may ignore the child or constantly criticize the parents' attempts to manage the condition. For some people, illnesses carrying a stigma, such as epilepsy, cancer, or AIDS, may lead to rejection rather than support from friends, or even family.

Informal support systems also may be stressors. Some friends or family members may have difficulty dealing with the chronic condition and withdraw support to the patient and family. Others may become "burned out" and need time before they can provide support again. Lay support that is inadequate, inappropriate, ineffective, or poorly timed may create added stress for families (Ayers, 1989).

Kazak and Wilcox (1984) reported that families of children with spina bifida had smaller social networks than a comparison group of families with healthy children. The primary difference was in the size of friendship networks, not family networks: The families of children with spina bifida had less well-developed networks of friends. It was also noted that the social networks of families of children with spina bifida were more dense, indicating that the people in the network were more apt to know and interact with one another than people in less-dense networks. Higher levels of density were associated with higher levels of parental stress. These findings, if supported by other studies, would raise the issue of how to help families increase friendship networks or to identify other sources of support, perhaps professional services, that might be useful to them.

For various reasons, some people with chronic conditions may not have a support system because they cannot maintain relationships. In other instances, the condition may interfere with a person's ability to get out. In a sample of incontinence in the elderly, Harris (1986) reported that three-fourths of the incontinent persons reported limitation of activity. Over 57% of those with incontinence had telephone or personal contact with relatives and friends but were less likely to participate in other outside activities like social events and church functions. "Loners" who are chronically ill comprise another group who may be without support systems. As people age, their social network decreases and the amount and quality of social support is likely to diminish. Lambert & Lambert (1985) found that as women with rheumatoid arthritis aged, their support system decreased and the supporting persons were less able to help as they became more vulnerable and fragile themselves.

The person with acquired immunodeficiency syndrome (AIDS) must face a multitude of difficult psychosocial issues, such as stigma, isolation, change in cognitive functioning, inadequate social support, financial worry, job discrimination, debilitation, an uncertain future, and an untimely death. Since the majority of persons with AIDS are gay men or intravenous drug users, there is social devaluation of the victims and, in many instances, a lack of traditional family support. Because of misinformation, the public has reacted with fear, panic, hatred, prejudice, and social ostracism (Halloran, Hughes, & Mayer, 1988). It is not surprising that persons with AIDS have a much higher risk of suicide than do persons with other serious chronic conditions.

Support during transitions.

Obtaining formal support can be problematic at various times during the course of the chronic condition. For example, the young adult moving from the pediatric to the adult setting will have to establish relationships with a new set of professionals. Survivors of cancer and youngsters with cystic fibrosis, spina bifida, or diabetes may be faced with such changes. Patients moving from an acute care setting to a rehabilitation center or a chronic care facility, as well as families moving to a new location, also may face this transition. Others likely to encounter such transitions are patients who must travel to new hospitals or other institutions for a period to receive required medical or rehabilitative care. The wife of a young man going to another hospital for a bone marrow transplant commented on how difficult it would be for her husband to get used to the new staff and doctors who would be caring for him.

Life-Style Adjustment Stressors

There are numerous stressors associated with adjustment to the diagnosis of a chronic condition and learning to live with it on an ongoing daily basis. Statements of families regarding these stressors are in Box 10–7.

Autonomy and independence People with chronic diseases or physical handicaps are often faced with some state of dependency (Zola, 1982),

---

> ### Box 10–7 *Statements Reflecting Life-style–Adjustment Stressors*
>
> "None of our vacations are taken together." (Parent)
>
> "Not too long ago I went to my sister's and I couldn't even climb up the stairs. I used to be very active. Now, we think twice before we go anywhere." (Patient)
>
> "We've never been away from her for more than perhaps two weekends in our whole married life." (Parent)
>
> "Our social life is incredibly changed. . .I can't tell you how many social engagements we've called off at the last minute or just haven't shown up because she'd get a little cough." (Parent)
>
> "Our whole life revolves around Sam." (Spouse)
>
> "Just when something is going well, I'm reminded that our life is so incredibly different. I can't do half the things I used to." (Patient)

---

either because of the condition or necessary treatments. Motor skills are essential for mobility and independence and are closely associated with social and friendship patterns. Self-care is hindered when body control is limited. Immobility can be a result of pain, restraint, paralysis, casts, or traction. When immobility occurs, normal discharge of energy and aggression is inhibited, self-preservation is threatened, and anxiety and depression are likely to result. Of particular concern is the threat to personal privacy and opportunities to be alone. When mobility is severely limited, people cannot move away from those who are around them; rather, they are dependent on them for such movement.

Children.
Conditions associated with limited movement contribute to delayed or distorted development. Motor skills are central to a child's ability to explore the environment and are the foundation for cognitive development in infancy (recall that infants learn through use of their senses). Infants generally respond to immobility by becoming dull and apathetic. Toddlers generally take pride in developing control over their bodies. As their motor skills increase, there is greater independence and exploration of the environment, thus fostering a developing sense of autonomy. At this stage children want to do everything for themselves. When mobility is limited, this developing sense of autonomy will be hindered. Physical restrictions, limited strength and agility, repeated episodes of enforced passivity or painful experiences associated with the condition may limit the preschoolers' capability for goal directed efforts. Immobility may foster passivity and dependence against which the normal child struggles (Lewis, 1982), hampering development of initiative. Older children become frustrated, depressed (unable to work out aggressive feelings), compliant, or stoic.

Chronic conditions may delay a child's reaching developmental milestones at the appropriate time. For example, limitations in activities of daily living were studied for 202 children with spina bifida (McCormick, Charney, & Stemmler, 1986). Activities studied were the child's ability to (1) take part in physical activities, (2) walk, (3) toilet self, (4) take part in ordinary play, (5) bathe self, (6) dress self, and (7) attend school. Limitations in six or more activities were noted for 40% of the children. Only 13% had no limitation in activities of daily living.

The presence of a chronic condition interferes with adolescent struggles for independence. If the youngster is under 18 years of age, parents are regarded as the legal guardians; they sign the papers and make decisions, thus threatening the youth's self-determination (Bru, 1985). Career decisions may have to be altered. Illness leads to increased tension between parents and adolescent and may increase the adolescent's refusal to comply with regimens. On the other hand, some adolescents may have closer relationships with their parents and not experience struggles for independence to the same extent as their healthy peers (Blum, 1983).

Experiences may be somewhat limited for those who are deaf, blind, bedridden, or in a wheelchair; and the children lack experiences common to most youth: going to a supermarket or library, taking public transportation, or shopping. Things will need to be brought into the child's environment to provide missing experiences, and whenever possible the child's experience should be first hand. Language and speech may be affected by disabilities such as cleft palate or deafness.

Social Isolation Social isolation may develop as the demands of the disease limit activities. Other reasons for increasing social isolation include changes in physical appearance, embarrassment and reluctance to be seen by others because of symptoms such as coughing or flatulence. One of the first roles to change as energy decreases is the work role. Leisure activities may be curtailed or modified to accommodate the demands of the condition. Persons with urinary incontinence had lower participation in all social activities than those in the same age group without urinary problems (Harris, 1986). Mothers report being unable to travel outside of the city or having to change plans, sometimes at the last minute, because of their child's condition (Singer & Farkas, 1989). Three quarters of the mothers said the disability had not affected the desire to go out, and two thirds said they had not decreased the amount of time spent with family and friends.

Dilemmas in Adaptation

Register (1987) identifies some dilemmas the chronically ill person faces. These include decisions related to stigma: to act normally or like a sick person, remain apart from others with same condition or associate with them, ask for help or refrain from asking; reveal the presence of the condition or hide it from others. Specific decisions to be made are related to the following: how much to tell, when to ask for help, whom to ask for help, whether to seek alternative treatments or doctors, when to seek alternative treatments or doctors, how much energy to expend, when to complain, and what to complain about.

Summary

Stressors are contingency variables representing a major source of concern and difficulty for a system. Examples of the various definitions and conceptualizations of stressors were discussed in this chapter. As used in the Contingency Model of Long-Term Care, **stressors** are any stimuli, or the absence of stimuli, in the environment or internal to the system that can tax or exceed the system's resources for adapting and for accomplishing tasks, and that elicit a response from the system. Stressors may be actual (elicit a response) or potential (could elicit a response). **Potential stressors** are events or conditions known to be stressors that, for some individuals under certain circumstances, have a probability of becoming stressors. Stressors may be developmental or situational. **Developmental stressors** are stressful events that occur during the normal course of one's normal growth and development and can strain or surpass the system's ability to cope. **Situational stressors** are stressful events that arise as the result of a stressful event and can strain or surpass the system's ability to cope; they are superimposed on developmental stressors and tasks. Operationally, stressors are defined as any area individual or family systems indicate are problematic, or potentially problematic, for themselves or for members of the family.

Stressors associated with chronic conditions are related to (1) the condition and its management, (2) internal and external resources, (3) relationships and communication, and (4) life-style adjustment. Stressors related to the condition and its management include the nature of the condition, knowledge and information, technology, time, nutrition, and hospitalization. External resource stressors may be related to health care, education, occupation, finances, housing, and child care. Internal resource stressors are health, energy, self-concept, self-esteem, body image, feelings, and death. Relationships and communication stressors may occur within the family or outside of it. Life-style adjustment stressors are related to autonomy, independence, and social isolation.

References

Abramson, L.Y., Seligman, M.E.P., & Teasdale, J.L. (1978). Learned helplessness in humans: Critique and reformulation. *J Appl Abnorm Psychol, 87*, 49–74.

Adams, J., & Weaver, S. (1986). Self-esteem and perceived stress in young adolescents with chronic disease. *J Adolesc Health Care, 7*(3), 173–177.

Aldrich, K.C. (1963). The dying patient's grief. *J Am Med Assoc, 184*(5), 109–111.

Andrews, H., & Roy, C. (1985). *Essentials of the Roy adaptation model.* Norwalk: CT: Appleton-Century-Crofts.

Antonucci, T. (1985). Personal characteristics, social support, and social behavior. In R. Binstock & E. Shanas (Eds.), *Handbook of aging and social sciences* (2nd ed.). New York: Van Nostrand Reinhold.

Aquilera, D.C., & Messick, J.M. (1982). *Crisis intervention: Theory and methodology* (4th ed.). St. Louis: Mosby.

Armstrong, N. (1987). Coping with diabetes mellitus: A full-time job. *Nurs Clin North Am, 22*(3), 559–568.

Averill, J. (1973). Personal control over aversive stimuli and its relationship to stress. *Psychol Bull, 80*, 286–293.

Ayers, T.D. (1989). Dimensions and characteristics of lay helping. *Am J Orthopsychiatry, 59*(2), 215–225.

Bandura, A. (1977). Self-efficacy: Toward a unifying theory of behavioral change. *Psychol Rev, 84*, 195–215.

Baxter, R.T. (1981). Divorce: The second trauma. *Accent, 2*, 47–52.

Beck, C., Rawlings, R., & Williams, S. (1984). *Mental health-psychiatric nursing.* St. Louis: Mosby.

Benner, P., Roskies, E., & Lazarus, R.S. (1980). Stress and coping under extreme conditions. In J.E. Dimsdale (Ed.), *Survivors, victims, and perpetrators: Essays on the Nazi Holocaust* (pp. 219–258). Washington, DC: Hemisphere.

Bernheimer, L.P., Young, M.S., & Winton, P.J. (1983). Stress over time: Parents with young handicapped children. *J Dev Behavior Pediatr, 4*(3), 177–181.

Blum, R.W. (1983). The adolescent with spina bifida. *Clin Pediatr, 22*(5), 331–335.

Blum, R. (1984). *Chronic illness and disabilities in childhood and adolescence.* San Diego: Grune & Stratton.

Boyce, W.T. (1985). Stress and child health: An overview. *Pediatr Ann, 14*(8), 539–542.

Bradbury, A.J., & Smith, C.S. (1983). An assessment of the diabetic knowledge of school teachers. *Arch Dis Child, 58*, 692–696.

Bru, G. (1985). Adolescence and young adulthood. *Cancer Nurs, Suppl 1*, 21–24.

Burke, S.O., Costello, E.A., & Handley-Derry, M.H. (1989). Maternal stress and repeated hospitalizations of children who are physically disabled. *Child Health Care, 18*(2), 82–90.

Burns, W., & Zweig, A. (1980). Self-concepts of chronically ill children. *J Genet Psychol, 137*, 179–190.

Burr, W.R. (1973). *Theory construction and the sociology of the family.* New York: Wiley.

Cairns, N.U., Clark, G.M., Smith, S.D., & Lansky, S.B. (1979). Adaptation of siblings to childhood malignancy. *J Pediatr, 95*, 484–487.

Cannon, W.B. (1929). *Bodily changes in pain, hunger, fear and rage.* Boston: Branford.

Cannon, W.B. (1935). Stresses and strains of homeostasis (Mary Scott Newbold lecture). *Am J Med Sci, 189*, 1–14.

Caplan, G. (1961). *An approach to community mental health.* New York: Grune & Stratton.

Caplan, G. (1964). *Principles of preventive psychology.* New York: Basic Books.

Carandang, M.L.A., Folkins, C.H., Hines, P.A., & Steward, M.S. (1979). The role of cognitive level and sibling illness in children's conceptualizations of illness. *Am J Orthopsychiatry, 49*(3), 474–481.

Carpenito, L. (1989) (3rd ed.). *Handbook of nursing diagnoses.* Philadelphia: Lippincott.

Cassileth, B.R., Volckmar, D., & Goodman, R.L. (1980). The effect of experience on radiation therapy patient's desire for information. *Radiat Oncol, Biol Phys, 6*(4), 493–496.

Chesler, M.A., & Barbarin, O.A. (1987). *Childhood cancer and the family: Meeting the challenge of stress and support.* New York: Brunner/Mazel.

Clarke, M. (1984a). Stress and coping: Constructs for nursing. *J Adv Nurs, 9*(1), 3–13.

Clarke, M. (1984b). The constructs of 'stress' and 'coping' as a rationale for nursing activities. *J Adv Nurs, 9*(3), 267–275.

Coddington, R.D. (1972a). The significance of life events as etiological factors in the diseases of children. I. A survey of professional workers. *J Psychosom Res, 16*, 7–18.

Coddington, R.D. (1972b). The significance of life events as etiological factors in the diseases of children. II. A study of a normal population. *J Psychosom Res, 16*, 205–213.

Comarr, A.E., & Vigue, M. (1978). Sexual counseling among male and female patients with spinal cord and/or cauda equina injury. *Urol Surv, 10*, 107–122.

Damrosch, S.P., & Perry, L.A. (1989). Self-reported adjustment, chronic sorrow, and coping of parents of children with Down syndrome. *Nurs Res, 38*(1), 25–30.

Daniels, D., Miller, III, J.J., Billings, A.G., & Moos, R.H. (1986). Psychosocial functioning of siblings of children with rheumatic disease. *J Pediatr, 109*, 379–383.

Darling, R.B. (1979). *Families against society.* Beverly Hills, CA: Sage.

DeJong, G., Branch, L.G., Corcoran, P.J. (1984). Independent living outcomes in spinal cord injury: Multivariate analyses. *Arch Phys Med Psychol, 65*, 66–73.

DeLongis, A., et al. (1982). Relationship of daily hassles, uplifts, and major life events to health status. *Health Psychol, 1*(2), 119–136.

Dixon, J.K. (1981). Group-self identification and physical handicap: Implication for patient support groups. *Res Nurs Health, 4*, 299–308.

Dohrewend, B.S., & Dohrewend, B.P. (Eds.). (1974). *Stressful life events: Their nature and effects.* New York: Wiley.

Dolgin, M.J., et al. (1986). Caregivers' perceptions of medical compliance in adolescents with cancer. *J Adolesc Health Care, 7*, 22–27.

Douglas, J.W.B. (1975). Early hospital admission and later disturbances of behavior and learning. *Dev Med Child Neurol, 17*, 456–480.

Droske, S. (1978). Children's behavioral changes following hospitalization—Have we prepared the parents. *J Assoc Care Child Hospitals, 7*(2), 3–7.

Eiser, C. (1980). How leukemia affects a child's schooling. *Br J Soc Clin Psychol, 19*(Part 4), 365–368.

Elliott, G.R., & Eisdorfer, C. (1982). *Stress and human health.* New York: Springer.

Engel, G. (1968). A life setting conducive to illness: The giving-up given-up complex. *Ann Intern Med, 69*, 293.

Engel, G.L. (1962). *Psychological development in health and disease.* Philadelphia: Saunders.

Engel, G. (1971). Sudden and rapid death during psychological stress: Folklore or folkwisdom? *Ann Int Med, 74*, 771–782.

Erikson, E. (1965). *Childhood and society.* New York: Penguin Books.

Erikson, E. (1968). *Identity: Youth and crisis.* New York: Norton.

Evans, R.L., et al. (1987). Family interaction and treatment adherence after stroke. *Arch Phys Med Rehabil, 68*, 513–517.

Falvo, D.R., Allen, H., & Maki, D.R. (1982). Psychosocial aspects of invisible disability. *Rehabil Lit, 43*, 2–6.

Ferrari, M. (1987). The diabetic child and well siblings: Risks to the well child's self-concept. *Child Health Care, 15*(3), 141–148.

Fife, B.L., Huhman, M., & Keck, J. (1986). Developmental of a clinical assessment scale: Evaluation of the psychosocial impact of childhood illness on the family. *Issues Compr Pediatr Nurs, 9*, 11–31.

Fink, S.L. (1967). Crisis and motivation: A theoretical model. *Arch Phys Med Rehabil, 48*, 592–597.

Friedland, J., & McColl, M. (1987). Social X and psychosocial dysfunction after stroke: Buffering effects in a community sample. *Arch Phys Med Rehabil, 68*, 475–480.

Friedman, M.M. (1987). Intervening with families of school-aged children with cancer. In M. Leahey & L.M. Wright (Eds.), *Families & life-threatening illness* (pp. 219–234). Springhouse, PA: Springhouse.

Fuchs, J. (1987). Use of decisional control to combat powerlessness. *ANNA Am Nephrol Nurses Assoc J, 14*(1), 11–13, 56.

Gatchel, R.J., & Baum, A. (1983). *An introduction to health psychology.* Reading, MA: Addison-Wesley.

Gething, L. (1985). Perceptions of disability of persons with cerebral palsy, their close relatives and able bodied persons. *Soc Sci Med, 20*(6), 561–568.

Gogan, J. (1977). Childhood cancer and siblings. *Health Soc Work, 2*, 42–57.

Green, C.P. (1986). Changes in responsibility in women's families after the diagnosis of cancer. *Health Care Wom Int, 7*, 221–239.

Greenspan, S. (1979). Intelligence and adaptation: An integration of psychoanalytic and Piagetian developmental psychology. *Psychol Issues, Monogr 47/48.*

Greer, B. (1985). Children of physically disabled parents: Some thoughts, facts, and hypotheses. In S.K. Thurman (Ed.), *Children of handicapped parents* (pp. 131–143). San Francisco: Academic Press.

Gull, H.J. (1987). The chronically ill patient's adaptation to hospitalization. *Nurs Clin North Am, 22*(3), 593–601.

Gurklis, J.A., & Menke, E.M. (1988). Identification of stressors and use of coping methods in chronic hemodialysis patients. *Nurs Res, 37*(4), 236–239, 248.

Halloran, J., Hughes, A., & Mayer, D.K. (1988). Oncology Nursing Society position paper on HIV-related issues. *Oncol Nurs Forum, 15*(2), 206–217.

Hamburg, D.A. (1982). Forward: An outlook on stress research and health. In G.R. Elliott & C. Eisdorfer (Eds.), *Stress and human health* (pp. ix–xxii). New York: Springer.

Harder, L., & Bowditch, B. (1982). Siblings of children with cystic fibrosis: Perceptions of the impact of the disease. *Child Health Care, 10*(4), 116–120.

Harris, T. (1986). Aging in the eighties, prevalence and impact of urinary problems in individuals age 65 years and over. *Advancedata*, No. 121, August 27, 1986. USDHHS.

Harvey, D.H.P., & Greenway, A.P. (1984). The self-concepts of physically handicapped children and their non-handicapped siblings: An empirical investigation. *J Child Psychol Psychiatry, 25*(2), 273–284.

Hayden, P., Davenport, S., & Campbell, M. (1979). Adolescents with myelodysplasia: Impact of physical disability on emotional maturation. *Pediatrics, 64*, 53–59.

Heisel, J.S., Ream, S., Raitz, R., Rappaport, M., & Coddington, R.D. (1973). The significance of life events as contributing factors in diseases of children. III: A study of pediatric patients. *J Pediatr, 83*, 119.

Hill, R. (1949). *Families under stress.* New York: Harper & Row.

Hodges, L.C., & Parker, J. (1987). Concerns of parents of diabetic children. *Pediatr Nurs, 13*(1), 22–24, 68.

Holmes, T.H., & Rahe, R.H. (1967). The social readjustment rating scale. *J Psychosom Res, 11*, 213–218.

Horowitz, A. (1985). Sons and daughters as caregivers to older patients: Differences in caregiver role performance. *Gerontologist, 25,* 612–615.

Hymovich, D.P. (1977). The hospitalized child: A sociological perspective. *Clinical nursing specialist symposium, 1976.* (pp. 21–35), Rochester, NY: University of Rochester.

Hymovich, D.P. (1981, May 13). Chronic childhood illness: Family impact and parent coping. Association for the Care of Children's Health, Toronto, Canada.

Hymovich, D.P. (1982, April 30). Chronic childhood illness: Family impact and parent coping. Sigma Theta Tau Research Conference, Akron, OH.

Hymovich, D.P., & Baker, C. (1985). The needs, concerns and coping of parents of children with cystic fibrosis. *Fam Relat, 34,* 91–97.

Iles, J.P. (1979). Cancer with children: Healthy siblings' perceptions during the illness experience. *Cancer Nurs, 2,* 371–377.

Jacobsen, A.M., Hauser, S.T., Wolfsdorf, J.I. et al. (1987). Psychological predictors of compliance in children with recent onset of diabetes mellitus. *J Pediatr, 100,* 805–811.

Jamison, R., Lewis, S., & Burish, T. (1986). Psychological impact of cancer on adolescents: Self-image, locus of control, perception of illness and knowledge of cancer. *J Chronic Dis, 39*(8), 609–617.

Jessop, D.J., & Stein, R.E.K. (1985). Uncertainty and its relationship to the psychological and social correlates of chronic illness in children. *Soc Sci Med, 20*(10), 993–999.

Kanner, A.D., Coyne, J.C., Schaefer, C., & Lazarus, R.S. (1981). Comparison of two modes of stress management: Daily hassles and uplifts versus major life events. *J Behav Med, 4,* 1–39.

Kazak, A., & Wilcox, B. (1984). The structure and function of social support networks in families with handicapped children. *Am J Community Psychol, 12,* 645–661.

Kerr, M.E., & Bowen, M. (1988). *Family evaluation: An approach based on Bowen theory.* New York: Norton.

Knox, J.E., & Hayes, V.E. (1983). Hospitalization of a chronically ill child: A stressful time for parents. *Issues Compr Pediatr Nurs, 6,* 217–226.

Kobassa, S.C. (1979). Stressful life events, personality and health: An inquiry into hardiness. *J Pers Soc Psychol, 37,* 1–11.

Koch-Hattem, A. (1986). Siblings' experience of pediatric cancer: Interviews with children. *Health Soc Work, 11*(2), 107–117.

Korn, S.J., Chess, S., & Fernandez, I. (1978). The impact of children's physical handicaps on marital quality and family interaction. In R.M. Lerner & G.B. Spanier (Eds.), *Child influences on marital and family interaction.* New York: Academic Press.

Korsch, B.M., Fine, R.N., & Negrete, V.F. (1978). Noncompliance in children with renal transplants. *Pediatrics, 61,* 872–876.

Kramer, R.F. (1981). Living with childhood cancer: Healthy siblings' perspectives. *Issues Compr Pediatr Nurs, 5,* 155–165.

Lambert, V., & Lambert, C. (1985). The relationship between social support and psychological well-being in rheumatoid arthritic women from two ethnic groups. *Health Care Wom Int, 6,* 405–414.

Langner, E.J. (1975). The illusion of control. *J Pers Soc Psychol, 32,* 311–328.

Lavigne, J., & Ryan, M. (1979). Psychological adjustments of siblings with chronic illness. *Pediatrics, 63,* 616–627.

Lawson, B.A. (1977). Chronic illness and the school-aged child: Effects on the total family. *Maternal Child Nurs, 2,* 49–55.

Lazarus, R.S. (1966). *Psychological stress and the coping process.* New York: McGraw-Hill.

Lazarus, R.S. (1971). The concepts of stress and disease. In L. Levy (Ed.), *Society, stress and disease: The psychosocial environment and psychosomatic diseases. Vol. 1.* (pp. 53–58). London: Oxford University Press.

Lazarus, R.S., & Cohen, J.B. (1977). Environmental stress. In I. Altman & J.F. Wohlwill (Eds.), *Human behavior and the environment: Current theory and research.* New York: Plenum.

Lazarus, R.S., & Folkman, S. (1984). *Stress, appraisal, and coping.* New York: Springer.

Lewis, M. (1982). *Clinical aspects of child development* (2nd ed.). Philadelphia: Lea & Febiger.

Lipsky, D.K. (1985). A parental perspective on stress and coping. *Am J Orthopsychiatry, 55*(4), 614–617.

McAnarny, E., Pless, B., Satterwhite, B., & Friedman, B. (1974). Psychological problems of children with chronic juvenile arthritis. *Pediatrics, 53*(4), 523–528.

McCormick, M.C., Charney, E.B., & Stemmler, M.M. (1986). Assessing the impact of a child with spina bifida on the family. *Dev Med Child Neurol, 28,* 53–61.

McCubbin, M.A., & Huang, S.T.T. (1989). Family strengths in the care of handicapped children: Targets for intervention. *Fam Relat, 38,* 436–443.

McCubbin, M.A., & McCubbin, H.I. (1987). Family stress theory and assessment. In H.I. McCubbin & A.L. Thompson (Eds.), *Family assessment inventories for research and practice* (pp. 1–25). Madison, WI: University of Wisconsin—Madison.

McCubbin, H., & Patterson, J. (1983). The family stress process: The double ABCX model. In H. McCubbin, M. Sussman, & J. Patterson (Eds.), *Social stress and the family: Advances and developments in family stress theory and research* (pp. 7–37). New York: Haworth Press.

McCubbin, H.I., & Thompson, A.L. (Eds.). (1987). *Family assessment inventories for research and practice.* Madison, WI: University of Wisconsin—Madison.

McKeever, P. (1981). Fathering the chronically ill child: A neglected area in family research. *Am J Maternal-Child Nurs, 6*(2), 124–128.

McKeever, P. (1983). Siblings of chronically ill children: A literature review and implications for research and practice. *Am J Orthopsychiatry, 53*(2), 209–218.

McNaull, F. (1981). The costs of cancer: A challenge to health care providers. *Cancer Nurs, 4*(3), 207–212.

MacVicar, M.G., & Archibald, P. (1976). A framework for family assessment in chronic illness. *Nurs Forum, 15*(2), 180–194.

Mailick, M. (1984). The impact of severe illness on the individual and family: An overview. In E. Aronowitz, & E.M. Bromberg (Eds.), *Mental health and long-term physical illness* (pp. 83–94). Canton, MA: Prodist.

Massie Jr., R. (1981). Personal perspectives on health care. In S. Francis (Ed.), *Children in health care: Ethical perspectives* (pp. 16–18). Washington, DC: Association for the Care of Children's Health.

Meisenhelder, J. (1985). Self-esteem: A closer look at clinical interventions. *Int J Nurs Stud, 22*(2), 127–135.

Meldman, L.S. (1987). Diabetes as experienced by adolescents. *Adolescence, 22*(86), 433–444.

Miller, B. (1990). Gender differences in spouse caregiver strain: Socialization and role explanations. *J Marr Fam, 52,* 311–321.

Miller, J.F. (1983). *Coping with chronic illness: Overcoming powerlessness.* Philadelphia: F.A. Davis.

Miller, K., & Iscoe, P. (1963). The concept of crisis: Current status and mental health implications. *Hum Organ, 22,* 195–201.

Mishel, M.H. (1981). The measurement of uncertainty in illness. *Nurs Res, 30,* 258–263.

Mishel, M.H., & Braden, C.J. (1988). Finding meaning: Antecedents of uncertainty in illness. *Nurs Res, 37*(2), 98–103, 127.

Moen, J., Wilcox, R., & Burns, J. (1977). PKU as a factor in the development of self-esteem. *J Pediatr, 90*(6), 1027–1029.

Molleman, E., Krabbendam, R.J., Annyas, A.A., Koops, H.S. et al. (1984). The significance of the doctor-patient relationship in coping with cancer. *Soc Sci Med, 18,* 475–480.

Moos, R.H., & Schaefer, J.A. (1986). Life transitions and crises. In R.H. Moos (Ed.), *Coping and life crisis* (pp. 3–21). New York: Plenum.

Murphy, L.B. (1962). *The widening world of childhood: Paths toward mastery.* New York: Basic Books.

Neugarten, B.L. (1979). Time, age and the life cycle. *Am J Psychiatry, 136,* 887–894.

Neumann, B. (1980). The Betty Neumann health-care systems model: A total person approach to patient problems. In J.P. Riehl & Sr. C. Roy (Eds.), *Conceptual models for nursing practice* (2nd ed.) (pp. 119–134). New York: Appleton-Century-Crofts.

Olshansky, S. (1962). Chronic sorrow: A response to having a mentally defective child. *J Pediatr, 43,* 190–193.

Parmelee, P. (1983). Spouse versus other family caregivers: Psychological impact on impaired aged. *Am J Community Psychol, 11,* 337–349.

Patton, A.C., Ventura, J.N., & Savedra, M. (1986). Stress and coping responses of adolescents with cystic fibrosis. *Child Health Care, 14*(3), 153–156.

Pearlin, L.I., & Schooler, C. (1978). The structure of coping. *J Health Soc Behav, 19*(March), 2–21.

Peters-Golden, H. (1982). Breast cancer: Varied perceptions of social support in the illness experiences. *Soc Sci Med, 16,* 483–491.

Quinton, D., & Rutter, M. (1975). Early hospital admissions and later disturbances of behavior: An attempted replication of Douglas' findings. *Dev Med Child Neurol, 18,* 447–459.

Register, C. (1987). *Living with chronic illness: Days of patience and passion.* New York: Free Press.

Ritchie, J.A., Caty, S., & Ellerton, M.L. (1984). Concerns of acutely ill, chronically ill, and healthy preschool children. *Res Nurs Health, 7,* 265–274.

Rodin, J., Rennert, K., & Solomon, S.K. (1980). Intrinsic motivation for control: Fact or fiction. In A. Baum & J.E. Singer (Eds.), *Advances in environmental psychology: Applications of personal control* (Vol. 2). Hillsdale, NJ: Erlbaum.

Roy, O. (1984). *Introduction to nursing: An adaptation model.* Englewood Cliffs, NJ: Prentice-Hall.

Rubenstein, B. (1984). When a child has a serious illness: Psychiatric aspects of chronic handicaps. In E. Aronowitz & E.M. Bromberg (Eds.), *Mental health and long-term illness* (pp. 45–65). Canton, MA: Prodist.

Sabbeth, B.F., & Leventhal, J.M. (1984). Marital adjustment to chronic childhood illness: A critique of the literature. *Pediatrics, 73*(6), 762–768.

Savedra, M.K. (1977). The severely burned child: Moving from hospital to home. *Maternal Child Nurs, 1,* 220–222.

Scharer, K., & Dixon, D.M. (1989). Managing chronic illness: Parents with a ventilator dependent child. *J Pediatr Nurs, 4*(4), 236–247.

Schilder, P. (1964). *The image and appearance of the human body.* NY: Wiley.

Schmale, A., & Iker, H. (1966). The psychological setting of uterine cervical cancer. *Ann NY Acad Sci, 125,* 807–813.

Select Panel for the Promotion of Child Health. (1981). *Better health for our children: A national strategy.* Washington, DC: Department of Health and Human Services.

Selekman, J. (1983). The development of body image in the child: A learned response. *Top Clin Nurs, 5*(1), 12–21.

Seligman, M. (1975). *Helplessness: On depression, development, and death.* San Francisco: W.H. Freeman.

Selye, H. (1975). Stress and distress. *Compr Ther, 1,* 9–13.

Sexton, D.L., & Munro, B.H. (1985). Impact of a husband's chronic illness (COPD) on the spouse's life. *Res Nurs Health, 8,* 83–90.

Shapiro, J. (1983). Family reactions and coping strategies

in response to the physically ill or handicapped child: A review. *Soc Sci Med, 17,* 913–931.

Shekleton, M.E. Coping with chronic respiratory difficulty. (1987). *Nurs Clin North Am, 22* (3), 569–581.

Singer, L., & Farkas, K.J. (1989). The impact of infant disability on maternal perception of stress. *Fam Relat, 38,* 444–449.

Sourkes, B. (1980). Siblings of pediatric cancer patients. In J. Kellerman (Ed.), *Psychological aspects of childhood cancer* (pp. 47–69). Springfield, IL: Charles C Thomas.

Spielberger, C.D. (1983). *Manual for the state-trait anxiety inventory.* Palo Alto, CA: Consulting Psychologists Press.

Spinetta, J.L., & Deasy-Spinetta, P. (Eds.). (1981). *Living with childhood cancer.* St. Louis: Mosby.

Stam, H.J., Bultz, B.D., & Pittman, C.A. (1986). Psychosocial problems and interventions in a referred sample of cancer patients. *Psychosom Med, 48* (8), 539–548.

Stapleton, S. (1983). Recognizing powerlessness: Causes and indicators in patients with chronic renal failure. In J.F. Miller (Ed.), *Coping with chronic illness: Overcoming powerlessness* (pp. 135–148). Philadelphia: F.A. Davis.

Stein, R.E.K. (Ed.). (1989). *Caring for children with chronic illness.* New York: Springer.

Strauss, A.L., Corbin, J., Fagerhaugh, S., Glaser, B.G. et al. (1984). *Chronic illness and the quality of life* (2nd ed.). St. Louis: Mosby.

Strax, T.E., & Wolfson, S.D. (1984). Life cycle crises of the disabled adolescent and young adult. In *Chronic illness and disabilities in childhood and adolescence* (pp. 47–57). New York: Grune & Stratton.

Swift, C., Seidman, F., & Stein, H. (1967). Adjustment problems in juvenile diabetes. *Psychosom Med, 29* (6), 555–571.

Tache, J., & Selye, H. (1985). On stress and coping mechanisms. *Ment Health Nurs, 7* (4), 3–24.

Taylor, S.C. (1980). The effect of chronic childhood illness upon well siblings. *Maternal-Child Nurs J, 9* (2), 109–116.

Tenbrink, M., & Brewer, P. (1976). The stages of grief experienced by parents of handicapped children. *AZ Med, 33,* 712–714.

Tew, B., & Lawrence, K.M. (1973). Mothers, brothers, and sisters of patients with spina bifida. *Dev Med Child Neurol, 15,* 69–76.

Thompson, R.H. (1986). Where we stand: Twenty years of research on pediatric hospitalization and health care. *Child Health Care, 14,* 200–210.

Thorne, S.E. (1989). Helpful and unhelpful communications in cancer care: The patient perspective. *Oncol Nurs Forum, 15* (2), 167–172.

Turk, J. (1964). Impact of cystic fibrosis on family functioning. *Pediatrics, 34,* 67–71.

Urey, J.R., & Henggeler, S.W. (1987). Marital adjustment following spinal cord injury. *Arch Phys Med Rehabil, 68,* 69–74.

Versluys, H.P. (1980). Physical rehabilitation and family dynamics. *Rehabil Lit, 41* (3–4), 58–65.

Waechter, E.H. (1971). Children's awareness of fatal illness. *Am J Nurs, 71,* 1168–1170.

Walker, A.J. (1985). Reconceptualizing family stress. *J Marr Fam, 47,* 827–837.

Weinberg, N., & Williams, J. (1978). How the physically disabled perceive their disabilities. *J Rehabil, Nos. 11–12,* 31–33.

Weisman, A.D., & Worden, J.W. (1976). The existential plight in cancer: Significance of the first 100 days. *Int J Psychiatr Med, 7,* 1–15.

White, R.W. (1959). Motivation reconsidered: The concept of competence. *Psychol Rev, 66,* 297–333.

Wickler, L., Wasco, N., & Hatfield, E. (1981). Chronic sorrow revisited: Parent vs. professional depiction of the adjustment of parents of mentally retarded children. *Am J Orthopsychiatry, 51,* 63–67.

Worden, J.W., & Sobel, H.J. (1978). Ego strength and psychosocial adaptation to cancer. *Psychosom Med, 40,* 585–592.

World Health Organization. (1980). *International classification of impairments, disabilities, and handicaps.* Geneva: World Health Organization.

Wortman, C.B., & Brehm, J.W. (1975). Responses to uncontrollable outcomes: An integration of reactance theory and the learned helplessness model. In L. Berkowitz (Ed.), *Advances in social experimental psychology* (Vol. 8) (pp. 277–336). New York: Academic Press.

Young, R.K. (1977). Chronic sorrow: Parents' response to the birth of a child with a defect. *Maternal Child Nurs, 2,* 38–42.

Zeltzer, L., et al. (1980). Psychological effects of illness in adolescence. II. Impact of illness in adolescents—crucial issues and coping styles. *J Pediatr, 97* (1), 132–138.

Zola, I.K. (1982). Denial of emotional needs in people with handicaps. *Arch Phys Med Rehabil, 63,* 63–67.

11 Coping Strategies

Coping is the process of responding to stressors or potential stressors. It involves any combination of cognitive, affective, or behavioral responses to any stressor. Coping with stress basically refers to a self-regulatory process by which a person reduces or prevents those responses that would normally occur under stress. People respond to stressful situations depending upon their perceptions of the event. Perceptions are determined by the cognitive processes of appraisal and reappraisal, through which

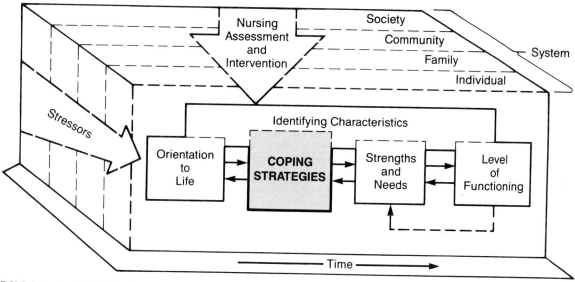

FIGURE 11—1 The Coping Strategies Component of Hymovich's Contingency Model of Long-Term Care

events take on personal meaning in relation to their impact on the individual or family system. Among the primary areas of concern in appraising an event are the person's survival, self-esteem, close attachment with significant others, and sense of belonging to a values group (Hamburg, 1982). The process of coping with a chronic condition entails a complex mixture of personality style, family influences, and life experiences, as well as factors related to the disease itself (Pinkerton et al, 1985).

Coping strategies to decrease focal stressor events are aimed at converting an unfamiliar situation to one that is familiar and thus more predictable. The more predictable the event and subsequent responses to it become, the more feasible it is for the person to take adaptive measures. This chapter provides a brief overview of the coping concept, followed by a discussion of coping as it pertains to the Contingency Model of Long-Term Care. Included in this chapter are the various coping strategies used by children and adults as they adapt and readapt to a chronic condition. The relationship of coping to other components of the model is shown in Figure 11–1.

Definition of Coping

The conceptual definition of coping depends on one's theoretical orientation. As with stressors, various conceptualizations and definitions of coping

appear in the literature. Regardless of the specific definition, coping basically refers to a self-regulatory process that is purposeful and intentional. By coping, the individual or family system reduces or prevents the responses that normally occur under stress (Burish & Bradley, 1983). Often, especially in the popular lay literature, coping is equated with adaptational success. Comments like "She coped well" or "He coped poorly" suggest either a successful or an unsuccessful outcome.

Several definitions of coping frequently appear in the chronic-illness and disability literature. The first is that of Lazarus and Launier (1978), who defined coping as "efforts, both action-oriented and intrapsychic, to manage (i.e., master, tolerate, reduce, minimize) environmental and internal demands, and conflicts among them, which tax or exceed a person's resources" (p. 311). As defined here, coping is a purposeful and intentional act, involving effort; it is a process independent of outcome. From this perspective, it refers to **efforts** to manage the stressful event, regardless of the outcome. This means that no single coping strategy is better than any other one; the strategy's effectiveness depends upon its effects in the immediate situation **and** in the long term. Murphy (1974) also views coping in children as a process that involves effort. Some authors (Haan, 1977; Menninger, 1963; Vaillant, 1977) describe a hierarchy of coping and defense processes, suggesting that some methods are automatically better than others. However, it is possible that

Table 11—1 Definitions of Coping

Definition	Source
". . . a process of constantly changing cognitive and behavioral efforts to manage specific external and/or internal demands that are appraised as taxing or exceeding the resources of a person"	Lazarus & Folkman, 1984, p. 141.
"a matter of flexible management of different devices for dealing with challenges from the environment"	Murphy, 1974, p. 273
". . . what one does about a perceived problem in order to bring about relief, reward, quiescence, or equilibrium"	Weisman & Worden, 1976–77, p. 3
". . . any response to external life-strains that serves to prevent, avoid, or control emotional distress"	Pearlin & Schooler, 1978, p. 3
". . . a strategic effort to master a problem, overcome an obstacle, answer a question, dissipate a dilemma—anything that impedes our progress"	Weisman, 1984, p. 36
"The ability to acquire and use the resources needed for family adaptation"	Patterson & McCubbin, 1983, p. 30
A cognitive, affective, and behavioral process to manage perceived stressors or potential stressors in the environment or internal to the system that tax or exceed the system's current resources for responding.	Hymovich & Hagopian

either the coping or defense process can be effective or ineffective, depending upon the particular context of the situation. Murphy's definition of coping is in Table 11–1, along with other definitions commonly seen in the chronic-illness literature.

Coping, as defined in the Contingency Model of Long-Term Care is a cognitive, affective, and behavioral process to manage perceived stressors or potential stressors in the environment or internal to the

system that tax or exceed the system's current resources for responding. This definition has implications for clinical practice because it focuses on what the person actually does in a specific situation, and how strategies shift as the situation changes.

The Concept of Coping

The concept of coping is complex and difficult to study. There is no accepted unifying theoretical position or definition and no uniform way of measuring the concept. Although theorists and researchers have proposed stages in the coping process (Horowitz, 1982; Klinger, 1977; Kubler-Ross, 1969; Shontz, 1975; Wortman & Brehm, 1975), these sequences are often found to vary clinically (Lazarus & Folkman, 1984). Coping is not static; rather, it changes according to situational demands and how a person perceives the situation. The concept of coping used in the Contingency Model of Long-Term Care is derived from the work of Lazarus and his colleagues (Lazarus & Folkman, 1984).

Coping may be conceptualized as either a disposition (personality trait or style), a process (Averill & Opton, 1968), or as an outcome (Stewart, 1980). Coping can be considered in relation to the concept of stress, either as an endocrinologic and physiologic process (Selye, 1976) or as an interactionist, cognitively-oriented process (Folkman, Schaefer, & Lazarus, 1979). In the Contingency Model of Long-Term Care, coping dispositions (trait, style) are referred to as *coping patterns*, and coping behaviors as *coping strategies*.

Physiologic Model

There are two traditional ways of conceptualizing coping. The first, derived from the animal model, is basically a unidimensional concept of drive and arousal. In this classic view, coping is an endocrinologic and physiologic process within the context of stress (Selye, 1976). Although the term is rarely used in this context, coping is a process that regulates neuroendocrinologic functioning. The success of a coping strategy is measured in relation to the organism's recovery or survival. Proponents of the physiologic conception of stress and coping recently acknowledged that cognitive factors play a role in the process (Folkman, Schaefer, & Lazarus, 1979). The work of Obrist (1981) on the pathophysiology of coping and cardiovascular responses is an example of research related to this model. This work suggests that active rather than passive coping is an important mediator of sympathetically controlled cardiovascular changes.

Psychoanalytic Ego Psychology Model

The second traditional approach for conceptualizing coping has been the psychoanalytic ego psychology model that focuses on how people perceive or think about their relationship with the environment. With this model, more attention is given to the cognitive aspects of coping and less to the behavioral aspects. Cognitive styles refer to automatic responses, rather than those involving effort.

Coping dispositions Within the psychoanalytic ego psychology model, coping has been conceptualized as a disposition, that is, a personality trait or style. As a **trait or style,** coping refers to a person's relatively stable and consistent tendency to respond to a variety of stressors in a similar way. For example, people may deal with their problems primarily by either monitoring or blunting, suppressing or expressing anger, avoiding, or being vigilant. Traits are used to classify people to make predictions about how they will cope in various situations. Lazarus and Folkman (1984) consider type A pattern of behavior to be a coping style. The pattern of behavior associated with type A individuals is defined as a "chronic, incessant struggle to achieve more and more in less and less time, and if required to do so, against the opposing efforts of other things or persons" (Friedman & Roseman, 1974, p. 67). A relationship between a type A life-style and coronary heart disease has been found (Glass, 1977). "Coronary prone behavior" is a constellation of three interrelated concepts: (1) a set of beliefs about oneself and the world, (2) a set of values leading to a pattern of motivation or commitment (e.g., striving), and (3) life-style behavior (e.g., competitive).

In the past, the trait concept of coping was emphasized in research. However, assessment of coping traits has limited value in predicting actual coping processes, and process measures generally show stronger relationships to outcome than do trait measures.

Interactionist Cognitive Model

A third, more recent view of coping is the interactionist, cognitively oriented view, whose primary proponent is Richard Lazarus (Lazarus & Folkman,

1984). Lazarus' model of coping has influenced the thinking of many researchers, and is incorporated into the Contingency Model of Long-Term Care. Stress results from any event that has the capacity to threaten, harm, or exceed the response capacities of the person. The person responds by making a series of appraisals about the nature of the stressor and its potential effect on one's life. The consequences of the stress are not only neuroendocrine responses but also as behavioral, cognitive, and emotional responses. Cognitive processes determine the quality and intensity of an emotional reaction and underlie coping activities.

Cognitive appraisal People cope in response to a threat to their life, health, wealth, or important social relationships. They anticipate danger that will interfere with their goals. This process involves **cognitive appraisal,** a continuous evaluative process of categorizing the facts and significance of a transaction (person's encounter with the environment) (Lazarus & Folkman, 1984). Cognitive appraisals as they relate to the Contingency Model of Long-Term Care are defined as continuous evaluative processes of categorizing the facts and significance of the event to the person. Cognitive appraisal depends on one's subjective perception and interpretation of an encounter, and is therefore phenomenologic. An individual or family system appraises what is happening to it and uses the understanding to shape future events. The process involves primary and secondary appraisals, followed by reappraisals.

Primary appraisal.
Primary appraisal is the cognitive process of evaluating environmental stimuli and making a judgment as to their significance to the system's well-being, that is, to what is at stake for the system (Folkman et al, 1986). The event (encounter) may be judged **irrelevant** if it has no implication for the well-being. A **benign-positive** appraisal occurs if the encounter is believed to preserve or enhance well-being at the time or at some time in the future. Such an appraisal may result in pleasurable emotions such as happiness, love, or exhilaration, or in negative emotions such as guilt or anxiety. Negative emotions can occur when someone believes the positive situation will not last or that some harm will eventually occur because one must pay for feeling good.

Stress appraisals are of three types: harm/loss, threat, and challenge. With an appraisal of **harm or loss,** some damage has already occurred, such as the diagnosis of a chronic condition or the death of a loved one. An event appraised as a **threat** is one in which harm or loss is anticipated. Such an appraisal is associated with negative emotions (e.g., fear, anger, anxiety) and is significant because it permits anticipatory coping. When the appraisal is one of **challenge,** the focus is on the potential for growth rather than harm, and the emotions associated with it are pleasurable. A challenging event, such as a job promotion, can be appraised as having the potential for threat because of the new demands placed on the individual. People who feel challenged, rather than threatened, are likely to have higher morale and adapt better to their situation. The ability to cope with a situation gives one a feeling of personal control. A persistent feeling of lack of control can lead to feelings of helplessness and depression (Seligman, 1975).

Secondary appraisal.

Secondary appraisal involves evaluation of available coping resources and options, such as to engage, flee, or seek relief in some defense mechanisms. More recently, secondary appraisal has been defined as coping options in a stressful encounter (Folkman et al, 1986). The secondary appraisal process is also a complex evaluative one. It takes into account the coping options available to the system, their likely consequences (outcomes), and system ability to use them effectively.

Reappraisal.

Reappraisal is the process of changing an appraisal on the basis of new information. It serves to modify an earlier appraisal and can take place many times. **Defensive reappraisals** are a form of reappraisal that "consist of any effort made to reinterpret the past more positively, or to deal with present harms and threats by viewing them in less damaging and/or threatening ways" (Lazarus & Folkman, 1984, p. 38). They arise from needs within the system rather than from the environment. This notion may be similar to Taylor's (1983) concept of downward comparison, discussed later in this chapter.

Primary appraisals (what is at stake) and secondary appraisals (coping options) take place simultaneously and interact with one another in determining the degree of stress and type of emotional reaction. For example, a woman who discovers a lump in her breast (focal stressor event) may feel very threatened (primary appraisal) at first and deny (secondary appraisal) its existence. When denial no longer helps, or when new information is obtained (reappraisal),

the woman seeks medical assistance (outcome). The elderly woman with rheumatoid arthritis who fears she will be harmed by surgery (primary appraisal) may deny her pain, disfigurement, and functional loss (secondary appraisal) until she is no longer able to carry out activities of daily living on her own. Once the quality of her life is at stake and loss of independence becomes an issue (reappraisal), she decides to consent to surgery (outcome). A father whose son is diagnosed with diabetes (focal stressor event) seeks information (primary appraisal) about the condition because he is frightened (secondary appraisal) about its implications for the child's life. As the parent and child come to understand the condition and its effects on their lives (reappraisal), they decide they will be able to integrate it into their daily routines (reappraisal). In this last example, the father and son come to view (appraise) the condition as a challenge.

Outcome of Coping Appraisals.

Within the context of Lazarus's model, coping is not just a response to something that has happened; it is also an active force in shaping what is happening and what will happen in the future. The way a person appraises a situation influences the coping process and one's emotional reactions. Appraisals are inferred from what a person says. If a family member tells you the patient's chronic condition could jeopardize the family's financial security, it may be inferred that the person has appraised the event as a threat. A parent whose child was having an exacerbation of a chronic illness appraised the situation as a threat and coped by taking the child to the hospital. The child's hospitalization became a new focal stressor with which the family had to cope. In a study of maternal response to the birth of a child with thalidomide defects, Roskies (1972) found that when mothers responded by wanting to see and feed their children, physicians were more likely to tell them their babies were of normal intelligence and to encourage them to take their babies home. For mothers who did not wish to see their infants, physicians were more likely to suggest the child be institutionalized. Roskies concluded that the mother's coping behavior was likely to shape the future course of her child's care. This circular relationship between stressors, coping, and outcome is depicted in Figure 11–2.

Each person has unique motives, belief systems, and competencies to cope with problems that influence interpretation of interactions with the environ-

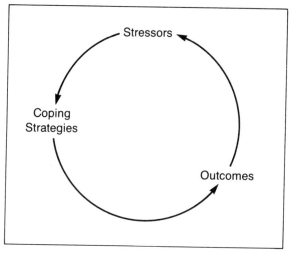

FIGURE 11–2 Circular Relationship Between Stressors, Coping, and Outcome. The arrows indicate that stressors lead to coping strategies, which in turn lead to outcomes that may then become sources of additional stressors.

ment. Coping is any action or belief that modifies some aspect of the appraisal and evaluation process. It is individual and related to one's perception of the stressful event and appraisal of the methods one selects. A person may elect to avoid a situation, confront it, or use self-deceptive activities.

A coping process can attempt to modify the stressor itself, modify the evaluation and appraisal, or change the person's reactions to it. The degree of success of a coping process will depend upon what is to be accomplished. If coping processes are successful, they would reduce the stress in very different ways, depending on the processes used.

Coping as a multidimensional phenomenon Some investigators believe that coping should be conceptualized as a multidimensional behavior or phenomenon (Fleishman, 1984; Pearlin & Schooler, 1978). From this perspective, coping includes a number of types of behaviors; functions at a number of levels; and is accomplished by many different behaviors, cognitions, and perceptions. As yet, there is no clear-cut typology of coping, and those typologies that have been proposed do not distinguish clearly among types of coping. Such distinctions are important because different types may differ in their antecedents and consequences (Fleishman, 1984).

Coping Functions

Coping functions refer to the purposes coping strategies serve for the system. Coping functions can be defined within specific contexts, that is, they are specific for the situation, such as performing a procedure or learning about a diagnosis. Or they can be defined in general terms derived from a theoretical perspective. Lazarus and his colleagues suggest that there are two major functions of coping: (1) managing or changing the problem causing distress (problem-focused) and (2) regulating the emotional response to the problem (emotion-focused). In earlier work, Lazarus (1977) called these functions direct-action (problem-focused) and palliative (emotion-focused) strategies. Box 11–1 illustrates these coping strategies as used by patients on dialysis.

Although both types of coping eventually relieve stress, attempts to cope with difficult situations are not always successful. People may be unsuccessful in coping if they find they are unable to eliminate, or even reduce, the threat, and they give up their efforts to achieve goals that are hindered by the stressor (Carver & Scheier, 1985). Although both types of coping can occur in relation to the same stressful event, problem-focused coping is generally used in situations where people believe that something can be done to change the situation.

Problem-Focused Coping

Problem-focused coping refers to actions taken to remove or alleviate the source of stress. These strat-

---

Box 11–1 Coping Strategies Used by Patients on Dialysis

The coping strategies used most often in a study of patients on hemodialysis were prayer, maintaining control, acceptance, and hope. Both affective (emotion-focused) and problem-focused coping were related significantly to psychosocial stressors, while only affective coping was related to physiological stressors. Problem-oriented strategies were used significantly more than affective-oriented ones. Patients coped with uncertainty by taking one day at a time.

Source: Gurklis & Menke, 1988.

egies are similar to those used for solving problems. They may be directed toward altering environmental stressors (pressures, barriers, resources, procedures) or internal stressors (changing levels of aspiration, decreasing ego involvement, learning new skills or procedures). It has been suggested that these strategies are used more often when a positive change is expected (Scheier, Weintraub, & Carver, 1986). See Table 11–2 for some statements of problem-focused strategies. For example, a 55-year-old firefighter who had a heart attack and decided to take early retirement and a concert pianist who developed arthritis and eventually became a music teacher both used problem-focused coping strategies. Changing one's level of aspiration is not easy but does allow coping with the current stressor. A woman whose 58-year-old mother required daily radiation therapy treatments but did not drive solved the transportation problem by forming a car pool. A 32-year-old woman recently diagnosed with multiple sclerosis searched the library for information to facilitate an understanding of her initially vague symptoms.

Ayers (1989) identified two dimensions of coping to relieve problems, both related to the source of assistance to be provided and the focus of the coping strategy used. Sources may be natural (oneself or persons in one's social network) or supplemental, that is, from outside the social circle (e.g., peer sup-

port groups). Focus may be individual, that is, on helping oneself with minimal assistance from others, or interpersonal, on seeking assistance through the actions of others.

Emotion-Focused Coping

Emotion-focused coping refers to attempts to reduce or eliminate the emotional distress associated with the stressful event, that is, to make the person feel better. Emotion-focused coping can either facilitate or inhibit problem-focused coping. Emotion-focused coping is likely to be used when people believe they cannot change the situation and must endure it. There is also evidence that these strategies are used by people who expect the outcome of the event to be unfavorable. They tend to focus on their negative expectations and on the subjective (emotional) distress associated with the stressors.

Emotion-focused coping is a broad category with several subcategories. The strategies are cognitive processes to lessen emotional distress, change the meaning of the distress, or increase emotional distress. Some people may increase their distress because they need to feel worse before they can feel better, or because they may need to "psych" themselves up before they are mobilized to action. Strategies that change the meaning of the situation without changing it objectively are cognitive reappraisals. It does not matter whether these reappraisals are based on a realistic interpretation of cues or on a distortion of reality. Certain forms of emotion-focused coping strategies are reappraisals while others are not, or they may be appraisals at one time but not at another. People use emotion-focused strategies to maintain hope and optimism, deny both fact and implication, or refuse to acknowledge the worst. Deception can be successful only if it is unconscious; people cannot deceive themselves and simultaneously be aware that they are doing so. Specific emotion-focused coping strategies are listed in Table 11–3.

Table 11–2 Problem-Focused Coping Strategies to Remove or Alleviate Stress

Sources of Stress	Coping Strategies
External	Alter external environment Remove pressure Remove barriers Gather resources
Internal	Alter internal environment Change level of aspiration Decrease ego involvement Learn new skills
Internal or external	Disregard problem Find distraction in some other interest Seek contact with others Actively gather relevant information

Source: Scheier, Weintraub, & Carver, 1986.

Mediators Influencing Coping Strategies

Psychosocial responses to illness are largely subjective. Therefore, people who face similar stressors may cope with them in different ways that lead to different outcomes. Multiple coping strategies may be used at varying levels of awareness as people at-

Table 11–3 Emotion-Focused Coping Strategies

To lessen emotional distress
  Avoidance
  Minimization
  Distancing
  Selective attention
  Positive comparisons
  Wresting positive value from negative events

Change meaning of situation (reappraisal)
  Decide more important things to worry about
  Consider how much worse things can be

Other (may or may not lead to reappraisal)
  Engage in physical exercise to get mind off
    problem
  Meditating
  Having a drink
  Venting anger
  Seeking emotional support

Strategies aimed at increasing emotional distress
  Self-blame
  Self-punishment

Source: Lazarus & Folkman, 1984, pp. 150–151.

tempt to accomplish their developmental and situational tasks. The strategies used reflect the system's developmental history, the circumstances surrounding the illness event, and the cultural influences that play a role in defining preferred strategies (Hamburg, 1982). According to Barofsky (1981), two sets of factors influence the coping strategies people use. The first set includes sociodemographic or personal characteristics such as age, sex, education, income, temperament, personality, and previous ways of coping with stressors. These are the same as the identifying characteristics of the Contingency Model of Long-Term Care. Commitment and beliefs are other individual factors that influence cognitive appraisal. Commitment defines what is meaningful or important for a person and serves as a motive for behavior. Beliefs are personally formed notions and meanings an individual has about the environment (Lazarus & Folkman, 1984). These identifying characteristics and orientations to life were discussed more fully in previous chapters.

The second set of variables influencing coping are aspects of the stress-producing situation itself, such as the stage of the person's chronic disease. Appraisal of potential stressors and coping strategies are also affected by a person's access to environmental resources, such as social, economic, educational, or other important resources (Lazarus, 1980). Additional situational factors influencing cognitive appraisal are novelty, predictability, event uncertainty, and temporal factors (imminence, duration, uncertainty, ambiguity, timing). For example, a young boy paralyzed by a bullet was told he would be confined to a wheelchair for the rest of his life. His initial response, "Oh boy, I always wanted to ride in a wheelchair," was related to the novelty of the situation. With time the boy asked, "When will I be able to walk?"

Family Relationships and Support

Communication and cooperation within the family are important in enhancing one's ability to cope with a chronic condition and in reducing family stress. Family adjustment and intimacy are enhanced by communication around religious affairs, philosophy of life, friends, in-laws, finances, and recreation. Also contributing to adjustment are joint decision making, division of household tasks, and leisure interests and activities.

Parents form the executive unit in directing family functions and determining the emotional environment. Their role is crucial in establishing how the family unit will handle the crisis (Minuchin, 1974). Parental agreement on a philosophy of child rearing is considered valuable for effective coping. According to Rubinstein (1984), parents who do not have a philosophy or who do not agree on a philosophy seem to have more difficulty coping with their child's condition. A significant variable in determining family ability to cope in a positive way with stressors imposed by a childhood chronic condition is a mutually supportive marital relationship (Fife, 1978; Howarth, 1972). Unfortunately parents often cope with the condition by failing to take time to meet their own individual or relationship needs. In fact, Hymovich and Baker (1985) found that the majority of 161 parents of children with cystic fibrosis did not believe it was necessary to take care of their own needs before those of their children.

In families of children with cancer, communication was found to be related to child happiness, closeness to parents, and a nondefensive family atmosphere (Spinetta & Maloney, 1978). It appears from current research, that open communication with children about parental chronic illness also facilitates family closeness (Hymovich, 1990). Studies of children with fatal illnesses revealed that protecting the child and concealing the severity of the condition seems to intensify feelings of loneliness and anxiety. On the other hand, freedom in communication relieves children of feelings of isolation and abandonment and promotes relationships in which sharing and mutual support can take place (Share, 1972).

Patterson and McCubbin (1983) identified coping patterns used by parents of children with cystic fibrosis, cerebral palsy, and myelomeningocele. One pattern was to maintain family integration, cooperation, and an optimistic definition of the situation. Mothers tended to use strategies that focused on the interpersonal dimensions of family life (expressiveness, cohesion). The strategies used by the fathers complemented those of the mothers in facilitating family cohesiveness. Fathers also supported the system-maintenance dimensions of family life by maintaining organization with rules and procedures. Over 90% of the mothers of children with long-term tracheostomies reported sharing problems with their spouse (Singer & Farkas, 1989).

Walker (1988) identified coping strategies used by siblings of children with cancer and has begun to develop a taxonomy of sibling coping. She suggested two major domains of coping activities (cognitive and behavioral), 12 themes (e.g., processing information, seeking support, escaping, soothing self), and 33 categories of coping. Her findings appear in Box 11–2. She discovered less than 50% agreement between parent and child perceptions of these strategies. In another study, chronically ill children and their siblings indicated they used the following strategies to modify their environment, relationships, and life-styles: refusing, complaining, moving, stealing, fighting, locking one's door, and making money (Hymovich, 1984).

Age

The manner in which coping changes with age is controversial. Some research supports the notion that people become more passive with age, while other studies indicate that people become more realistic and effective. Lazarus and Folkman (1984) conclude their review of the changing nature of coping with age by saying that "as sources of stress

> **Box 11–2   Coping Strategies Used by Siblings of Children with Cancer**
>
> Walker (1988) studied siblings of children with cancer. She identified three domains of sibling cognitive coping strategies and two domains of behavioral coping strategies. The cognitive strategies were (1) intrapsychic, either deliberate (thought stopping, wishful thinking) or subconscious (denial), (2) interpersonal, either supportive (talking or being with others) or substitute (lost relationship), and (3) intellectual, either seeking information (media, school projects) or processing information (analyzing, learning). The behavioral domains were (1) self-focusing, either attention-seeking (being nice, acting out), or self-soothing (repetitive actions, eating), (2) distraction, either solitary (play alone) or group (quiet or strenuous activities), and (3) exclusion in the form of time out (quiet place) or escape (special place).

Source: Walker, 1988.

change with stage of life, coping will change in response" (p. 172). Neugarten (1979) suggested that traditional views of psychologic health are not applicable to the elderly population who develop different processes of coping. For example, the combativeness of the elderly may become an asset to survival.

Variables mediating a child's coping strategies include temperament, age, previous experiences with stress and coping (also related to age and developmental level), mobility, cognitive level, and support system. Other variables important to coping include speed of orientation, ability to establish social relations, amount of autonomy, capacity to use help, cooperation with authority, and feelings about self (Heider, 1966; Moriarty, 1961). Coping strategies change as the youngster's cognitive, motor, and social skills develop.

Even young infants have the capacity to control stressful events through self-regulation (Murphy & Moriarty, 1976, p. 72). The ability to cope with threatening situations is present at birth and has been demonstrated in infants as young as 2 days (Brazelton, 1973). At this age, infants can shut out sound, withdraw from painful stimuli, respond to being uncovered or undressed, and console themselves. Coping behaviors in infancy are mainly through motor activity that is either impulsive, to release tensions, or goal directed. The amount, intensity, tempo, and quality of incoming stimuli can be controlled somewhat by the infant's narrowing focus and by concentrating on only one area while ignoring the rest. This self-regulation may break down in situations of acute anxiety or severe threat. A basic task of the infant is to manage stimuli by (1) evoking enough and sufficient stimuli, (2) protecting against excessive or painful stimulation, and (3) selecting stimuli needed for gratification (Murphy, 1974). Some infant tension-releasing strategies are crying, fussing, thumb sucking, and crib rocking. The first two strategies tend to bring help to the infant, whereas the latter two provide pleasurable sensory gratification for the baby.

By 6 to 8 months, infants develop coping activities to help them deal with anxiety related to strangers. They either withdraw or use elaborate ways to increase contact, usually with the mother, by turning or moving toward her, clutching her leg, or climbing into her lap.

Time

Many studies have identified phases or stages, each with different coping strategies, throughout the course of an illness. In an early study of severely burned adults, Hamburg and Adams (1967) concluded that although there was considerable variation in individual coping, a general sequence was present for all. During the acute initial phase, attempts to minimize the impact of the event included the use of extensive denial about the nature and seriousness of the condition and its likely consequences. Patients gradually sought information about factors relevant to their recovery and assessed probable long-term effects. During this time, periods of depression were observed as they faced the reality of the condition. Some form of meaningful group membership was important in the resolution of problems. People most helpful in the problem-solving efforts were other patients on the ward, some staff, the family, and some community people, such as close friends.

Early studies of parents of children with leukemia suggested three phases of parental adaptation. These studies of parents were related to coping with the death or impending death of children with malignant diseases (Chodoff, Friedman, & Hamburg, 1964; Friedman, Chodoff, Mason, & Hamburg, 1963; Knudsen & Natterson, 1960). The first phase included disbelief and denial, expression of anger and bitterness, disregard for needs of other family members, and concentration on satisfying immediate personal needs. In the intermediate phase, parents tried to integrate the meaning of the crisis into their lives and accept its reality. They could deal with concrete problems unrelated to the child and do what was necessary for their child. In the final stage, that of the child's relapse, parents reacted with intensified emotion and finally were able to engage in anticipatory grieving.

Stewart and Sullivan (1982) identified three stages, each with different coping strategies, experienced by patients with multiple sclerosis (MS). During the nonserious phase, 85% of the patients interpreted their symptoms as nonserious and attributed them to (1) ailments that were not illnesses but slight changes in physical status caused by nonmedical conditions, personal situations such as overwork or social stress, personal limitations such as an "innately weak constitution," poor personal health (out of shape or run down), or getting older; (2) minor illnesses such as arthritis, poor circulation, or anemia; or (3) side effects of other illnesses, such as hypertension or injuries. They responded to most of these ailments and minor illnesses by home treatments or a combination of home treatment and consulting a physician. During this period their physicians either supported their self-diagnosis or found nothing physically wrong.

During the serious phase, the 60 study participants consulted 227 different physicians and had a total of 407 diagnostic appointments plus appointments for follow-up treatments and tests. Because treatments were not effective, patients quickly lost faith in their doctors and moved on to others. Patients played an increasingly active role in their therapeutic relationships with their physicians; either they returned to the same physician for further action after initial misdiagnosis and treatment, or they searched for a new physician. They also tried self-diagnosis by reading popular and scientific medical books and consulting with friends and relatives in the medical and nursing professions. As this phase progressed, changes in relationships with family and friends occurred for two thirds of the patients. They began to discuss their symptoms less frequently as the phase progressed. They assumed everyone was tired of hearing about them, and they felt they received less support from them over the course of this phase. These patients were

> in a very ambiguous situation in which they were unable to accomplish social consensus and an integrated role structure. They were pushed, on the one hand, by the increasing seriousness and discomfort of their symptoms toward an effort to adopt the sick role. They were prevented from successfully adopting the sick role, on the other hand, by their diagnostic uncertainties, the refusal of physicians to legitimize their sick role adoption and negative reactions of relatives and friends. (Stewart & Sullivan, 1982, p. 1402)

The outcome of this ambiguity for over half the patients was abnormal emotional conflict and tension, with feelings of frustration, worry, anxiety, moodiness, irritability, and intermittent depression. Less frequent problems (1% to 13%) were social withdrawal, sleep difficulties, weight loss over 30 pounds, regressive behavior, mental confusion and memory loss, increased alcohol consumption, suicidal thoughts, and stomach aches.

Eventually, physicians began to suspect something serious. Most patients were then hospitalized for about 3 weeks for diagnostic tests and within 6 months they had a definitive diagnosis of MS. Nearly all patients reported a decrease in stress during the diagnostic phase and reported being more relieved than upset by the diagnosis. Their positive response to the diagnosis was attributed to pleasure at having a name for their symptoms; receiving greater support from friends, relatives, and physicians; and being relieved to know they were not going to die if that threat had been a concern. In addition they felt encouraged about the future course of the illness, mainly because of "unrealistic optimism" on the part of their physicians.

Coping and Chronic Conditions

The way people cope with illness in general and with specific medical procedures may affect their recovery (Cohen & Lazarus, 1979). People who refuse to be passive patients often have difficulty in adjusting to hospitals. On the other hand, the same people are likely to show better long-term rehabilitation after a serious condition than do patients who accept the sick role (Elliott & Eisdorfer, 1982). In diseases like chronic obstructive pulmonary disease or asthma, expressing emotion can exacerbate respiratory symptoms and hasten decompensation. At the same time, it may attract the attention of physicians to medical problems, resulting in increased treatment efforts that may prolong survival, suggesting the likelihood that "the squeaky wheel gets greased."

Various lists of coping strategies have been proposed (e.g., Pearlin & Schooler, 1978; Sidle et al, 1969; Weisman, 1974; Weisman & Worden, 1976–1977). Mages & Mendelsohn (1979) reduced some of these lists to three broad categories: (1) techniques designed to minimize stress, (2) activities that attempt to deal with specific issues, and (3) activities that involve others. Techniques to deal with distress may involve efforts to avoid certain situations or feelings, to control events, and to detach oneself from potentially upsetting situations. Efforts to deal with specific issues may include seeking information, participating in decision making, or learning new skills to compensate for lost functions. Others with whom one may become involved include the person's family and friends or self-help groups.

Lazarus (1982) identified four main coping modes that can serve either problem-focused or emotion-focused functions. These four modes are information seeking, direct action, inhibition of action, and intrapsychic processes. Hymovich (1984) identified seven categories of coping strategies used by parents of chronically ill children: (1) seeking information and resources, (2) utilizing information and resources, (3) managing stressors, (4) modifying strategies, (5) anticipatory planning, (6) educating others, and (7) helping and supporting others.

Coping strategies are a set of behaviors used under stress in an attempt to improve the situation. Coping styles are the manner in which the person generally responds to stressors. Coping styles described by various investigators can be divided into three categories: approach, nonspecific defenders, and avoidance that occur along a continuum (Cohen & Lazarus, 1973; Miller, 1983). This continuum is depicted in Figure 11–3. People who practice avoidance use repression, denial, projection, and any strategy that minimizes the seriousness of the threat. Intellectual strategies like selective inattention, ignoring, and rationalizing are other avoidance strategies. Approach behaviors include talking, vigilant focusing, and sensitizing. Vigilant focusing refers to an obsessional alertness and compulsive attention to

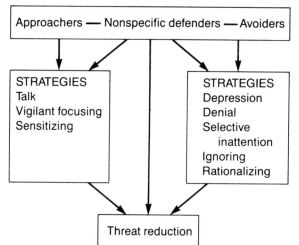

FIGURE 11—3 Three Categories of Coping Styles
Source: Modified from Miller, 1983, p. 25.

details. These are the people who need detailed explanations of their condition and therapy. They clearly have anxiety, readily acknowledge threatening emotions of hate, fear, and disgust, and directly confront their emotional states. The nonspecific defenders, or neutrals, use a combination of approach and avoidance strategies.

Managing the Condition

Strategies for managing chronic conditions fall into five broad categories: seeking and using information, performing skills, seeking and using resources, monitoring, and incorporating the condition into family life-style. These categories and their subcategories are described below and listed in Table 11—4.

Table 11—4 Categories and Subcategories of Managing the Condition

Seeking information	Incorporating the condition
Performing skills	into family life-style
Seeking and using	Changing location
resources	Modifying dietary
Monitoring and	patterns
self-monitoring	Maintaining normalcy
Adhering to	Modifying roles
therapy	Modifying the environment

Seeking information The amount and type of information people want about their own or their family member's chronic condition vary with one's coping style and the context of the situation. Patients and family members generally want information that is of primary importance to them at the time (Forsyth, Delaney, & Gresham, 1984). The patient in pain wants information about pain relief, and the parent about to administer insulin to a child wants to know how to perform the procedure properly. Hymovich (1981) identified seeking and using information as a major strategy of parents of chronically ill children.

Lenz (1984) suggests six steps in the search for information: (1) presence of a stimulus, (2) goal setting, (3) a decision regarding whether to seek information actively, (4) search behavior, (5) information acquisition and codification, and (6) a decision regarding the adequacy of the information. Information may be sought through personal or impersonal methods. Impersonal information is sought from an inanimate source, such as publications, referral sources, or someone unknown to the person. Major impersonal sources of self-help information are the popular media (newspapers, magazines, television, books, and video- or audiotapes). Unfortunately, some of the information patients read may be inaccurate or misinterpreted. Consequently, it behooves nurses to determine what their patients or families are reading and to clarify when necessary.

The personal method of obtaining information is from an individual known to the person. Studies of health-related information seeking suggest that the personal method is preferred over the impersonal method (Lenz, 1984). Huag and Lavin (1983) report trial and error as the most common pattern of learning for persons with chronic conditions. In one study, family members who reported learning new skills by trial and error reported the greatest dissatisfaction with that method of learning (Grobe, Illstrub, & Ahmann, 1981).

Children obtain information by watching television; talking with parents, siblings, and peers; asking questions; observing; going to church; and looking at pictures (Hymovich, 1984; Pelletier, 1981). When hospitalized, children seek information about their bodies (intrusions, mutilation, sensations, and functioning) and about their environment (Pelletier, 1981).

A study of the preferred source of information of 11- to 20-year-old adolescents was reported by

Levenson et al (1982). Sixty-eight percent of these youngsters preferred private discussions, primarily with their physicians. Another 68% wanted their parents included in the discussions. Patients under age 15 years were likely to prefer information from their parents only. Newly diagnosed patients and those in relapse preferred to avoid group discussions and did not want friends to receive additional information. Also it was found that the information needs of Hispanic adolescents were not being met adequately, which was attributed to the language barrier and difficulties in using the health care system.

Caty, Ellerton, and Ritchie (1984) reviewed 39 articles describing the coping behaviors of hospitalized children between the ages of 20 months and 10 years. Their classification of coping strategies is similar to Lazarus' four modes of coping. Caty et al's classification was information exchange (giving and seeking information), action/inaction, and intrapsychic. Information-exchange behaviors increased with age, with preschoolers giving more information and older children seeking more information.

Performing skills   Skills needed to manage the condition are learned through experience. The more quickly people can apply these skills or coping strategies automatically, the more effectively and efficiently they can manage or adapt to the environment. Some of the skills needed include manipulating a wheelchair; suctioning; administering insulin; and recognizing the signs and symptoms of an insulin reaction. Early stages of skill acquisition require enormous effort and concentration, whereas in later stages skills have become automatic (Lazarus & Folkman, 1984). Transition from effort-intensive to automatic is gradual. Once a skill has become automatic, it can no longer be considered coping because it no longer taxes or exceeds the person's usual available resources.

Children can become increasingly involved in self-care endeavors as they develop, thus providing themselves with increasing opportunities to participate in normal activities without needing adult intervention. Children's actions to manage stressors include specific actions to manage their condition, such as helping with postural drainage, giving their own insulin, and taking pills. Parental management of the disease includes strategies the children may be too young or ill to do for themselves, including giving medications, performing treatments (e.g., postural drainage), providing appropriate nutrition, and preventing complications.

Seeking and using resources   Studies based on data from the Health Belief Model indicate that prevention and detection as well as diagnostic and treatment services are most often used by younger or middle-aged white females who have better-than-average education and income. Mental health and social service services were found to be utilized by about only one quarter of children with chronic health problems and psychiatric disorders (Cadman et al, 1987).

Hymovich (1981) identified seeking and using support services as a major parental coping strategy. The services sought and used included health care (e.g., consulting with specialists), financial assistance (e.g., getting the drug store to reduce prices because patient buys frequently and in quantity); and material resources (sheepskin and clothes that snap). Support services included baby sitting and organizational support (e.g., joining groups or forming groups if unavailable). In addition, the parents were actively involved in finding programs for their children (e.g., home stimulation, day care) and seeking to alter public policy related to their children's needs.

Family and friends are important resources for support. People are likely to turn to family and friends for advice, reassurance, and other kinds of support, rather than to professional service organizations (Gourash, 1978).

Monitoring and self-monitoring   "Self-monitoring is a necessary part of self-care" (Tobin et al., 1986). Self-monitoring involves assessment methods whereby the person observes and records his or her own behavior or physiological condition. The same strategies can be used by parents caring for (monitoring) their chronically ill youngsters and by care givers of adults unable to care for themselves, although in these instances self-monitoring becomes monitoring. Monitoring strategies include checking blood glucose levels, blood pressure, weight, or symptoms; observing environmental stimuli that precipitate the onset of symptoms or increased risk factors associated with health problems; using cognitive processes that guide self-care behaviors, such as self-instruction; and behaviors that reduce risk factors (e.g., removing food from house) and manage symptoms (e.g., muscle relaxation to reduce pain).

Self-monitoring may serve a number of purposes for the patient. For example, Miller, Summerton, and Brody (1988) found that monitoring was initiated to reduce uncertainty and its accompanying arousal rather than for controlling actions. However, Braden (1990) found that monitoring was significantly related to enabling skills for patients who attended self-help classes but not for those who did not attend them.

In collaboration with the nurse or physician patients can begin to recognize the effect of their behavior on various symptoms, such as the effect of diet and exercise on glucose levels or the effect of stressful situations on blood pressure. Monitoring has advantages, such as learning more about one's disease, as well as disadvantages, such as an exaggerated concern about bodily functions (urine, blood, bowel movements). Some research suggests that self-monitoring strategies are effective for increasing adherence to regimens, whereas other studies show no effect (Johnson et al, 1986; Kirscht & Rosenstock, 1979).

Adhering to therapy.

Many factors have been studied in relation to a person's adherence behaviors (Kirscht & Rosenstock, 1979). Among them are personality (e.g., locus of control) and social characteristics (e.g., age, sex, educational level), neither of which has been found very helpful for predicting adherence to a regimen. Studies of general knowledge of the medical condition have shown inconsistent findings regarding adherence. However, as the patient's knowledge increases with respect to required behavior, frequency and time to perform it, the more likely becomes the person's adherence to it.

Generally the more complex the regimen and the longer its duration, the less likely is the person to follow through. Adherence to one aspect of the regimen is not likely to be related to performance of another. For example, failure to keep appointments may show little association with failure to take medications. Also, adhering to one aspect of a diabetic regimen does not preclude adhering to other aspects (Johnson et al, 1986). Therefore, health care providers need to be careful about generalizing from one aspect of the patient's behavior to others (the notion of spread). There is increasing evidence that social support and family stability are positively associated with adherence to medical regimens.

Illness behavior has three components (Mechanic, 1986): (1) attention to physical symptoms, (2) processes affecting how symptoms are defined and accorded significance, and (3) extent to which help is sought, life routine is interrupted, and so forth. People differ in their sensitivity to symptoms,

in the likelihood of defining them as serious when they are present, and in the frequency with which they seek medical assistance. It also has been shown that cultural differences exist in the way bodily symptoms such as pain are interpreted and presented (Zborowski, 1952). People of Irish descent describe symptoms with calm restraint, whereas those of Italian descent give vividly dramatic descriptions (Zola, 1966).

Compliance has been defined as "the extent to which a person's behavior (in terms of taking medication, following diets, or executing lifestyle changes) coincides with medical advice" (Haynes, 1979, cited in Cromer & Tarnowski, 1989, p. 207). Ability to predict one's own level of compliance and previous history of compliance have been reported to be reliable predictors of future compliance (Cromer & Tarnowski, 1989). Quality of patient-physician relationship (Haynes, Taylor, Sackett, 1980; Jones & Caldwell, 1981) and cultural differences between patient and physician (Kleinman, 1978) also contribute to patient compliance.

The average level of compliance in children, adolescents, and adults has been estimated at 50%, with a range between 10% and 80% in the pediatric population, depending on the disease, its treatment, characteristics of the study sample, definition of compliance, and methods of measurement (Dunbar, 1983). There is some evidence that adolescents are less compliant than younger children (Jacobson, Hauser, Wolfsdorf et al, 1987; Pidgeon, 1989; Tebbi et al, 1986). Studies of adolescents with asthma (Spector, 1985), juvenile diabetes (Wilson & Endres 1986), scoliosis (Eliason & Richman, 1984), juvenile rheumatoid arthritis (Litt & Cuskey, 1981), and obesity (Harris, Sutton, Kauffman et al, 1980; McClaran, 1983) report noncompliance rates ranging from 40% to 55%. Family characteristics and the patient's locus of control and previous history of compliance have been associated with adolescent adherence. Poor communication and dysfunctional interaction have been consistently associated with poor compliance in adolescents with chronic disorders including renal transplants (Korsch, Fine, & Negrete, 1978), diabetes (Babrow, Ruskin, & Siller, 1985), and seizure disorders (Friedman, Litt, & King, 1986).

Johnson and colleagues (1986) measured 13 aspects of adherence to a child's diabetic regimen. They found daily diabetes management was influenced by the youngster's age, with adolescents significantly less adherent on eight of the measures than were younger children. Adolescents ate, monitored their glucose, and exercised less often than those who were younger. They also had more variable injection times, deviated more from the ideal intervals, and often took their injections with or following meals. These findings were consistent with those of Christensen et al (1983).

Families play an important role in patient adherence to therapy. Clear and direct communication and exchange of information were found to be associated with families of patients following stroke who adhered to their therapy (Evans et al, 1987). Among the family variables associated with compliance in school-age children and adolescents were family harmony, interaction, and support.

Incorporating the condition into family life-style　Life-style modifications are frequently necessitated by the presence of a chronic condition in a family. These modifications take many forms and vary in degree, and at times, family life may become organized around the needs of the affected family member. The entire family system is involved in incorporating the condition into their life-style. The process involves the individual members of the system as well as the family as a unit and may include modifying roles, relationships, dietary patterns, work hours, and vacation plans. Making modifications are strategies to alter conditions or situations affecting family functioning. Fagerhaugh (1975) described how people with emphysema coped by changing their life-style and daily schedule to conserve their energy. Examples of modifying the environment include fixing up a camper to accommodate a mist tent, moving to a ranch house, and remodeling the home. Modifying family life-style includes obtaining knowledge and skill for continuing care; maintaining a sense of normalcy by trying to preserve usual patterns or taking a chance and letting the child participate in family activities; hiding or minimizing the condition; living normally despite therapy and symptoms; giving up activities, such as camping; and modifying the daily routine.

Parents of a chronically ill child may have to change their own or their child's behavior, alter expectations of their child, and modify their values, attitudes, and beliefs. Knafl (1982) reported that parents perceive their healthy children as adjusting well to a sibling's condition and hospitalization unless they had to change routines or care givers drastically. With major changes, healthy siblings do not adjust so well. Cooper (1984) identified coping strat-

---

> **Box 11–3　*Coping Strategies Used by Female Spouses***
>
> In a study of 15 wives of men with lung cancer, Cooper (1984) found that spouses voluntarily limit their activities to only those husband or wife can tolerate. They spend progressively less time maintaining social ties, thereby reducing their circle of friends. This leads to increasing isolation from support systems. In addition, there is loss of freedom, relinquishing of recreational and social activities and spending more time in the house for longer hours. Shopping trips are timed because the spouse worries when away. Some spouses assumed new roles and responsibilities, obtained jobs, or continued to work longer than they had planned to because of decreased family income.

Source: Cooper, 1984.

egies used by wives of men with lung cancer to modify their life-style. A summary of this study is in Box 11–3.

Managing Time.

The symptoms of a chronic condition and their treatment interfere with the patient's time schedule and often with that of the entire family. Symptoms and treatments complicate time management "because they consume time, preempt time, and interfere with the structuring of time" (Reif, 1975, p. 83). People with chronic conditions and their families must figure out how to manage symptoms and treatment so that the least amount of available time is used and time is left for other activities.

Time-conserving tactics include budgeting time for treatment; routinizing and streamlining condition-related activities (e.g., using time- and labor-saving devices, storing everything in one place, and omitting selected aspects of the regimen); and "piggybacking" normal activities onto those related to the disease, such as reading during rest periods. Scheduling strategies include monitoring the condition so that disease-related, social, and occupational activities can be planned, and working with family and friends so that last minute changes in social activities can be made. Some people have worked out a buddy system so that the buddy can take over if necessary. Another scheduling strategy is to regulate or delay treatments to coordinate them with a conventional social and occupational schedule (Reif, 1975).

Changing location.

Chronic conditions may necessitate moving elsewhere either because someone must change occupation or because the family needs to be near hospital and treatment facilities. In some cases, the decision to move the entire family, temporarily or permanently, is made to avoid long separations.

Modifying dietary patterns.

Many conditions require dietary modifications, and families may cope by changing the dietary pattern of the whole family (Anderson, 1981). The entire family, or at least those responsible for grocery shopping and meal planning and preparation, should be educated about the diet restrictions.

Maintaining normalcy.

Normalization is a term to describe the response of the family to negate illness or abnormal behavior in order to maintain valued social roles. The concept has been associated with patients with mental illness (Schwartz, 1957), polio (Davis, 1963), thalidomide malformation (Roskies, 1972), and disability or retardation (Birenbaum, 1970). Normalization allows the family to acknowledge the abnormality while denying its social significance (Knafl & Deatrick, 1986). Families use various strategies to convey an impression of normalcy to others. Such strategies include minimizing abnormalities in physical appearance, participating in usual activities, maintaining usual social ties, limiting contacts with those in similar circumstances, avoiding embarrassing situations, and controlling information. It is assumed that normalization is good, but this area has not been fully explored.

Coping strategies to normalize life-style are developed in an attempt to make the experience of the condition as much a part of everyday life as possible. These strategies help to deemphasize family vulnerability and emphasize the development and use of personal strengths (Anderson, 1981; Knafl & Deatrick, 1990). Normalization comes, in part, when the condition becomes peripheral and is no longer the central organizing theme in the person's life (Mechanic, 1986). Therefore, it may not be possible in some situations. Anderson (1981) provides an excellent example of how a parent attempted to normalize the insulin injections her child would need.

I said, 'You must brush your teeth every morning, and he said 'ya' and I said, 'Why do you brush your teeth every morning?' and he says, 'To keep them healthy.' So I said, 'From now on you're going to have a needle every morning to keep your body healthy and that's the way it's going to be, let's not make any fuss about it . . .' (p. 429)

A mother with cancer tried to normalize her crying for her children. She explained to them that she needed to cry sometimes just as they did.

Parents are likely to face a double bind: They have their own conceptions of normality, yet their child's life cannot be normal. Parents may give their child two different messages: one that the child is well and normal, the other that the child is not well and different. Bateson's double-bind theory is analogous (Bateson et al, 1956) to this. The person in a double-bind situation must choose between two alternatives, neither of which is completely satisfactory, and leaving the situation is not allowed. Inconsistencies are likely to exist between the normalization process and everyday practices. For example, a parent may keep a child home to prevent infection during the flu season rather than send the child to school and risk getting the flu.

"Although parents might present their child as 'just an ordinary child,' and endeavor to normalize their child's everyday experiences, social reality for the sick child must of necessity be different from that of the 'well' child . . . Two different world views are constructed . . ." (Anderson, 1981, p. 432). For example, play for the sick child might emphasize cognitive skills while for healthy children it might emphasize cognitive, physical, and social skills.

Normalization or minimization is also a strategy adults use with chronic obstructive pulmonary disease (COPD) (Chalmers, 1984). Thorne (1985) interviewed eight chronically ill persons and their spouses or partners. Although these families admitted that living with the disease had its ups and downs, and had caused changes in their emotional state, roles, communications, and social lives, they maintained a positive attitude and adapted by maintaining normalcy and personal dignity.

Aspects of self-care pertinent to chronically ill and disabled youngsters need to take into account the importance of household responsibilities. Healthy adolescents normally have household chores, but Hayden and colleagues (1979) report that only 50% of adolescents with spina bifida participate in household chores. Blum (1983) notes that assignment of home chores to youngsters with cerebral palsy was a major way parents conveyed a sense of competence to their disabled children.

Modifying roles.

The presence of a chronic condition may necessitate role changes for all or some family members, either temporarily or permanently. Gervasio (1989) notes times when roles should be shifted to alleviate strain for the chronically ill person, but the person refuses to give up the usual role performance.

Parent roles may shift when a child has a chronic condition. For example, Kazak (1986; Kazak & Marvin, 1984) describes how financial stressors experienced in families of chronically ill children may require a division of labor somewhat more pronounced than in families without a handicapped child. In these families the father may become the exclusive breadwinner while the mother manages the care-giving needs.

Modifying the environment.

Modifying the environment involves making alterations in order to facilitate functioning. Environmental manipulations may be minor, such as removing throw rugs or using assistive devices. Sometimes they may involve major modifications such as installing wheelchair ramps, lowering counters, adding an air conditioner, or building a first-floor addition. When modifying the environment is not possible, patients may try to avoid precipitants that are present in the environment (Chalmers, 1984).

Coping with Feelings

As noted in Chapter 10, uncomfortable feelings associated with chronic conditions may be experienced by the patients as well as other family members.

Coping with uncertainty and anxiety   The combination of means for coping with uncertainty and anxiety depends on the characteristics of the patients and their individual situations. If people are available for discussion and answering questions, the person whose usual coping method is to discuss problems (social means) is more likely to follow this tactic than is someone who tends not to discuss personal matters. The approach to problem solving depends on both the person's characteristics and the situation (Folkman & Lazarus, 1980).

Molleman and colleagues (1984) identified four ways in which adults with cancer cope with uncertainty and anxiety: self-instruction, direct action, social means, and ego defense. Self-instruction was the most commonly identified strategy. However, neither self-instruction, direct action, nor social means significantly reduced uncertainty for patients; only help from experts (nurses, physicians) was effective for reducing uncertainty. Contact with partner, family, friends, and other patients was not effective in reducing uncertainty, although it was important for reducing anxiety.

Coping with grief   Lindemann (1944, 1965) described the "grief work" of the normal individual, delineating the intrapsychic tasks of "working through" the loss. The process of coping is evident in the duration of grief work following diagnosis of a chronic condition or loss of a loved one (Lazarus & Folkman, 1984). The initial period is one of shock and disbelief or denial of the traumatic event. Behaviors during this time include activity, crying, struggling to carry on normal activities, and detachment. Eventually there is acceptance of the loss and reengagement. This process may last for a few months or several years. Some of the classic work on the grieving process was done by Lindemann (1944) and Bowlby (1969). The grieving process is often prolonged, and symptoms of grief such as anxiety, somatization, depression, and interpersonal sensitivity may persist for at least 2 years (Miles, 1985; Moore, Gillis, Martinson, 1988). With chronic conditions, it may last longer.

Searching for meaning   When a focal stressor event occurs such as being diagnosed with a chronic condition, there is a threat to one's self-esteem and social value. Taylor (1983) believes adjustment to such threatening events centers around three themes. The first is a search for meaning in the experience. This search involves the need to understand why the event occurred and what the impact has been. According to attribution theory, people will make attributions following a threatening event to understand, predict, and control their environment (Wong & Weiner, 1981). In seeking the meaning of an illness or injury, people try to ascertain the causes. Their formulations shape the meaning of the situation and can open or close options for actively dealing with it or the feelings it evokes. Patients may suffer especially when they interpret their physical status as threatening self-worth. In such cases they become sensitive to criticism or rejection in a manner that interferes with more active and open coping. Such patients need continued support and reassurance that their problems are not reflections on their personal worth. Individuals with a sense of their own coping capacity are more confident and open, setting the stage for successful adaptation (Mechanic, 1986, p. 116).

A major pattern of coping identified for parents of children with cystic fibrosis was "endowing the illness with meaning" (Venters, 1981). This strategy enabled parents to interpret their condition-related difficulties positively rather than negatively and to define the condition within a previously existing religious or medical-scientific philosophy of life. Families who used this coping strategy had a significantly higher level of functioning than those who did not.

Attributing causes and outcomes to chronic conditions People often try to make sense of and control their lives by using causal thinking after an important life event. Engaged in a causal search they often ask, "Why me?" Lowery and her colleagues have been studying causal attributions of chronically ill adults for a number of years. In a recent study, Lowery and Jacobsen (1985) reported that patients with arthritis, diabetes, and hypertension tended to attribute successful outcomes internally, i.e., to their efforts, and failures externally, that is, to task difficulty. Patients doing poorly tended to hold no commitment to any cause for the condition. The authors suggest that factors other than causal attributions may mediate patients' responses to their condition. They do not recommend programs to modify attributions until further research identifies the other factors that may be mediating patients' responses to their condition.

Making downward comparisons Taylor, Lichtman, and Wood (1983) studied how people adjust to threatening events. Many of the mental mechanisms are founded on illusions or social comparisons. Examples of illusions people create are: attributing a cause to their condition when the true cause remains unknown; believing they can control their disease when in fact they cannot; and making up a person worse off than themselves when none exists. These illusions are considered beneficial because they are protective and allow the person to come to terms with information that is difficult to accept, thus allowing psychological adaptation.

To cope with a threatening experience or victimization, people enhance their subjective well-being by comparing themselves to those less fortunate (Affleck et al, 1987; Wills, 1981). They may create hypothetical worst-world scenarios of what could have happened; selectively focus on one aspect of the stressful event and view it in a more favorable light; or manufacture normative standards of adjustment that make their own adjustment appear exceptional (Taylor, Lichtman, & Wood, 1983). In some instances they may speak of the benefits that resulted from the experience. Both the victimization and the appraisal are important in influencing how well a person will function. This process, "downward comparison," is evoked by a situation where frustration or misfortune has occurred and well-being has been decreased. The solution is to compare oneself with another who is worse off, thus enabling the victim to feel better about his or her own situation (see Figure 11–4). This comparison is usually made early in the stages of adaptation and is similar to Lazarus and Folkman's (1984) notion of defensive reappraisal (reinterpreting an event as less damaging or threatening).

Downward comparison has been documented in a number of studies with chronically ill adults, including patients with cancer (Wood, Taylor, & Lichtman, 1985), spinal cord injury (Schultz & Decker, 1985), arthritis (Affleck et al, 1987), COPD (Chalmers, 1984), and mothers of children in an intensive care unit (Affleck et al 1987). Statements expressing downward comparison are in Box 11–4.

Coping with ambiguity A chronic condition tends to put one in an ambiguous state regarding interactions with others. Two strategies are generally used for coping with this ambiguity surrounding one's marginal status (Sussman, 1977). One is confrontation, whereby the person or an organized group of people use defiance to effect change. For example, a 43-year-old man confined to a wheelchair because of severe arthritis volunteered to take charge of the Rhododendron Society's annual show and sale. He announced to the group, "What you see is what you get. If you think you can get anything better, go ahead and try." The group accepted his offer.

A second approach involves a "putting-on" technique. The person who is putting on publicly acknowledges the power, wisdom, and superiority of the other by becoming the "model" client. At the same time, the person privately rejects this state of affairs and works in subtle ways to subvert power and authority. "'Putting-on' is basically accommodation to the realities of power and control in order to

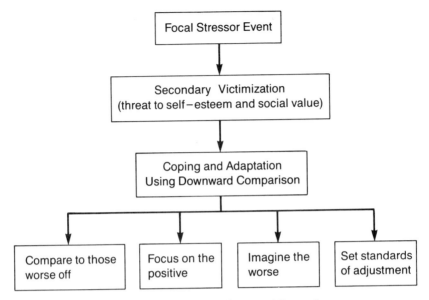

FIGURE 11—4   Coping and Adaptation Using Downward Comparison

---

Box 11—4   *Examples of Downward Comparison Statements*

"I live in the city, but they live 2 hours away."

"I was lucky. I only had to have a lumpectomy and radiation therapy. My neighbor needed a mastectomy and chemotherapy."

"It could have been worse. She could have had brain damage."

---

handle threats to one's self-respect, image, maintenance, and physical and psychological safety. The trick is to 'put on' someone without his knowing it" (Sussman, 1977, p. 251). Putting-on techniques include playing dumb, trying, acting uninterested, selectively hearing and perceiving situations, acting out the disabled roles, and abusing privileges.

"Passing," closely related to putting on, is another technique for moving out of the ambiguous situation (Roberts, 1983). Passing involves not appearing to be different from the dominant group so that one is included with them "by mistake." The notion of marginality is reserved for those who cannot pass because of their physically obvious or revealed characteristics. Marginality refers to adopting enough of the values, attitudes, and behaviors of the dominant group to be conditionally accepted by them as one of the "good ones."

Maintaining hope   Many people with chronic disease must face the reality of a downward physical course. Maintaining hope is one way of coping with this situation and sustaining a system through stressful periods (Skolny & Riehl, 1974). Hope is a temporary coping strategy built on the notion that the future can be better. It helps one come to terms with misfortune and stress and is a defense against despair. A distinction needs to be made between wishing and hoping (Pruyser, 1963). Wishing tends to focus on "specific objects or desirable things" whereas "hoping does not deal with objects at all, but is focused on global or existential conditions" (p. 164).

Hope is defined as a multidimensional construct (Miller & Powers, 1988). The process of hoping involves four cognitive-affective tasks: Reality surveillance, encouragement, worrying, and mourning (Wright & Schontz, 1968). Reality surveillance is a cognitive function that grounds one's hopes in a phenomenal (subjective) reality as opposed to objective reality. As long as the person believes it is reality, it gives one grounds for hoping. Encouragement is the affective component of reality surveillance that occurs when the person finds some reality base for hoping. It serves as a motivator to continue striving, thus sustaining the person's hope. Worrying occurs when uncertainty exists; it forces the person to reexamine reality. When reality is reexamined, the person may find new supports for hoping or may find that hoping has to be abandoned for "wishful expectation," in which even remote possibilities are taken as evidence for continued hope. The final process involved in hoping is mourning. Mourning occurs when the person is forced to relinquish original hopes and prepares the person to reappraise values and accept substitutions for hope. Selected definitions of hope appear in Table 11–5.

McGee (1984) proposed a model of hope-hopelessness as polar opposites with hope and despair as overlapping concepts. In her model, despair causes a loss of hope whereas hopelessness is an extreme state of despair. She also proposes that hope has a component as both a trait and state, similar to the concept of state-trait anxiety of Speilberger (1966). She believes that individuals are predisposed toward either a hopeful or a pessimistic approach to

life (trait). The level of hopefulness at any one time is influenced by the situation variables such as probability of goal achievement, sources of support, and importance of the goal. If one believes a goal can be accomplished, has support, and believes the goal is important, the level of hope increases.

Miller (1983) defined three levels of hope. The first level is elementary and includes superficial wishes. Level two includes hoping for relationships, self-improvement, and self-accomplishments. The third level involves hoping for relief from suffering, personal trial, or entrapment. Hope differs from the intrapsychic activity of wishing. A person wishes something desirable might happen but does not organize personal behavior with the expectation that it must happen. In hope, a person believes that the event must happen (Korner, 1970). For example, a person may hope the symptoms of COPD will get better; however, wishing the COPD would go away is not likely to make that happen.

Hinds and Martin (1988) explored the process through which adolescents with cancer move toward achieving hopefulness. The process consists of four variant phases, each with specific coping strategies. The first phase is cognitive discomfort, a state of mental uneasiness and desire to be relieved of it. Two coping strategies, thought stopping and thought reflection, are associated with this phase.

The second phase, distraction, involves cognitive and behavioral activities to promote concentration on something neutral or positive. Associated coping strategies are (1) doing something, (2) acknowledging that the situation could always be worse, (3) stating they had made it this far, (4) looking forward to normalcy, (5) cognitive clutter (thinking about other things), (6) reminding oneself that God will take care of one, (7) looking back, (8) gaining knowledge of survivors, and (9) finding comfort in knowing that others have hope for them.

Cognitive comfort, the third phase, is the extent to which periods of solace and lifting of spirits are experienced. The two coping strategies used during this period are forgetting about the cancer and hopefulness.

The final phase is personal competence, or the extent to which the adolescents perceive themselves as resilient, resourceful, and adaptable. Coping strategies associated with this phase are commitment to treatment, adaptation to symptoms, and taking care of problems.

A coping strategy of parents that has helped some families includes maintaining hope, optimism,

Table 11–5 Definitions of Hope

Definition	Source
"the expectation greater than zero of achieving a goal"	Stotland, 1969, p. 2
"a temporary measure of relief, a sustaining power in coping with permanent stress"	Korner, 1970, p. 134
"a sense of the possible"	Lynch, 1974, p. 32
"the capacity to anticipate that even though one feels uncomfortable now, one may feel better in the future"	Peretz, 1970, p. 8
"the degree to which a personal tomorrow exists"	Hinds, 1984, p. 360
"subtle, if not unconscious, expectation of an abstract but positive aspect of the future"	Stoner & Keampfer, 1985, p. 269
"a temporary measure of relief, a sustaining power in coping with permanent stress"	Scanlon, 1989, p. 134

faith, courage, and an altruistic view of the situation. This strategy enables parents to find a philosophic or religious framework for understanding the condition (Patterson & McCubbin, 1983).

Using defense mechanisms Investigators differ on the relationship between "defenses" and "coping." Hann (1977) views defense mechanisms as rigid patterns of behavior that distort reality, whereas coping is seen as behavior that is adaptive and oriented to reality. Cohen and Lazarus (1973) believe that the relationship reflects a value judgment on the part of the observer and involves inferences that may not be based on adequate data. They assume that defenses are unconscious mechanisms that are one part of the coping process. It is important to recognize that these mechanisms are attempts to protect oneself from the threat of ego disorganization under the impact of the condition, and that they are not likely to be used in isolation from other coping strategies (Mailick, 1984). Discussion of some common defense mechanisms follows.

Denial.

Denial is a defense mechanism adults and children use to avoid anxiety resulting from inner conflict and external stress (Kaplan, Freedman, & Sarock, 1980). It is the subconscious blocking out of emotional experiences. The outcome of denial as a coping strategy may be positive or negative. Some studies that show people who deny or avoid threats are worse off than those who deal with them; other studies suggest that denial is associated with positive outcomes. Denial or avoidance can lead to ineffective consequences if the person fails to engage in appropriate problem-focused coping to decrease the actual danger or damage from the condition (e.g., failing to seek medical attention or adhere to medical regimen). Weisman (1974) differentiates between denial of fact and denial of implication; for example, it may be more dangerous to deny the fact that one has cystic fibrosis than to deny the implication that this implies an early death. Denial of implication may be similar to illusion, positive thinking, or hopefulness. Denial can be constructive when it provides temporary protection from a threatening event or unpleasant reality until the person is ready to cope with it. Denial can be harmful or destructive when it interferes with ability to take steps to ensure health; for example, a man with hypertension may take antihypertensive drugs to control his blood pressure, but may deny the additional need to reduce sodium intake, lose 20 pounds, or avoid stressful situations.

Denial or avoidance may be adaptive modes of coping for people who are chronically ill with diseases that are not life threatening. By denying they are ill, they are able to maintain and enhance those parts of themselves that are healthy, without giving in to the sick role (Burke, 1987). For example, adults requiring renal dialysis and those with coronary disease report using denial to decrease feelings of anxiety and dependency (Cromer & Tarnowski, 1989). Many people with conditions classified as chronic illnesses by health care professionals do not perceive themselves as being ill or sick. Rather, they perceive themselves as basically healthy even though they have an illness that is stable, treatable, and manageable. People may negate or minimize the seriousness of a problem and go from doctor to doctor seeking a cure for an illness that cannot be cured.

Avoidance and suppression.

Avoidance refers to an unconscious shunning of situations, activities, or objects that might arouse unwanted sexual or aggressive impulses (Barry, 1984). Suppression differs from avoidance in that it is a conscious decision to delay paying attention to an unwanted conflict or impulse until a later time. It allows one to postpone dealing with an anxiety-provoking situation until it can be handled properly. A person may accept the reality of a threat by making a deliberate effort not to think about it. For example, the person may not ask for information or may not listen to that which is offered.

In some circumstances there may be tunneling of vision or restriction of focus to small segments of reality. Roskies (1972) reported that mothers of children deformed by thalidomide said they could continue to function only by forgetting the painful past, ignoring the uncertain future, and concentrating on living day by day. Mages and Mendelsohn (1979) noted that patients with cancer often narrowed their interests when they felt overwhelmed by the many physical, emotional, and practical burdens of their disease. Avoidance behaviors of children include withdrawing from the situation (flight), isolation, and regression. Clinging and crying may be temporary avoidance behaviors: A child who clings to her parent and cries may get a short reprieve before the nurse performs a procedure.

Intellectualization.

Intellectualization helps to separate facts from emotions. People pay close attention to details, often talk in the abstract, and tend to generalize about everything. Intellectualization tends to occur in people who have difficulty dealing with feelings. For example, when a patient who was undergoing radiation therapy was asked how she was doing, she replied, "I'm up to 7,000 rads and I have to go to 8,000 rads. I get 200 rads a day, so I'll finish on Friday. Most people with this type of cancer only have 5,000 rads, so I've had a big dose."

Acting out.

Acting out is another defense mechanism that may be used by the chronically ill person. In this case, the person gives into impulses to avoid tensions that would result if their expression were postponed (Kaplan, Freedman, & Sarock, 1980). Children of chronically ill parents and siblings of chronically ill children have used this defense mechanism. They may run away from home, begin to use drugs, smoke, drink alcohol, or play hooky from school. Adults, too, may use smoking, drinking, and drugs as forms of acting out.

Regression.

Regression is a defense mechanism used by people of all ages when the ego is severely threatened by stress. Personality functioning returns to an earlier level where needs were met and modes of gratification were more satisfying. For example, a toddler who had been toilet trained may regress to soiling his pants when parents are busy with a sibling newly diagnosed with leukemia. In the adult, any internal or external stressor, such as hospitalization or the occurrence of a new symptom, can cause regression. It may be manifested by quiet, uncommunicative behavior, sleeping more than usual, or not being able to comprehend what is spoken. The family may also regress due to the stress caused by a chronic condition in one of its members.

Identification.

Identification is another mechanism used by healthy adults to deal with stressful experiences. The person accepts the thoughts, attitudes, experiences, or feelings of other people as though they are actually his or her own. A young woman about to undergo surgery and radiation therapy for breast cancer had a very positive attitude because she identified with an aunt who had breast cancer 7 years before and was now considered cured.

Using Humor.

Humor is a mature defense mechanism used when a difficult situation cannot be fully acknowledged without expense to self or others (Barry, 1984). Humor has been psychologically beneficial in reducing feelings of anxiety, tension, and anger (Robinson, 1977). Studies of patients with cancer (Frank-Stromberg, 1986), nurses, and other hospital personnel (Hutchinson, 1987) indicate that humor is frequently used to reduce stress. Cousins (1983) used humor to assist in the recovery of his illness, believing it reduced stress and improved his psychologic well-being.

Anticipation.

Anticipation is a healthy defense mechanism used at all but the most stressful times. Anticipation used when an approaching situation is expected to be anxiety provoking allows some of the anxiety to be resolved in advance. For example, Hymovich (1981; Hymovich & Baker, 1985) identified anticipatory planning for potential stressors as a major coping strategy of parents of chronically ill children. Specific strategies included family planning, and making financial plans, and asking school teachers to watch the child closely.

Communicating thoughts and feelings

Degree of communication falls along a continuum: from people who verbally share most if not all of their thoughts and feelings, to those who share little or nothing. However, Walzlawick, Beavin, and Jackson (1967) argue that "one cannot **not** communicate" because all verbal and nonverbal responses, as well as silences, are meaningful communications. The communication rules adopted by the family determine how and what information can be exchanged.

Most (73%) patients report that discussing their problems with friends and families who provide reassurance support, empathy, and information helps alleviate fears or tensions and is generally helpful (Stam, Bultz, & Pittman, 1986). Patterns of communication within the parental and spousal dyad are important in shaping responses to events (Cook, 1983; Rando, 1985). Although communication may not eliminate or resolve differences, it may establish the ability to respond with more empathy because sensitivity to the partner's experience is increased.

Synchrony of response occurs when each partner takes on the role of comforter, reassurer, decision maker, or instrumentalist as necessary (Benfield, Leib, & Reuter, 1976; Drotar, Baskewwicz et al, 1975).

Understanding the medical situation through communication with others facing similar circumstances and consultation with the medical staff is a major coping strategy used by many patients and family members (Patterson & McCubbin, 1983). Venters (1981) identified "sharing the burdens of the illness" as an important strategy in family functioning in families of children with cystic fibrosis. Families who were able to share their burdens with someone outside of the family (e.g., psychologist, clergy) had significantly higher levels of functioning than those who could not. Similar strategies are also noted for chronically ill adults and their spouses (Baider & De-Nour, 1984; Northouse, 1988).

Accepting, refusing, and giving support   Parents give their time, energy and money to support individuals, groups or organizations related to their child's condition. Children mention assisting others by giving advice and help with schoolwork, or refusing to help by withholding information. Patients or family members may give emotional support to others in waiting rooms and hospital rooms. Strong bonds are often formed between patients in clinic waiting rooms, dialysis centers, rehabilitation centers, radiation therapy departments, and chemotherapy departments. For some patients and families, participation in formalized support groups provides a mechanism to cope with the disease and its problems. Thorne (1985) reports that families who have experienced chronic conditions welcome the chance to turn their experiences into ways of helping others. These families were willing participants in research studies and hospital visitation programs.

Outcome of Coping Strategies

Coping is a process that involves the recognition of a problem, a specific response to the problem, and the outcome of the response (Barofsky, 1981). The outcomes of coping strategies are relevant concerns of nurses and other health care personnel. Coping behaviors can be evaluated according to the effectiveness with which a task is accomplished or the cost of this effectiveness to the individual (Silber

et al, 1961a, 1961b). Cost can be divided into two components. The physiologic cost is the toll taken on the body, whereas the psychologic cost is the emotional toll or violation of the person's value integrity (Lazarus, 1984).

Effective coping can have a strong influence on health. For example, Weisman and Worden (1975) found that the type of coping strategies used by patients with advanced cancer was related to patient survival. Patients able to maintain active and mutually responsive relationships were likely to survive longer than those without such relationships. Interestingly, this is contrary to the finding of Reiss and colleagues (1986) who noted that patients on renal dialysis had a shorter survival when they had strong family relationships.

According to Roskies and Lazarus (1980), there are at least three ways that ineffective coping can add to the risk of illness or death. First, strategies such as drinking, smoking, overeating, or reckless driving can cause direct tissue damage. Second, a more indirect way than the first of contributing to the risk of illness or death relates to the physiologic effects of sympathetic arousal (e.g., hypertension, massive hormonal activity) that give a person the extra energy needed to complete some task. Third, failure to employ adaptive coping behaviors that could help preserve life or well-being are another danger. Denying the presence of a breast lump that might signify cancer or of chest pain that could indicate heart attack exemplify ineffective coping. In these instances, denial may reduce the immediate emotional distress, but it could be at the cost of seeking needed medical care.

Pinkerton and associates (1985) studied adult patients with cystic fibrosis, classifying them as good, poor, or intermediate copers. There were twice as many hospital admissions for the poor copers over a 1-year period than for the good copers, despite the fact that the poor copers had better pulmonary function tests.

Although people may have the skills necessary to cope competently with situations, they also must believe they have them in order to actually function effectively. This is Bandura's (1977) notion of self-efficacy, an expectation that one can achieve personal mastery. Having a conviction that one can be effective will determine whether or not the person even tries to cope with a given situation. People who are afraid they will not succeed tend to avoid threatening situations they believe exceed their coping skills. For example, an adolescent with cystic fibrosis

(CF) who felt she had no social skills frequently turned down invitations to participate in activities because she did not believe she would be able to handle them. Her sister, who also had CF, felt confident in her ability to cope with new situations and rarely turned down invitations unless she did not feel well.

Summary

The process of coping with and adapting to a chronic condition is ongoing and developmental. Coping enables one to gain control, to regain a positive self-concept. Everyone copes in his or her own way. Coping strategies are a set of behaviors used under stress to improve the situation. Four major categories of coping and their accompanying strategies are discussed: (1) managing the condition; (2) coping with feelings; (3) communicating thoughts and feelings; and (4) accepting, refusing, and giving support. Managing the condition involves seeking and using information and resources, performing condition-related skills, monitoring or self-monitoring, and incorporating the condition into one's family life-style. Among the feelings with which chronically ill persons and their families must cope are uncertainty, anxiety, grief, and ambiguity. A major role of nurses is to serve as family facilitators; that is, to support the family and patient and to help them to cope more effectively with stressors arising from the chronic condition. We need to recognize that how an individual or family copes with a chronic condition at one point will not necessarily be the way they cope with it at a later time.

References

Affleck, G., Tennen, H., Pfeiffer, C., Field, J., & Rowe, J. (1987). Downward comparison and coping with serious medical problems. *Am J Orthopsychiatry, 57* (4), 540–578.

Anderson, J.M. (1981). The social construction of illness experience: Families with a chronically-ill child. *J Adv Nurs, 6,* 427–434.

Averill, J.R., & Opton, E.M., Jr. (1968). Psychophysiological assessment: Rationale and problems. In P. McReynolds (Ed.), *Advances in psychological assessment* (Vol. 1). Palo Alto: Science and Behavior.

Ayers, T.D. (1989). Dimensions and characteristics of lay helping. *Am J Orthopsychiatry, 59*(2), 215–225.

Babrow, E.S., Ruskin, T.W., & Siller, J. (1985). Mother-daughter interaction and adherence to diabetes regimens. *Diabetes Care, 8,* 146–151.

Baider, L., & De-Nour, K.A. (1984). Couples' reactions and adjustment to mastectomy: A preliminary report. *Int J Psychiatry Med, 14,* 265–276.

Bandura, A. (1977). Self-efficacy: Toward a unifying theory of behavioral change. *Psychol Rev, 84,* 195–215.

Barofsky, I. (1981). Issues and approaches to the psychosocial assessment of the cancer patient. In K. Proktop & L.A. Bradley (Eds.). *Medical psychology: Contributions to behavioral medicine.* (pp. 55–65). New York, Academic Press.

Barry, P.D. (1984). *Psychosocial nursing assessment and intervention.* Philadelphia: Lippincott.

Bateson, G., et al. (1956). Toward a theory of schizophrenia. *Behav Sci, 1,* 251–264.

Benfield, D.G., Leib, S.A., & Reuter, J. (1976). Grief responses of parents after referral of the critically ill newborn to a regional center. *N Engl J Med, 294*(18), 975–978.

Birenbaum, A. (1970). Managing a courtesy stigma. *J Health Soc Behav, 12,* 55–65.

Blum, R.W. (1983). The adolescent with spina bifida. *Clin Pediatr, 22*(5), 331–335.

Bowlby, J. (1969). *Attachment and loss* (Vol. 1). New York: Basic Books.

Braden, J. (1990). A test of the self-help model: Learned response to chronic illness experience. *Nurs Res, 39*(1), 42–47.

Brazelton, T. (1973). *The neonatal behavioral assessment scale.* Philadelphia: Lippincott.

Burish, T.G., & Bradley, L.A. (1983). Coping with chronic disease: Definitions and issues. In T.G. Burish & L.A. Bradley (Eds.)., *Coping with chronic disease* (pp. 3–12). New York: Academic Press.

Burke, S.O. (1987). Assessing single-parent families with physically disabled children. In L.M. Wright & M. Leahy (Eds.), *Families and chronic illness* (pp. 147–167). Springhouse, PA: Springhouse.

Cadman, D., Boyle, M., Szatmari, P., & Offord, D.R. (1987). Chronic illness, disability, and mental and social well-being: Findings of the Ontario child health study. *Pediatrics, 79*(5), 805–813.

Carver, C.S., & Scheier, M.F. (1985). Self-consciousness, expectancies, and the coping process. In T. Field, P.M. McCabe, & N. Schneiderman (Eds.), *Stress and coping* (pp. 305–330. Hillsdale, NJ: Erlbaum.

Caty, S., Ellerton, M.L., & Ritchie, J.A. (1984). Coping in hospitalized children: An analysis of published case studies. *Nurs Res, 33*(5), 277–282.

Chalmers, K.I. (1984). A closer look at how people cope with airflow obstruction. *Can Nurse, 80,* 35–38.

Chodoff, P., Friedman, S.B., & Hamburg, D.A. (1964). Stress, defenses and coping behavior: Observations in children with malignant disease. *Am J Psychiatry, 120,* 743–749.

Christensen, N.K., Terry, R.D., Wyatt, S., Pichert, J.W., & Lorenz, R.A. Quantitative assessment of dietary adherence in patients with insulin-dependent diabetes mellitus. (1983). *Diabetes Care, 6*(3), 245–250.

Cohen, R., & Lazarus, R.S. (1973). Active coping processes, coping dispositions, and recovery from surgery. *Psychosom Med, 35,* 375–389.

Cohen, R., & Lazarus, R.S. (1979). Coping with the stresses of illness. In G.C. Stone, F. Cohen, & N.E. Adler (Eds.). *Health psychology: A handbook,* San Francisco: Jossey-Bass.

Cook, J. (1983). A death in the family: Parental bereavement in the first year. *Suicide Life Threat Behav, 13*(1), 42–61.

Cooper, F.T. (1984), Pilot study on the effects of the diagnosis of lung cancer on family relationships. *Cancer Nursing, 7*(4), 301–308.

Cousins, N. (1983). *The healing heart.* New York: Norton.

Cromer, B.A., & Tarnowski, K.J. (1989). Noncompliance in adolescents: A review. *J Dev Behav Pediatr, 10*(4), 207–215.

Davis, F. (1963). *Passage through crisis: Polio victims and their families.* Indianapolis: Bobbs-Merrill.

Drotar, D., et al. (1975) The adaptation of parents to the birth of an infant with a congenital malformation: A hypothetical model. *Pediatrics, 56*(5), 710–717.

Dunbar, J. (1983). Compliance in pediatrics populations: A review. In P.J. McGrath & P. Fireson (Eds.), *Pediatric and behavioral medicine issues in treatment* (210–230). New York: Springer.

Eliason, M.J., & Richman, L.C. (1984). Psychological effects of idiopathic adolescent scoliosis. *J Dev Behav Pediatr, 5,* 169–172.

Elliott, G.R., & Eisdorfer, C. (Eds.). (1982). *Stress and human health.* New York: Springer.

Evans, R.L., Bishop, D.S., Matlock, A., et al. (1987). Prestroke family interaction as a predictor of stroke outcome. *Arch Phys Med Rehab, 68,* 508–512.

Fagerhaugh, S. (1975). Getting around with emphysema. In A.L. Strauss & B.G. Glaser (Eds.), *Chronic illness and the quality of life* (pp. 99–107). St Louis: Mosby.

Fife, B. (1978). Reducing parental overprotection of the leukemic child. *Soc Sci Med, 12,* 117–122.

Fleishman, J.A. (1984). Personality patterns and coping patterns. *J Health Soc Behav, 25,* 229–244.

Folkman, S., & Lazarus, R.S. (1980). An analysis of coping in a middle-aged community sample. *J Health Soc Behav, 21,* 219–239.

Folkman, S., Schaefer, C., & Lazarus, R.S. (1979). Cognitive processes as mediators of stress and coping. In V. Hamilton & D.M. Warburton (Eds.), *Human stress and cognition: An information processing approach.* London: Wiley.

Folkman, S., Lazarus, R.S., Gwen, R.J., & Delongis, A. (1986). Appraisal, coping, health status and psychological symptoms. *J Pers Soc Psychol, 50*(3), 571–579.

Forsyth, G.L., Delaney, K.D., Gresham, M.L. (1984). Vying for a winning position: Management style of the chronically ill. *Res Nurs Health, 7,* 181–188.

Frank-Stromberg, M. (1986). Health promotion behaviors in ambulatory cancer patients: Facts or fiction? *ONF, 13*(4), 37–43.

Friedman, I.M., Litt, I.F., King, D.R. et al. (1986). Compliance with anticonvulsant therapy by epileptic youth: Relationships to psychosocial aspects of adolescent development. *J Adolesc Health Care, 7,* 12–17.

Friedman, M., & Roseman, R.H. (1974). *Type A behavior and your heart.* New York: Alfred A. Knopf.

Friedman, S.B., Chodoff, P., Mason, J.W., & Hamburg, D.A. (1963). Behavioral observations of parents anticipating the death of a child. *Pediatrics, 32,* 610–625.

Gervasio, A.H. Family relationships and compliance (1989). In K.E. Gerber & A.N. Nehemkis (Eds.), *Compliance: The dilemma of the chronically ill* (pp. 98–127). New York: Springer.

Glass, D.C. (1977). *Behavior patterns, stress and coronary disease.* Hillsdale: Lawrence Erlbaum.

Gourash, N. (1978). Help seeking: A review of the literature. *Am J Community Psychol, 6,* 413–423.

Grobe, M.E., Ilstrup, D.M., Ahmann, D.L. (1981). Skills needed by family members to maintain the care of an advanced cancer patient. *Cancer Nurs, 4*(5), 371–375.

Gurklis, J.A., & Menke, E.M. (1988). Identification of stressors and use of coping methods in chronic hemodialysis patients. *Nursing Research, 37*(4), 236–239, 248.

Hamburg, D.A. (1982). Forward: An outlook on stress research and health. In G.R. Elliott & C. Eisdorfer (Eds.), *Stress and human health* (pp. ix–xxii). New York: Springer.

Hamburg, D., & Adams, J. (1967). A perspective on coping behavior: Seeking and utilizing information in major transitions. *Arch Gen Psychiatry, 17,* 227–284.

Hann, N. (1977). *Coping and defending: Process of self-environment organization.* New York: Academic Press.

Harris, M.D. et al. (1980). Correlates of success and retention in a multi-faceted, long-term, behavior modification program for obese girls. *Addict Behav, 5,* 25–34.

Haynes, R.B., Taylor, D.W., Sackett, D.L. (Eds.). (1980). *Compliance in health care.* Baltimore: Johns Hopkins University Press.

Hayden, P. Davenport, S., & Campbell, M. (1979). Adolescents with myelodysplasia: Impact of physical disability on emotional maturation. *Pediatrics, 64,* 53–59.

Heider, G.M. (1966). Vulnerability in infants. *Genet Psychol Monogr, 73,* 1–216.

Hinds, P.S. (1984). Inducing a definition of hope through the use of grounded theory methodology. *J Adv Nurs, 9*, 357–362.

Hinds, P.S., & Martin, J. (1988). Hopefulness and the self-sustaining process in adolescents with cancer. *Nurs Res, 37*(6), 386–340.

Horowitz, M.J. (1982). Psychological processes induced by illness, injury, and loss. In T. Millon, C. Green, & R. Meagher (Eds.), *Handbook of clinical health psychology* (pp. 63–68). New York: Plenum.

Howarth, R. (1972). The psychiatry of terminal illness in children. *Proc R Soc Med, 65*, 1039–1042.

Huag, M., & Lavin, B. (1983). *Consummerism in medicine: Challenging physician authority.* Beverly Hills: Sage.

Hutchinson, S. (1987). Self-care and job stress. *Image: J Nurs Scholarship, 19*(4), 192–196.

Hymovich, D.P. (1981). Assessing the impact of chronic childhood illness on the family and parent coping. *Image, 13*, 71–74.

Hymovich, D.P. (1984, April 24). Assessment of families with a chronically ill child: Report of a research study. University of Illinois, Chicago.

Hymovich, D.P. (1990, January). The impact of cancer in a parent on family functioning. Presentation. University of Pennsylvania.

Hymovich, D.P., & Baker, C.D. (1985). The needs, concerns and coping of parents of children with cystic fibrosis. *Fam Relat, 34*, 91–97.

Jacobsen, A.M., Hauser, S.T., Wolfsdorf, J.I., et al. (1987). Psychological predictors of compliance in children with recent onset of diabetes mellitus. *J Pediatr, 100*, 805–811.

Johnson, S.B., Silverstein, J., Rosenbloom, C., et al. (1986). Assessing daily management in childhood diabetes. *Health Psychol, 5*(6), 545–564.

Jones, F.A., & Caldwell, H.S. (1981). Factors affecting patient compliance with diagnostic recommendations. *Am J Orthopsychiatry, 51*, 700–709.

Kaplan, H.I., Freedman, A.M., & Sarock, B.J. (1980). *Comprehensive textbook of psychiatry/III.* Baltimore: Wilkins & Wilkins.

Kazak, A. (1986). Families with physically handicapped children: Social ecology and family systems. *Fam Process, 25*, 265–281.

Kazak, A., & Marvin, R. (1984). Differences, difficulties and adaptation: Stress and social networks in families with a handicapped child. *Fam Relat, 33*, 66–77.

Kirscht, J.P., & Rosenstock, I.M. (1979). Patients' problems in following recommendations of health experts. In G.C. Stone, F. Cohen, N.E. Adler (Eds.). *Health psychology—A handbook* (pp. 189–215). San Francisco: Jossey-Bass.

Kleinman, A. (1978). Clinical relevance of anthropological and cross-cultural research: Concepts and strategies. *Am J Psychiatry, 135*, 427–431.

Klinger, E. (1977). *Meaning and void.* Minneapolis: Minneapolis University Press.

Knafl, K.A. (1982). Parent's views of the response of siblings to pediatric hospitalization. *Res Nurs Health, 5*(1), 13–20.

Knafl, K.A., & Deatrick, J.A. (1986). How families manage chronic conditions: An analysis of the concept of normalization. *Res Nurs Health. 9*, 215–222.

Knafl, K.A., & Deatrick, J.A. (1990). Family management style: Concept analysis and development. *J Pediatr Nurs, 5*(1), 4–14.

Knudsen, A., & Natterson, J. (1960). Participation of parents in the hospital care of fatally ill children. *Pediatrics, 26*, 482.

Korner, I.N. (1970). Hope as a method of coping. *J Consult Clin Psychol, 34*(2), 134–139.

Korsch, B.M., Fine, R.N., & Negrete, V.F. (1978). Noncompliance in children with renal transplants. *Pediatrics, 61*, 872–876.

Kubler-Ross, E. (1969). *On death and dying.* New York: Macmillan.

Lazarus, R.S. (1977). Cognitive and coping processes in emotion. In A. Monat & R.S. Lazarus (Eds.), *Stress and coping* (pp. 145–158). New York: Columbia University Press.

Lazarus, R.S. (1980). Cognitive behavior therapy as psychodynamics revisited. In J. Mahoney (Ed.), *Psychotherapy process: Current issues and future directions.* (pp. 121–126). New York: Plenum.

Lazarus, R.S. (1984). The costs and benefits of denial. In S. Breznitz (Ed.), *Denial of stress.* New York: International Universities Press.

Lazarus, R.S. (1982). Stress and coping as factors in health and illness. In J. Cohen, J.W. Cullen, & L.R. Martin (Eds.), *Psychosocial aspects of cancer* (pp. 163–190). New York: Raven Press.

Lazarus, R.S., & Folkman, S. (1984). *Stress, appraisal, and coping.* New York: Springer.

Lazarus, R.S., & Launier, R. (1978). Stress-related transactions between person and environment. In L.A. Pervin & M. Lewis (Eds.), *Perspectives in international psychology* (pp. 287–327). New York: Plenum.

Lenz, E.R. (1984, April). Information seeking: A component of client decisions and health behavior. *Adv Nurs Sci, 6*, 59–72.

Levenson, P.M., et al. (1982). Information preferences of cancer patients ages 11–20 years. *J Adolesc Health Care, 3*, 9–13.

Lindemann, E. (1944). Symptomatology and management of acute grief. *Am J Psychiatry. 101*, 141–148.

Lindemann, E. (1965). Symptomatology and management in acute grief. *Crisis intervention.* New York: Family Service Association of America.

Litt, I.F., & Cuskey, W.R. (1981). Compliance with salicylate therapy in adolescents with juvenile rheumatoid arthritis. *Am J Dis Children, 135*, 434–481.

Lowery, B.J., & Jacobsen, B.S. (1985). Attributional analysis of chronic illness outcomes. *Nurs Res, 34*(2), 82–88.

Lynch, W.F. (1974). *Images of hope.* Baltimore: Notre Dame Press.

McClaran, D.M. (1983). Nutritional factors affecting patient attrition in a weight reduction program. *J Am Coll Health, 32,* 236–239.

McGee, R.F. (1984). Hope: A factor in influencing crisis resolution, *Adv Nurs Sci, 6,* 34–44.

Mages, N.L., & Mendelsohn, G.A. (1979). Effects of cancer on patients' lives: A personological approach. In G.C. Stone, F. Cohen, & N.E. Adler (Eds.). *Health psychology: A handbook,* San Francisco: Jossey-Bass.

Mailick, M. (1984). The impact of severe illness on the individual and family: An overview. In E. Aronwitz, & E.M. Bromberg (Eds.), *Mental health and long-term physical illness* (pp. 83–94). Canton, MA: Prodist.

Mechanic, D. (1986). *Medical sociology* (2nd ed.). New York: Free Press.

Menninger, K. (1963). *The vital balance: The life process in mental health and illness.* New York: Viking.

Miles, M.S. (1985). Emotional symptoms and physical health in bereaved parents. *Nurs Res, 34,* 76–81.

Miller, J.F. (1983). *Coping with chronic illness: Overcoming powerlessness.* Philadelphia: F.A. Davis.

Miller, J.F., & Powers, M.J. (1988). Development of an instrument to measure hope. *Nurs Res, 37*(1), 6–10.

Miller, S.M., Summerton, J., & Brody, D.S. (1988). Styles of coping with threat: Implications for health. *J Pers Soc Psychol, 54,* 142–148.

Minuchin, S. (1974). *Families and family therapy.* Cambridge, MA: Harvard University Press.

Molleman, E., Krabbendam, P.J., Annyas, A.A. et al. (1984). The significance of the doctor-patient relationship in coping with cancer. *Soc Sci Med, 18,* 475–480.

Moore, I.M., Gillis, L.L., & Martinson, I. (1988). Psychosomatic symptoms in parents two years after the death of a child with cancer. *Nurs Res, 37*(2), 104–107.

Moriarty, A. (1961). Coping patterns of preschool children in response to intelligence test demands. *Genet Psychol Monog, 64,* 3–127.

Murphy, L. (1974). *The widening world of childhood: Paths toward mastery.* New York: Basic Books.

Murphy, L.B., & Moriarty, A.E. (1976). *Vulnerability, coping, and growth: From infancy to adolescence.* New Haven, CT: Yale University Press.

Neugarten, B.L. (1979). Time, age and the life cycle. *Am J Psychiatry, 136,* 887–894.

Northouse, L.L. (1988). Social support in patients' and husbands' adjustment to breast cancer. *Nurs Res, 37*(2), 91–95.

Obrist, P.A. (1981). *Cardiovascular psychophysiology: A perspective.* New York: Plenum.

Patterson, J.M., & McCubbin, H.I. (1983). Chronic illness: Family stress and coping. In C.R. Figley & H.I. McCubbin (Eds.), *Stress and the family: Vol. II. Coping with catastrophe* (pp. 21–36). New York: Brunner/Mazel.

Pearlin, L.I., & Schooler, C. (1978). The structure of coping. *J Health Soc Behav, 19*(March), 2–21.

Pelletier, L. (1981). Collecting information: A way to cope with cardiac surgery. *Matern Child Nurs J, 10*(2), 143–154.

Peretz, D. (1970). Development, object relationships and love. In B. Schoenberg, A.C. Carr, D. Peretz, et al (Eds.), *Loss and grief: Psychological management in medical practices* (pp. 3–19). New York: Columbia University Press.

Pidgeon, V. (1989). Compliance with chronic illness regimens: School-aged children and adolescents. *J Pediatr Nurs, 4*(1), 36–37.

Pinkerton, P., Trauer, T., Duncan, F. et al. (1985). Cystic fibrosis in adult life: A study of coping patterns. *Lancet, 2,* 761–763.

Pruyser, P. (1963). Phenomenology and dynamics of hoping. *J Sci Study of Religion, 3,* 86.

Rando, T. (1985). Bereaved parents: Particular difficulties, unique factors and treatment issues. *Soc Work, 30*(1), 19–23.

Reif, L. (1975). Beyond medical intervention strategies for managing life in the face of chronic illness. In M.C. Davis, M. Kramer, & A.L. Strauss (Eds.), *Nursing in practice: A perspective on work environments* (pp. 261–273). St. Louis: Mosby.

Reiss, D., Gonzalez, S., & Kramer, N. (1986). Family process, chronic illness and death: On the weakness of strong bonds. *Arch Gen Psychiatry, 43,* 795–804.

Robinson, V. (1977). *Humor and the health professions.* New York: Charles B. Slack.

Roskies, E. (1972). *Abnormality and normality: The mothering of thalidomide children.* Ithaca, NY: Cornell University Press.

Roskies, E., & Lazarus, R.S. (1980). Coping theory and the teaching of coping skills. In P.O. Davidson & S.M. Davidson (Eds.), *Behavioral medicine: Changing health life styles* (pp. 38–69). New York: Brunner/Mazel.

Rubinstein, B. (1984). When a child has a serious illness: Psychiatric aspects of chronic handicaps. In E. Aronowitz & E.M. Bromberg (Eds.), *Mental health and long-term illness* (pp. 45–65). Canton, MA: Prodist.

Scanlon, C. (1989). Creating a vision of hope: The challenge of palliative care. *Oncol Nurs Forum, 16*(4), 491–496.

Scheier, M.F., Weintraub, J.K., & Carver, C.S. (1986). Coping with stress: Divergent strategies of optimists and pessimists. *J Pers Soc Psychol, 51*(6), 1257–1264.

Schultz, R., & Decker, S. (1985). Long-term adjustment to physical disability: The role of social support, perceived control, and self-blame. *J Pers Soc Psychol, 48,* 1162–1172.

Schwartz, C. (1957). Perspectives on deviance-wives' definitions of their husbands' mental illness. *Psychiatry, 20*, 275–291.

Seligman, M. (1975). *Helplessness: On depression, development, and death.* San Francisco: W.H. Freeman.

Selye, H.L. (1976). *The stress of life* (rev ed.). New York: McGraw-Hill.

Share, L. (1972). Family communication in the crisis of a child's fatal illness: A literature review analysis. *Omega, 3*, 187–201.

Shontz, F.C. (1975). *The psychological aspects of physical illness and disability.* New York: Macmillan.

Sidle, A., Adams, J., Moos, R., & Cady, P. (1969). Development of a coping scale. *Arch Gen Psychiatry, 20*, 226–232.

Silber, E., Coelho, G.V., Murphy, E.B. et al. (1961a). Competent adolescents coping with college decision. *Arch Gen Psychiatry, 5*, 517–527.

Silber, E., Hamburg, D.A., Coelho, G.V. et al. (1961b). Adaptive behavior in competent adolescents. *Arch Gen Psychiatry, 5*, 354–365.

Singer, L., & Farkas, K.J. (1989). The impact of infant disability on maternal perception of stress. *Fam Relat, 38*, 444–449.

Skolny, M.A., & Riehl, J.P. (1974). Hope: Solving patient and family problems by using a theoretical framework. In J.P. Riehl & C. Roy (Eds.), *Conceptual models for nursing practice* (pp. 206–218). New York: Appleton-Century-Crofts.

Spector, S.L. (1985). Is your asthmatic patient really complying? *Ann Allergy, 55*, 552–556.

Spielberger, C.D. (Ed.). (1966). *Anxiety and behavior.* New York: Academic Press.

Spinetta, J.J., & Maloney, L.J. (1978). The child with cancer: Patterns of communication and denial. *J Consult Clin Psychol, 46*(6), 1540–1541.

Stam, H.J., Bultz, B.D., & Pittman, C.A. (1986). Psychosocial problems and interventions in a referred sample of cancer patients. *Psychosom Med, 48*(8), 539–548.

Stewart, A.L. (1980, October). *Coping with serious illness: A conceptual overview.* Santa Monica, CA: Rand Corporation.

Stewart, D.C., & Sullivan, T.J. (1982). Illness behavior and the sick role in chronic illness: The case of multiple sclerosis. *Soc Sci Med, 16*, 1397–1404.

Stoner, M.H., & Keampfer, S.H. (1985). Recalled life expectancy information, phases of illness, and hope in cancer patients. *Research in Nursing and Health, 8* 269–274.

Stotland, E. (1969). *The psychology of hope.* San Francisco: Jossey-Bass.

Sussman, M.B. (1977). Dependent disabled and dependent poor: Similarity and conceptual issues and research needs. In J. Stubbins (Ed.), *Social and psychological aspects of disability* (pp. 247–259). Baltimore: University Park Press.

Taylor, S.E. (1983). Adjustment to threatening events: A theory of cognitive adaptation. *Am Psychol, 38*, 1161–1173.

Taylor, S., Lichtman, R., & Wood, J. (1983). It could be worse: Selective evaluation as a response to victimization. *J Soc Issues, 39*, 19–40.

Tebbi, C., Cummings, K.M., Zeron, M.A. et al. (1986). Compliance of adolescent cancer patients. *Cancer, 58*, 1179–1184.

Thorne, S. (1985). The family cancer experience. *Cancer Nurs, 8*(5), 285–291.

Tobin, D.L., Reynolds, R.V.C., Halroyd, K.A. et al. (1986). Self-management and social learning theory. In K.A. Holroyd, & T.L. Creer (Eds.), *Self management of chronic disease* (pp. 29–55). Orlando, FL: Academic Press.

Vaillant G. (1977). *Adaptation to life.* Boston: Little Brown.

Venters, M. (1981). Familial coping with chronic and severe childhood illness: The case of cystic fibrosis. *Soc Sci Med, 15A*, 287–297.

Walker, C.L. (1988). Stress and coping in siblings of childhood cancer patients. *Nurs Res, 37*(4), 208–212.

Waltzawick, P., Beavin, J.H., & Jackson, D.D. (1967). *Pragmatics of communication.* New York: Norton.

Weisman, A.D. (1974). *The coping capacity. On the nature of being moral.* New York: Human Sciences Press.

Weisman, A.D. & Worden, J.W. (1976–77). The existential plight of cancer: Significance of the first 100 days. *Int J Psychiatry Med, 7*, 1–15.

Weisman, A., & Worden, J. (1975). Psychosocial analysis of cancer deaths. *Omega, 6* 61–75.

Wills, T. (1981). Downward comparison principles in social psychology. *Psycholog Bull, 90*, 245–271.

Wilson, D.P., & Endres, R.K. (1986). Compliance with blood load glucose monitoring in children with type 1 diabetes mellitus. *J Pediatr, 108*, 1022–1024.

Wong, P.T.P., & Weiner, B. (1981). When people ask "why" questions, and the heuristics of attributional search. *J Pers Soc Psychol, 40*, 650–663.

Wood, J.V., Taylor, S.E., & Lichtman, R.R. (1985). Social comparison in adjustment to breast cancer. *J Pers Soc Psychol, 49*(5), 1169–1183.

Wortman, C.B., & Brehm, J.W. (1975). Responses to uncontrollable outcomes: An integration of reactance theory and the learned helplessness model. In L. Berkowitz (Ed.), *Advances in experimental social psychology* (Vol. 8). New York: Academic Press.

Wright, B.A., & Schontz, F.C. (1968). Process and tasks in hoping. *Rehabil Lit, 29*(11), 322–331.

Zborowski, M. (1952). Cultural components in responses to pain. *J Soc Issues, 8*, 16–30.

Zola, I.K. (1966). Culture and symptoms—An analysis of patients' presenting complaints. *Am Sociolog Rev, 31*, 615–630.

12 Stressors and Coping Strategies: Nursing Assessment and Intervention

This chapter provides guidelines for assessing individual and family stressors and coping strategies, and selected nursing interventions to facilitate coping. Additional assessment and intervention strategies are discussed in Chapters 13 and 14.

Assessment

Stressors

Because appraisal of a situation has a strong effect on the coping strategies one uses, assessing client perceptions of events provides nurses with valuable information. Assessment of potential system stressors includes determining stressors of individual family members and those of the family as a whole. For example, self-concept concerns of a child with a chronic condition may differ from those of the siblings, but financial cutbacks faced by the family may be stressors for the entire family. Assessment involves identifying and differentiating between stressors associated with the chronic condition and those associated with the person's age, such as temper tantrums of toddlers or skin changes in the aged. Stressors related to internal and external resources are assessed. Potential internal resource stressors include the person's health and energy, knowledge and information, self-concept, feelings, and family. Potential external resource stressors are related to health care, social support, education, occupation, finances, child care, and housing.

Internal resource stressors

Health and energy.
Physical energy and strength needed to function on a daily basis and during times of crisis should be assessed for each family member. Include assessment of ability to sleep, new or chronic sleep problems, previous means of dealing with them, and measures that seem to induce sleep. Topics to cover in assessing individual and family health and energy stressors are included in Table 12–1.

Knowledge and information.
Careful assessment as to the amount of necessary information is essential before teaching is begun. Guidelines for information to be obtained are included in Table 12–1. In addition, questions asked by patients and families provide an indication of readiness to learn and areas of interest or concern. Determining whether they are asking about behavior, feelings, or diagnostic and treatment issues is important in selecting appropriate nursing intervention strategies. Areas of assessment pertaining to knowledge and information listed in Table 12–1 are discussed in Chapter 14.

Feelings.
Data regarding feelings can be gathered as other information is obtained and from the questions patients and family members ask. Guidelines for assessing uncertainty, helplessness, hopelessness, and chronic sorrow are presented in Table 12–1.

To understand the significance of findings regarding a helpless or hopeless person requires knowledge of the pathophysiology of the patient's illness and treatments, the person's developmental level, psychologic state, and level of functioning. Observations include whether the person initiates conversation and uses facial expressions.

Sexuality.
Health professionals often avoid sexual assessments and sexuality as a component of health teaching and counseling. Discomfort and lack knowledge of techniques of asking questions and of the effects of illness and drugs on sexual functioning contribute to this avoidance (Kerfoot & Buckwalter, 1985). Many health care providers are embarrassed or afraid to raise the subject and therefore do not discuss it with the patient or family. In addition, there is little research in the area of nursing and sexuality. Sexual assessment guidelines are in Table 12–2.

Family relationships and communication.
Whether or not assessing members of the family other than the patient is possible, it is still important to gather information about family relationships. Patient or care-giver (e.g., child's parent) perceptions of relationships and communication provide valuable information about available support. With this knowledge, nurses can gauge whether information, assistance with emotional responses, provision of resources and equipment, and teaching will be sufficient, or whether a stronger support system is needed. Information regarding boundary permeability, role flexibility, quality of relationships, communication patterns, tolerance for differences, and perceptions of events is useful. Guidelines for assessing family communication are in Table 12–1.

Table 12-1 Guidelines for Assessment of Individual and Family Stressors

Topic	Assessment*
INTERNAL RESOURCES	

Focal stressor event(s)
  Developmental
  Situational
	Onset
	Manifestations
	Duration
	Intensity

Health and energy	Current health status Rest and sleep patterns Current difficulties (new, chronic) Available energy

Knowledge and information
  Name of illness
  Etiology
  Onset of symptoms
	General knowledge about disease
	Name of present illness
	What caused it
	Initial thoughts

Pathophysiology	What illness does to self
Course of disease	Severity Expectations re course: short, long
Treatment	Purpose Possible side effects, complications Skills needed Unanswered questions about treatment
Resources	What is available How to use
Feelings	Self-efficacy (control) Hopeful Uncertainty

Family	Knowledge of condition and treatment
	Relationships (supportive)
	  Changes
	Responsibilities
	  For care of ill person
	  Other
	Role changes and flexibility
	Communication (open, closed)
	Boundary permeability
	Recreation activities
	Hobbies
	Tolerance for differences
	Necessity for respite care

Table 12-1 Guidelines for Assessment of Individual and Family Stressors   *Continued*

Topic	Assessment*
EXTERNAL RESOURCES	
Informal support systems	People who provide help when needed
Feeling about support	Comfort in asking or accepting it
Types of help (used, available, needed)	Listen
	Information
	Problem solving
	Tangible: food, money
	Child care
	Household tasks
	Errands
	Transportation
	Social support outside family
Formal support services	Educational
	Occupational
	Financial
	Housing
	Child care
	Respite care
	Recreational
Satisfaction with support	No
	Yes

Strengths (developmental, situational)	Needs (developmental, situational)

*Instruments to assess stressors: Parent Perception Inventory: Concerns (PPICONC) (Hymovich, 1990); Parent Perception Inventory: Feelings (PPIFEEL) (Hymovich, 1990); Family Inventory of Life Events (FILE) for adults, and the Adolescent-Family Inventory of Life Events (A-FILE) (McCubbin & Thompson, 1987); Family Inventory of Resources Management (FIRM) (McCubbin & Comeau, 1987).
To assess social support: The Personal Resource Questionnaire (PRQ85) (Weinert, 1987); Inventory of Social Support (Dunst, Trivette, & Deal, 1988).

External resources   External resources to be assessed will depend on the particular needs of the patient and family. For example, for families with young children, availability of formal and informal child care resources will be important, whereas for families with only adults, assessment of respite resources may be necessary. Potential external resource stressors include social-support systems, health care, educational, occupational, financial, child care, and housing. The following section provides a brief discussion of these resources, and Table 12–1 includes guidelines for assessment.

Social support.
Considerable evidence suggests that the maintenance and use of social relationships facilitates effective coping for individuals and families when a chronic illness or disability is present. To facilitate development or maintenance of a support system, nurses should know who comprises the support network. Assessing this information provides a basis for helping clients mobilize their resources. Assess individual perceptions of the helpfulness of their support and satisfaction with the support received. The amount and type of social support being offered

Table 12–2   Guidelines for Sexual
Assessment

- The nature of the problem
- Previous ways of sexual expression
- Current and past health history that may impinge on sexual functioning (e.g., deformities, pelvic surgery, alcohol, medications)
- Quality of marital or interpersonal relationship
- Psychologic level of functioning (e.g., self-esteem, body image, depression)
- Energy level (fatigue, pain)
- Attitudes towards one's body
- Previous patterns of sexual activity
- Partner's understanding

Sources: Cohen (1986); Flodberg (1990).

needs to be considered. Instrumental supports (money, health services) and social supports may be useful only for certain situations. For example, having adequate health care resources are helpful when one is ill, but are not particularly useful to a person seeking employment.

There are a number of approaches to assessing support networks. One approach is to use a single specific question to identify network members. Another approach uses multiple items: First, the person names the people he or she talks to when concerned about a personal matter. Then the person names the people who help with specific tasks (e.g., household, child care), give advice on important decisions, lend large sums of money, or care for the home in person's absence. Information is also gathered about social and recreational activities to describe the person's "social worlds" and the "relative boundaries" of neighbors and community. Table 12–1 contains guidelines for assessing support systems.

Financial impact.

In assessing financial impact, it helps to keep in mind that economics often dictate outcomes and what patients are able to do and what health care they can accept. Patients do not usually bring up their financial concerns because they do not think nurses are interested in or concerned about financial matters.

Coping Strategies

Although insight into how the person usually copes with situations is useful, it is valuable to find out how the person is coping with current identified focal stressors. Whenever possible, coping strategies used by each family member should be assessed. If there is a primary care giver in the home (parent, adult child, spouse), assessing that person's coping strategies will be especially useful.

Because coping strategies are situation specific, there are times when problem-solving strategies are appropriate, whereas at other times defensive strategies such as denial may be appropriate. Including a history of coping with crises in general, as well as with unexpected ones, provides valuable information regarding possible future coping. Rolland (1987) believes that the family's history of dealing with moderately severe ongoing stressors is a good predictor of how it will adjust to a chronic illness.

Assessment becomes an ongoing process; assumptions cannot be made about what a person will do in a different situation unless a relatively stable pattern has been established over time. For example, Hymovich (1981) noted that parents used different coping strategies when upset about their child's chronic illness than when upset with their spouse. Since health care professionals work with clients in relation to specific situations, knowing the coping strategies used for those situations is important.

There are unresolved issues regarding the assessment of coping as it relates to chronic-disease research (Burish & Bradley, 1983) and some are relevant to clinical practice. First, coping may be evaluated either as a relatively stable disposition (trait, style) or as a process. However, the extent to which these dispositions can be linked to how one copes with a particular situation is questionable. Second, measurement is confounded by the fact that coping behaviors change in response to environmental demands over time. In addition, judgments of coping effectiveness may vary with different domains (e.g., social versus vocational domains) or across different time periods (e.g., immediately following a myocardial infarction or during the subsequent rehabilitation period). Consequently, assessment of coping needs to take place at selected times throughout the illness trajectory.

In addition, how coping behavior is determined to be effective or adaptive involves judging the intent or purpose of the behavior. It also requires making this judgment between different domains of the individual (physical, psychologic, social), over different periods of time (short term, long term), and as a function of different situations (e.g., diagnosis, hospitalization). Determining the outcome of coping also means imposing a set of value judgments. If different values are possible, then different outcomes will be attributed to the coping strategies. Finally, little is known about the relationships among various measures of coping (e.g., self-report, observer report, and physiologic measures).

Horowitz and Wilner (1980) suggest that once a coping strategy is effective, people tend to forget about it and only recall methods that have been ineffective. Consequently, be aware that when assessing coping strategies, people may not readily recall what they usually do because it has become automatic. Eliciting specific coping strategies may involve more direct questioning or listing strategies that may be used. Information to include in assessing coping is included in Table 12–3.

If coping is identified as a problem, then in-depth assessment of this area may be necessary. Several assessment instruments are available for assessing coping. The way coping is measured depends upon its theoretical orientation and definition (Barofsky, 1981). Currently, both self-reports and observer reports are used to measure coping, although the relationship between the two has not been extensively studied. Specific methodologies include in-depth interviews and observations of individuals in crisis, essay and sentence-completion techniques, and short-story and problem-situation techniques (Moos, 1974).

Table 12–3 Assessment of Individual and Family Coping Strategies

Topic	Assessment*
Usual way of coping	Satisfaction with previous coping Beliefs about ability to manage
Ability to cope with this event	Seek information Use information
Management of condition	Use of skills Seek resources Use of resources Monitor self or other Adhere to regimen
Incorporate illness into life-style	Manage time Maintain normalcy Modify roles Modify environment
Cope with feelings	Search for meaning Attribute causes and outcome Make comparisons Maintain hope Use defense mechanisms

Strengths	Needs

*Coping instruments: Hymovich's Parent Perception Inventory: Coping (PPI-COPE) (Hymovich, 1984, 1989, 1990); Family Crisis Oriented Personal Evaluation Scales (F-COPES) (McCubbin & Thompson, 1987); Coping Health Inventory for Parents (CHIP) (McCubbin & Thompson, 1987); Jalowiec Coping Scale (Jalowiec, Murphy, & Powers, 1984); Ways of Coping Scale (Folkman & Lazarus, 1980).

Instruments for assessing coping have been developed in disciplines including nursing, medicine, and psychology. They have been used in research and clinical situations with various patient populations. Questionnaires have been devised to measure coping in adults with specific chronic illnesses and in parents of chronically ill children. These instruments include Lazarus' (Folkman & Lazarus, 1980) Ways of Coping Scale, Hymovich's Parent Perception Inventory: Coping (PPI-COPE) (Hymovich, 1984, 1989, 1990), and McCubbin's F-COPES (McCubbin et al, 1981). Suggested instruments are included in Table 12–3.

Management of the illness Johnson and colleagues (1986) suggest multiple 24-hour recall interviews are an efficient way to obtain estimates of adherence behaviors, especially for children over 9 years of age. They have been used with children who have diabetes and their parents. This type of interview focuses on specific behaviors over a relatively brief time frame.

Clinical studies assess compliance in one of two ways: direct methods using biologic assays (e.g., body fluids such as blood, urine, or saliva) or indirect methods such as pill counts, self-reports, indexes of therapeutic outcome, and physician estimates (least accurate) (Cromer & Tarnowski, 1989). Large discrepancies have been found when self-reports of adherence are compared with more objective measures, indicating that self-reports are generally not very accurate, with patients tending to overestimate their compliance. Admissions of noncompliance are usually accurate, however. Self-reports and pill counts are generally inaccurate measures of compliance behavior when compared with bioassays.

Life-style Chronic illness often causes disruptions in daily living and normal routines. There are also competing demands for energy. Household members may try to carry out their old role responsibilities while assuming new roles imposed by the illness of a family member.

To facilitate self-care, the regimen should be tailored to the individual. Chewning (1982) suggests the following questions for assessing what is important for the person and what may be interfering with the quality of the person's life:

1. Does anything (or what things) get in the way of doing . . . ?
2. How often are you able to . . . ?

3. Some people say they have trouble . . . . Does this happen to you too?

Answers to these questions may identify problem areas interfering with the quality of life of both patient and family.

Intervention

Preparing for Stressful Events

It is important to prepare patients physically and psychologically for stressful events. Studies indicate that the more knowledge a person has prior to a stressful event, the less upsetting the stressor will be (Johnson, Kirchoff, & Enders, 1975; Skipper & Leonard, 1968). Researchers who classified patients according to coping style suggest that sensitizers should be prepared extensively, although patients who tend to repress information should be left alone (Shipley, Butt & Horowitz, 1979).

Studies suggest that presenting information about what will occur during a medical procedure is not necessarily useful for children who have already experienced the procedure (Faust & Melamed, 1984; Klorman et al, 1980). In fact, Melamed and colleagues (1983) found that both modeling and demonstration of information increased arousal and self-reported concerns of young, experienced surgical patients. They suggest that experienced children may benefit most from preparation that includes training in ways to cope with the procedure. Children with previous negative medical experiences demonstrated more behavioral distress during a throat culture examination than did children with previous positive or neutral medical experiences. In the control group that received attention (had a story read to them or discussed favorite activities), distress was increased for those children who previously had negative experiences. Amount of past exposure was not related to observed distress.

Stress inoculation training **Stress inoculation training** (SIT) is a cognitive-behavioral approach to prepare patients for upcoming stressful events (Kendall & Watson, 1981; Meichenbaum, 1985; Meichenbaum & Novaco, 1978). SIT provides the person with skills to use in the stressful situation. The technique enhances resistance to the event by "exposure to a stimulus strong enough to arouse defenses without being so powerful that it overcomes them" (Meichenbaum & Turk, 1987, p. 3). For example, high emotional distress in patients with cancer was reduced with brief directed therapy (Worden & Sobel, 1978). The goal of SIT should be to foster flexibility in the person's coping repertoire so that coping strategies can be adjusted to "situational demands and changing contexts and goals" (Meichenbaum, 1985, p. 17).

Stress inoculation training is not a single technique; rather, it refers to a treatment paradigm that may involve a number of elements. These elements are listed in Table 12–4. "SIT is designed to nurture and develop coping skills, not only to resolve specific immediate problems but also to apply to future difficulties" (Meichenbaum, 1985, p. 21). Training involves three phases:

1. The conceptualization phase focuses on establishing a collaborative relationship with clients and helping them understand the transactional nature of stress and coping.
2. The skill acquisition and rehearsal phase during which clients develop and rehearse various coping skills or remove obstacles that prevent them from using already available coping skills.
3. The application and follow-through phase includes booster sessions, follow-up assessments, and planning for the future. During this phase, the person tests the learned coping skills under stress conditions.

The number of SIT sessions varies from one, for patients about to undergo surgery, to as many as 40; the average is 12 to 15, each lasting an hour, plus booster and follow-up sessions that gradually decrease over the next 6 to 12 months. Laboratory research has demonstrated that SIT is effective in reducing anxiety, controlling anger provocation, and alleviating pain (Kendall & Watson, 1981).

Table 12–4 Elements of Stress Inoculation Training

Didactic teaching	Relaxation training
Socratic discussion	Self-monitoring
Cognitive restructuring	Self-instruction
Problem solving	Self-reinforcement
Behavioral and imaginal rehearsal	Efforts at environmental change

Graded exposure Graded, or gradual, exposure to new events or less threatening stressors "can potentiate new skills, enhance feelings of self-efficacy, and psychologically 'immunize' the individual or group . . . [It] can engender a client's sense of self-confidence, hope, perceived control, commitment, and personal responsibility" (Meichenbaum, 1985, p. 17).

Facilitate Stress Reduction

Stress management Stress management involves the teaching of specific coping skills, such as relaxation, problem solving, reality testing, or assertiveness (Meichenbaum, 1985). Although these techniques are useful, Lazarus (1984) urges caution because they could exacerbate stressful reactions. As noted earlier, there are times when strategies such as denial or disengagement are appropriate responses to a situation.

Behavior therapy.

Behavior therapy is an alternative to traditional psychodynamic therapy. Generally, behavioral changes are required for most treatment regimens. Behaviors can change the conditions of the environment, provide mastery experiences that raise feelings of self-efficacy, and effect physiologic processes (such as labored breathing). Its early narrow focus was centered on classical (S-R) and operant (S-O-R) conditioning. Gradually, its flexibility increased and eventually cognitive behavior therapy developed.

According to the behavioral model of intervention there is a sequential, continuing process of evaluation and intervention. The process involves identifying problems, developing goals, determining and implementing treatment methods, and collecting information to evaluate goal attainment (Taylor, Lieberman, Agras et al, 1982). Evaluation is made with the client at each session so that if techniques are not effective, they can be revised or discarded quickly.

Techniques of behavior therapy are being replaced with coping-skills training, involving self-initiation and self-application of behavioral interventions. Therapeutic goals of self-management of chronic disease are accomplished when "(1) Self-control skills are learned; (2) beliefs likely to promote changes in health behavior are enhanced (e.g., efficacy expectations); and (3) environmental conditions (including family and social networks) that promote self-control of a chronic condition are created"

(Tobin, Reynolds, Holroyd, & Creer, 1986, p. 32). Although the client may need training in only one coping skill, it is probably a variety of coping skills that will be needed. Based on social learning theory, these skills might include observing the environment, monitoring one's behavior, analyzing and planning new courses of action, and carrying out new behavioral activities. Behavioral techniques include relaxation strategies, assertiveness training, cognitive coping and problem-solving approaches, and communication skills training.

Relaxation training.

Relaxation training aims to alter perceptions of bodily experiences. As with other interventions, research indicates various responses to such therapy. For example, studies of relaxation techniques show a decrease in blood pressure in persons at risk for coronary heart disease (Patel et al, 1985) and patients following a myocardial infarction (MI) (Thoresen et al, 1985). Thoresen also reports improvement in psychological well-being in post-MI patients, although Munro and colleagues (1988) did not find this in a similar group of patients. Munro reports a decrease in diastolic blood pressure lasting at least 3 months in patients post-MI, whereas Pender (1985) reports a decrease in systolic blood pressure at a 4-month follow-up in patients with essential hypertension. A meta-analysis of 48 nonmechanically assisted relaxation techniques indicated that relaxation techniques are effective in alleviating clinical symptoms of the following chronic problems: hypertension, headaches, and insomnia (Hyman, Feldman, Harris et al 1989).

Relaxation techniques are also being taught to children and adolescents. These techniques have helped them cope with anxiety and pain. The techniques used often include behavioral counseling, relaxation training, and biofeedback (Spirito et al, 1987).

Cognitive therapy

The focus of cognitive intervention is to change thoughts as well as feelings and actions. Cognitive strategies include cognitive restructuring, problem solving, and guided self-dialogue (Meichenbaum, 1985). The central factor in cognitive behavior therapy is how the person interprets situations.

Cognitive restructuring.

Cognitive therapy, also known as cognitive reappraisal or cognitive restructuring, refers to a process whereby a nurse intervenes to help an individual deal with stress by changing the person's perception of the situation. Through therapy, a person's thoughts, beliefs, and attitudes may be changed by interpreting reality in a new and different way. Cognitive therapy is defined as "structured short-term treatment for depression and anxiety based on helping the client to identify and change distorted thought patterns that trigger and perpetuate one's distress" (Childress & Burns, 1981, p. 1024).

Cognitive theorists believe that maladaptive feelings are caused by maladaptive thoughts. These thoughts, often illogical, distorted, and unrealistic, then lead to anxiety. Some maladaptive, self-defeating, and distorted cognitions identified by Burns (1980) include:

- All-or-none thinking, or things are either black or white
- Overgeneralization
- Dwelling on a single negative event
- Eliminating positive experiences
- Jumping to conclusions
- Catastrophizing or minimizing
- Using "should" statements
- Labeling oneself negatively.

Beck identified **automatic thoughts,** those that occur spontaneously (out of the blue) and not in relation to any particular event, as negative and producing stress. Negative, stress-producing automatic thoughts include: "It is such an effort to do anything," "Life is just one string of problems," "Life has no meaning," and "Life is hopeless" (Meichenbaum, 1985, p. 59). Such thoughts can be elicited by asking clients what thoughts usually run through their heads.

In cognitive therapy, the individual is first taught to be aware of and recognize cognitive distortions and observe the reaction of one's body. Behavioral techniques are then taught to encourage self-control. Beck and his colleagues (1979) suggested (1) eliciting the person's thoughts, feelings, and interpretation of events, (2) gathering evidence with the person for and against such interpretations, and (3) setting up homework experiments to test the validity of the interpretations and to gather more data for discussion.

Cognitive-behavioral interventions.

Cognitive-behavioral interventions are strategies to affect cognitive functioning and behavioral adjustment (Kendall & Watson, 1981). Changes in cognitive functioning refer to changes in what the person says to oneself. An important component of this approach is modifying self-statements. Kendall and Watson's review of the research literature related to these approaches indicated a clear superiority of the coping interventions over information interventions. Among the findings were the trend toward reduced hospital stays for hospitalized children and adults.

Behavior management techniques allow the individual to gain self-control in situations that were previously stressful. In some instances, self-reward techniques can dramatically improve one's performance. Self-reward can include self-talk or self-praise, by which an individual gives positive messages to himself or herself to change thought patterns.

Cunningham and Tocco (1989) conducted a randomized trial to test the effectiveness of a psychoeducational program and a coping-skills program for adult patients with cancer. The coping-group intervention consisted of supportive discussion, ventilation of feelings, general problem solving, and information sharing. The psychoeducational group received similar supportive discussions plus coping-skills education (relaxation training, positive imagery, goal setting, and general life-style management). This study supports the trend towards greater improvements with brief, behaviorally-oriented programs than with purely supportive interventions. Both groups showed significant change in affective state, but the change in the psychoeducational group was about twofold greater.

Problem-solving training.

Problem-solving training is another method for helping clients cope with problems, and all programs have certain elements in common:

1. Defining the problem (stressor or stress reaction) to be solved
2. Setting realistic goals, stated in behavioral terms
3. Generating possible alternative courses of action
4. Considering the consequences of the alternatives
5. Deciding which alternative to try
6. Implementing the most acceptable and practical solution
7. Evaluating the effectiveness of the solution.

Wasik (1984) translated each step into a question one asks oneself, and clients use a problem-solving log. Clients themselves identify a stressful problem and try to answer the questions. The questions are:

- What is the concern? (Problem identification)
- What do I want? (Goal selection)
- What can I do? (Generation of alternatives)
- What might happen? (Consideration of consequences)
- What is my decision? (Decision making)
- Now do it! (Implementation)
- Did it work? (Evaluation)

Although some people may be able to talk about problem solving, they may not be able to implement their plans effectively. Role-playing, modeling, imagery rehearsal, and graduated practice may be useful in helping clients implement the problem-solving plans and evaluate the outcome (Meichenbaum, 1985). Graduated practice refers to giving clients realistic and relevant homework assignments for carrying out some of their coping skills in the actual situation.

Contingency management   **Contingency management** involves goal setting, contracting, reinforcement, and response-cost condition. These forms of contingency management are described below.

Contracting   **Contracts** are effective strategies for promoting positive health outcomes. They are mutually arrived at agreements between the client and the health provider about goals to be achieved. The purpose of contracts is to define who is responsible for what behavior. Contracts are usually designed to specify the behavior-consequence relationships and are signed by at least two parties. They may be agreements for doing or refraining from doing something. The signers may be the health care provider, the client, and a family member or some other significant person.

Several philosophic beliefs underlie the utilization of health contracts (Brykcznski, 1982). First is the belief that all people have the potential for growth and the right to self-determination. Second is a commitment to identifying and developing strengths, rather than emphasizing weaknesses and limitations. Third is the holistic view of individuals.

Fourth is the belief that the client and the health provider are equal partners.

Studies show that contracting is effective for improving patient outcome. In a study of patients with hypertension, no clients who developed contracts dropped out as compared with an 8% and 26% drop-out rate in two groups that did not develop contracts (Steckel & Swain, 1977). In addition, contract-group blood pressure stabilized by the second of four visits, while that of the others fluctuated throughout the four visits. In another study by the same researchers, only 3% of the persons with hypertension, diabetes, or rheumatoid arthritis failed to follow their contracts over a 3-year period (Swain & Steckel, 1981). The blood pressure of those who contracted dropped twice as fast as for those who did not, and their weight loss was also greater. In both studies the contracts included self-rewards for success, and in the 1981 study the contracts were renegotiated with each visit. Rewards were not included in Herje's (1980) study of contracting with clients having chronic low-back pain. Nevertheless, these clients made more short-term protective posture changes and did more low-back exercises than did clients who received an educational intervention without contracts. Other studies indicate the value of contracts when there is an occasional follow-up telephone call to check on progress (Etzwiler, 1974) or when a contract is witnessed or signed (Ureda, 1980) by a person significant to the client. Reported case studies demonstrate the successful use of contracts for a patient with burns (Simons et al, 1979) and one with cancer (Zangari & Duffy, 1980).

Key components to effective contracts with clients include (1) focusing on the behaviors that lead to the goal rather than on the goal itself; (2) identifying small steps the client believes can realistically be accomplished before the next visit; (3) describing a set of steps tailored for the client, which, over a series of contracts, lead to an end goal important to the client; (4) a means for recording client behaviors (e.g., exercise diary, blood pressure record, food diary, rest log); and (5) identifying a reward the client values, if rewards are involved. Rewards should be selected by the client and be personally meaningful, although the nurse may need to suggest a range of options for some people (Chewning, 1982). In addition contracts should be written, realistic, measurable, positive, time dated, rewardable, and evaluated (Herje, 1980).

If the client makes little progress in meeting the contract, the contract should be renegotiated so that it is more realistic with respect to the person's current strengths. Contracting is not recommended for patients with organic brain syndrome, the very young, or those who are severely retarded (Simons et al, 1979). Others may not be able to participate because of denial, confusion, or grief (Herje, 1980).

It is often time-consuming to enter into a contract, requiring commitment, responsibility, and follow-up for all involved. However, patients actively involved in planning and participation are more likely to internalize the new health behaviors.

Response-cost condition.

A response-cost condition is a method of contingency management in which there is a cost to the patient for noncompliance. Stimulus control strategies are aimed at intervening with the antecedents of the behavior. These strategies include cuing, self-talk, problem solving, and self-regulation of medication.

Cuing strategies might include setting an alarm clock to remind one to take pills, writing a note in the calendar to remember office or clinic visits, or putting pills in strategic places where they are taken, such as by the sink or on the dinner table. Needless to say, in families with young children who may get into the pills, such a strategy is not recommended.

Intervention for Selected Stressors

Crisis Situations

Contact with some clients may be infrequent except during periods of crisis, especially if the families are functioning well. Crisis theory implies difficulty in family functioning; therefore the focus of crisis intervention should be on the family system rather than on the individual system. Family vulnerability at various stages of the condition experience may necessitate periodic crisis intervention. During each crisis period, family members are faced again with the need to modify their roles and responsibilities and redefine their expectations and goals.

Crisis intervention is a process of short-term therapy focusing on rapid mobilization of emotional resources to resolve the immediate psychologic crisis and restore persons to their premorbid state (Capone et al, 1979).

> While crisis intervention may be useful in helping individual and family systems cope with an acute situation, it is not useful over the long-term when they are living with the condition on a day-to-day basis (Heinrich & Schag, 1984).

Crisis situations have been shown to have predictable outcomes, with timely intervention greatly influencing the predicted result. Relatively brief counseling is appropriate during the early weeks of a crisis. During this time, people are likely to be receptive to outside help and to accept and assimilate help quickly. Successful reduction of the crisis can mean an increase in the probability of successful resolution of the next crisis.

The goals of crisis intervention are to help people (1) return to the precrisis level, (2) grow and become stronger, more effective problem-solvers, (3) prevent a negative, destructive outcome, (4) relieve symptoms, (5) facilitate understanding of the precipitating events, and (6) identify remedial resources for the individuals involved in the crisis (Heinrich & Schag, 1984). The focus of crisis intervention is on the present problem and is a problem-oriented approach.

Approaches to intervention include manipulating the environment, enhancing coping, and modifying behavior to inhibit maladaptive responses and reinforce effective ones. Environmental manipulation involves reducing focal stressor events by offering direct services or making appropriate referrals. To facilitate coping, the nurse helps the person develop a cognitive understanding of the crisis, express feelings, and explore coping mechanisms.

A crisis-intervention plan is developed with the person in crisis and with others who are significant to the patient. The plan should be realistic, time limited, concrete, and consistent with the client's culture and life-style.

There are several steps or phases in crisis intervention (Aquilera & Messick, 1982). They include

1. Assessment of the individual, focal stressors, and coping strategies. If the individual represents a high suicidal or homicidal risk, referral to a psychiatrist and/or hospitalization may be necessary.
2. Planning of therapeutic intervention to restore a precrisis level of functioning. The

period of time in crisis, the amount of disruption in the life of the person and significant others, strengths, coping strategies, social supports, and alternative coping strategies are explored.

3. Intervention. This step consists of helping the person to gain an understanding of the crisis and to bring his or her present feelings into the open. Often, the person has suppressed feelings, and an emotional catharsis may reduce the overwhelming tension. Alternative ways of coping should be explored. In addition, reopening the social world can be an effective intervention, especially when the crisis has been precipitated by loss.
4. Resolution of the crisis and anticipatory coping. As the person tries new coping and problem-solving skills, tension and anxiety should be reduced and positive changes will occur. Realistic plans for the future should be discussed.

Specific techniques of crisis intervention are in Table 12–5. They should be dynamic (flexible) and negotiable (specific to the client).

Table 12–5   Crisis Intervention Techniques and Their Purposes

TECHNIQUE	PURPOSE
Sustainment	Lower anxiety, provide emotional support
Reassurance	Recognize responses are normal (if they are)
Encouragement	Counteract sense of helplessness and hopelessness
Sympathetic listening	Help person feel important
Ventilation	Encourage expression of feelings
Direct influence	Promote specific behavior changes
Advice giving	Help client figure out what to do when anxiety is high
Advocating	Give person a particular course of action
Warning	Know consequences or potential consequences

Hospitalization

For most persons, hospitalization is an emotion-laden and stressful event, and it is especially so for the chronically ill. For people with a long-term condition, hospitalization often means the condition is out of control or the disease has progressed and the individual's health is deteriorating. For others, it may mean respite or the possibility of improved functioning. Regardless of the anticipated outcome, hospitalization usually creates stress. Nurses, in addition to giving the patient and family control and allowing them to direct aspects of care, can employ other strategies to decrease the stress of hospitalization.

Use of humor   Humor, used appropriately, can help establish patient-caregiver relationships by providing a sense of familiarity needed in a strange setting. Situations in which surprise, ambiguity, or a feeling of relief is present, as well as uncertainty, will support humor (Robinson, 1977). Humor puts stressful situations into perspective and encourages a sense of trust (Simon, 1989). It can be destructive, however, if used in a way that ridicules the patient. Ways to foster humor appear in Box 12–1. Lieber (1986) identified timing, receptiveness, and content as appropriate criteria for determining the appropriate use of humor. Humor is inappropriate during times of high anxiety.

Preparing for discharge   Planning is the key to successful posthospital care. Preparing families for

---

changes at home includes letting them know the patient may have new needs and that responsibilities of family members may shift.

At times discharge from the hospital can be frightening. When nurses only talk about how "nice" it will be to go home, they are denying the child or adult the opportunity to express concerns and work through negative feelings and fears about the anticipated event. Care givers need instructions **and** practice in doing procedures before discharge. This experience helps reassure care givers and patients that they are capable of meeting the special needs.

Attention needs to be given to children who have an increasing focus on their altered body image and what it will mean to being accepted by family and friends. Making children aware they will be asked questions about appearance can help prepare them for the experience (Savedra, 1977).

Patients requiring technological support at home need additional consideration in planning for their discharge. Studies from the REACH Program in Gainesville, Florida, and the Pediatric Home Care Program in New York suggest the need for outreach to the home and family to make discharge successful for children with chronic conditions requiring complex care, and to support children in the community (Stein & Jessop, 1984). If home care efforts are to be effective, the family must be willing to care for the child at home. Most parents are ambivalent at first, and many are appropriately fearful of the responsibility and its impact on their lives. Parental involvement should start as soon as possible. Inpatient nursing staff are facilitators of a successful discharge plan and need to be parent trainers, not just givers of direct care. Each home care family should have a designated case coordinator—one person who helps put all the pieces together. A carefully thought out, flexible plan that covers many contingencies is required. The plan must be individualized and developed together by the family and team members. The same principles apply to adult patients and their care givers.

A back-up system for emergencies needs to be in place prior to discharge. Appropriate equipment must be in place and tested in the home prior to discharge. Families and other care givers should be trained to use the equipment that will be in the home. Alternative plans for respite care or long-term placement should be considered if home care does not appear to work for the benefit of the child and family.

Box 12–1   ***Strategies to Facilitate Humor with Hospitalized Patients***
• Share cartoons, jokes, humorous anecdotes
• Have funny videocassettes available
• Have visits by therapeutic clowns
• Use puppets to increase playfulness
• Create a photo album of humorous events on the unit
• Create a humor room with props to structure laughter
• Be creative; use imagination

Source: Adapted from Simon, 1989.

Uncertainty

According to findings of Molleman et al (1984), clients can be encouraged to seek answers to their questions about the condition and its therapy, especially from experts like nurses and physicians. Nurses can determine patients' unanswered questions by asking about them. Supplying information, giving attention, and showing understanding are activities that influence coping by adults with cancer. To reduce their anxiety, patients should be encouraged to discuss their problems with other clients, family, and friends. Mishel and Braden (1988) distinguish between external cues (knowledge of physical aspects of treatment, beliefs in the efficacy of treatment, relationships with health care providers, expectations about care outcomes and performance of health system) and internal cues (sensations representing physiologic states generated by the treatment). They suggest that health providers reduced uncertainty relative to the external cues but that friends and relatives were needed to support their personally constructed views of the condition (internal cues). When the prognosis is uncertain and expectations are unclear, nurses and patients have to try to find a middle ground for balancing optimism about the future with a healthy dose of realism.

Chronic Sorrow

If one accepts the view that chronic sorrow does exist, the implications for clinical practice are different than if one believes grief is a time-limited phenomenon. If it is time-limited, interventions include (Damrosch & Perry, 1989; Wikler, Wascow, & Hatfield 1981)

1. Facilitating clients as they work through each stage of the grief process
2. Discontinuing services at the conclusion of the adjustment period
3. Identifying those clients who did not go through all the stages as dysfunctional.

If sorrow is believed to be chronic or ongoing, nursing interventions include

1. Telling clients chronic sorrow is a normal, natural response to a chronic illness
2. Offering ongoing support
3. Permitting clients an opportunity to express their feelings.

When a Person Is Dying

Hull (1980) reviewed 13 studies of patients dying of cancer to determine family members' perceptions of supportive nursing behaviors. Least supportive were behaviors to encourage ventilation of family members' own feelings. Although families identified a need for emotional support, they did not rate specific behaviors generally considered as emotionally supportive to be so. Among these behaviors were encouragement to talk about negative feelings, holding the person's hand, or encouraging sharing of feelings. Family members thought the nurse's responsibility was toward the dying patient rather than to them, especially when nurses were busy and time was limited. Relatives and friends were considered more appropriate sources of family support at this time than were nurses.

Hull (1980) also found that family members wanted assurance that their loved one was comfortable (free of pain) and receiving good nursing care, and they wanted to be physically close to hospitalized patients. Therefore, comfortable and adequate accommodations for family members are needed. Families caring for the patient at home needed information on how to perform the necessary procedures, especially comfort measures.

Nurses can help relatives through the mourning process. To do this, the nurse can explain the usual stages of mourning, being careful to point out that each person reacts somewhat differently and may move between the stages. Explanation should include the value of mourning—it is itself healthful and an adaptive process necessary for psychological health.

Children select the person with whom they feel comfortable discussing their fears and concerns (Kikuchi, 1975). Generally, this is someone who is honest and willing to discuss difficult subjects. Nurses need to be sensitive enough to pick up indirect cues, such as talking about someone else who is very ill, dying, or who died. Children and adults test the nurse's reactions, as well as their own, to be sure both of them can actually talk about a sensitive subject. Responding to the person with honesty, clarity, and support facilitates open communication.

Life review Butler (1963) described **life review** as a "naturally occurring, universal mental process characterized by the progressive return to the consciousness of past experiences and particularly, the resurgence of unresolved conflicts" (p. 65). Life review provides the opportunity to reminisce and finish any unfinished business of life. It allows one to maintain self-esteem, reaffirm a sense of identity, reduce feelings of loss and isolation, and emphasize the accomplishments of life. By verbalizing memories, it gives a person a chance to grieve in anticipation of impending death. According to Butler (1974) reminiscence can be stimulated by

1. Encouraging writing
2. Taping the session
3. Asking the family to bring in photographs
4. Helping the patient organize memorabilia in an album
5. Having the patient start a family tree
6. Encouraging the patient to write letters to old friends.

Hamilton (1985) says "the elderly are living historical novels who have written and acted out their past" (p. 146). She believes the nurse's role is to provide reminiscence therapy, which involves tapping memories to stimulate a higher level of wellness. Reminiscence can be verbal, written, or silent musings of the past and has three components: memory, experiencing, and social interaction. During reminiscence therapy the nurse is an active listener who shows caring. Being a supportive listener and remaining nonjudgmental are important according to deRaymon (1983), who suggests several points to make the process work:

- Make yourself genuinely available.
- Do not violate the confidentiality of the interaction.
- Help the person take satisfaction in the life he or she has led.
- Use silence.
- Encourage self-expression.
- Time your intervention appropriately.
- Involve family members.
- Use touch.
- Allow the patient to retreat.
- Suggest the patient seek help from a counselor if you cannot help or work with the patient.

Helplessness

Seligman (1975) raised the possibility of reversing helplessness. Studies have found that when children believe failure is their own fault, they work harder at subsequent tasks than when they attribute it to some external cause (Gatchel & Baum, 1983). These data suggest that helping people to reevaluate their strengths, in addition to understanding the condition, may be beneficial. However, further research is needed to determine if such intervention strategies are indeed effective, and under what circumstances they are effective. Seligman (1975) believed care should be goal-oriented and should provide experiences that facilitate the patient's movement from a passive helpless orientation to one of active mastery. Another approach to reversing helplessness is to attempt to "immunize" people against the effects of exposure to uncontrollable events. Seligman suggested that prior experience with success might immunize the person against learned helplessness. However, Douglas & Anisman (1975) found that when the task was unlike the one causing helplessness, immunization was not effective.

Schneider (1980) suggested helplessness could be prevented by allowing the client to control as many events as possible within the constraints imposed by treatment needs and the patient's energy level. Most patients should be able to control whether to have the radio or television on or off, keep the drapes open or closed, or add or remove blankets on the bed. It is sometimes difficult for nurses when patients make requests that, on the basis of clinical knowledge, nurses know are potentially detrimental to well-being. When requests must be denied, it is important to explain tactfully and honestly why they cannot be carried out. The patient, for example, who must turn or be turned at specified intervals may request to remain in the most comfortable position. While this request cannot be met, it might be possible to engage the patient in suggesting another position for greater comfort.

Hopelessness

It has been suggested that nurses can help patients maintain hope while avoiding unrealistic hopefulness or unjustified hopelessness (Miller, 1983; Vaillot, 1970). However, Pruyser (1987) questions the possibility of being able to give or foster someone else's hope because hope is an existential condition rather than a specific object.

Potentially helpful nursing intervention strategies include helping the patient set realistic goals, participate in decision making, and direct thoughts to maximize experiences (Miller, 1983). Once the patient is oriented to reality, the nurse can provide information the patient needs to participate actively in self-care. Proper management of symptoms may help alleviate feelings of helplessness caused by symptoms that are out of control. Strategies for moving a patient from hopelessness and despair to hope include

1. Engaging in reality surveillance or searching for clues that hope (a feeling that one will achieve a goal) is possible
2. Devising and revising goals that are achievable and mobilizing hope
3. Hoping in God or discovering a sustaining supernatural love

Vaillot (1970) suggested the primary function of nurses was to inspire hope by trusting the patient's will to live and mobilizing forces that might work for the patient (e.g., supportive family or important goals). Strategies for reversing hopelessness require considerable patience and energy on the part of the nurse because the hopeless person may not try to exert any control over his life (Schneider, 1980). Being available and showing genuine concern for the patient as a person are suggested as ways of helping negate the patient's feelings of worthlessness.

In caring for the hopeless patient, the nurse must hope for the patient. This hope need not be unrealistic. Even a patient with no chance for recovery can still be offered the hope of relief from pain, comforting touches, a change of position, and a concerned, caring voice . . . The hopeless patient is caught in one perspective of time. He sees no past or future (except past misery), only the present. The nurse should direct the patient's thoughts beyond his present state to the future. (Schneider, 1980, p. 18)

Suggestions that a family member is coming tomorrow or that the intravenous will be removed the next day are examples of directing the patient to think beyond the present. Any statements made about the future, however, must be realistic and not contrived. Because hopeless patients also feel helpless, nursing actions to reverse helplessness are appropriate. Hopeless patients are not likely to attempt to exert any control over their situation, so it may be more difficult to help them see how previous attempts have been successful.

The suggestions presented above are useful interventions for assisting patients suffering from chronic disorders. The extent to which they actually inspire hope remains to be documented.

Sexuality

Sexual counseling is neither age nor gender specific: It is needed for men and women, young girls and young boys. Sexual counseling, assessment and provision of information about sexual feelings, behaviors, and myths, is an intervention that registered nurses can provide. Sexual therapy focusing on sexual disorders such as impotence, organismic dysfunctions, and other complicated sexual problems should be provided by registered nurses with advanced training in sex education and counseling.

Counseling about the effects of the chronic condition on sexuality is essential because, in many instances, patients may blame their sexual alteration on themselves, when a disease or medication may be causing their problem. Some patients may need education about alternative forms of sexual expression or assistance with working out relationships with significant others.

Factors to consider in sexual counseling include physical status of the patient, the physiologic effects of sexual activity, and psychologic effects of the condition on the patient and significant other. Guidelines for sexual counseling include (1) maintaining a nonjudgmental attitude, (2) using behavioral cues to identify when the patient is ready to discuss sexual concerns, (3) keeping the issue of sexuality in perspective for patient and partner, (4) providing a conducive environment for counseling, and (5) seeking feedback to determine whether counseling has been effective. The goals of counseling are to keep sexuality in perspective with the rest of one's life; reassure the patient that thoughts and feelings about sexual activity are normal; and provide information to dispel myths and correct misinformation (Annon, 1976). Nurses can suggest some strategies for persons having sexual difficulties. McCann (1989) suggests the following:

1. Encourage open communication about sexuality between partners.
2. Encourage partner to become involved in care activities such as washing and grooming to provide intimacy.
3. Encourage touching between partners.
4. Discuss energy-saving positions.
5. Discuss the use of imagery for sexual fantasy.
6. Discuss alternative means of sexual pleasure.

Katzin (1990) described insidious changes in sexual functioning that develop with certain chronic conditions and suggested that planning ahead may solve some of the sexual problems patients experience. For example, common problems for patients with chronic obstructive pulmonary disease are dyspnea and coughing. Katzin suggests sex in the late morning or early afternoon, when energy levels are at their peak, and engaging in activities to increase tolerance for activity (e.g., an exercise program). Other suggestions included taking bronchodilators before sex, using oxygen and inhalers, having a comfortable room temperature and humidity, and using positions that make breathing easier. For the person with arthritis, pain and stiffness can be problematic. Planning to have sex at a time when medications are at their peak effect, after a warm bath, and after simple range of motion exercises may add to comfort. With diabetes, peripheral neuropathy may interfere with a man's ability to have an erection. Good diabetic control and good psychosocial health may help. For women with diabetes, vaginal dryness or infection may be problematic, but medication may help. Some medications for hypertension and depression may cause diminished libido. Patients should be aware of this possibility, and if it is problematic, medications may be adjusted to reduce or eliminate the problem.

Pain

Patients with chronic conditions may experience acute (e.g., following surgery) or chronic pain (e.g., arthritis, cancer). Pain of varying intensity is experienced by at least 30% of our population (Rosomoff & Steele-Rosomoff, 1988), and chronic pain is a major cause of disability in the United States (Osterweis et al, 1987). The experience of pain is a highly personal one (Melzak, 1973), and it is often undertreated (Angell, 1982; McCaffery & Bebee, 1989). Although it is beyond the scope of this book to discuss the various theories and methods of treatment, we urge the reader to attend to the large body of literature on pain and to take an active role in alleviating pain. Intervention strategies include pharmacological management (narcotics and nonnarcotics) and noninvasive methods such as distraction, relaxation, and imagery. Negative cognitions (inability to control pain and catastrophizing) are associated with depression in patients with pain as well as those without pain (Turner & Clancy, 1986). Attention diversion, praying, and hoping may be useful in decreasing experimental pain, but it is not likely to be effective for chronic pain. Distraction may be less effective for chronic pain than it is for acute severe pain. Whether distraction techniques should be included in chronic pain treatment programs is still unknown.

Coping skills training was demonstrated to be effective in controlling pain (Turner & Clancy, 1986). Programs emphasize teaching cognitive and behavioral skills. A cognitive control program involves training in systematic progressive muscle relaxation, imagery, covert assertion, identification, and modification of distorted maladaptive thoughts related to pain and stressful events. Operant-behavior therapy involves aerobic walking, training patients and spouses to identify pain behaviors, for patient to decrease pain behaviors and spouse not to reinforce them and to reinforce well behaviors, and communication training. Outcome is measured by patient's perceptions of control over pain and ability to decrease pain.

Additional Interventions with Children

There are various approaches to helping children cope with their stressors. Nurses can draw on the child's previous experiences by relating new and unfamiliar situations to something that is familiar. Examples might include reminding children of previous experiences, such as the doctor listening to their chest, or comparing an anesthesia or aerosol mask with a space mask.

Vocabulary level and amount and type of material presented should be appropriate to the child's cognitive level. To be certain children understand what has been said, and to correct any misconceptions, ask children to explain to you what you told them. For example, a 9-year-old boy was told that the intravenous (IV) liquid he was having was to give him food that he couldn't eat yet. When the trays arrived for the other children, he asked the nurse how she was going to get a meatball into the IV tubing. Determine what a child knows verbally and understands conceptually. It is easy to be misled by children's verbalizations. Their words often indicate little in the way of real understanding. Take cues from the children, tell them what they want to know, and answer questions on their level.

Nurses can help children learn how to modify favorite activities to make them more appropriate for the demands of the condition. A child with asthma may be able to play goalie rather than a line position, or a child who has difficulty running could still play baseball by hitting the ball and having someone else run.

An innovative summer program at Downstate Medical Center in Brooklyn, New York, (Mogtader & Leff, 1986) applies the "peer-helping peer" principle. The program employs chronically ill adolescents as child-life assistants. In this position they are helped in coping with their own condition while allowing them to help other adolescents. The youngsters learn play skills (e.g., water, music, dramatic play, arts, crafts) and have pre- and postconferences, when they talk about the patients they are helping and about their own feelings and interactions.

One way children cope with their stressors is by telling stories. By carefully listening to the content of these stories, the nurse can gain insight into the children's fears and fantasies. Parents may be upset by their children's stories because they may feel they have failed the child. It can be helpful to explain to them that story telling is a coping mechanism for the child, not a reflection on their parenting ability.

Specific interventions to facilitate infant coping include rocking, stroking, holding, cuddling, changing position, providing a pacifier, initiating self-comforting measures (e.g., bringing fingers to mouth), and allowing infants to comfort themselves (Vipperman & Rager, 1980). To help toddlers and preschoolers cope with their chronic conditions the nurse can set realistic limits; provide for self-expression (e.g., play, puppets, opportunities for role reversal with hospital equipment, drawing) and release of aggression (hammer, water play, clay, ball throwing); provide books about children overcoming obstacles; touch the child to convey warmth and understanding; ensure access to such things as transition objects, family photographs, and parent rooming-in; provide opportunities to practice for potentially stressful situations; make reality oriented statements about fears (e.g., procedures are not punishment); allow time to rest between stressful procedures; hold and cuddle after stressful experiences, and provide diversional play opportunities for self-expression and action-oriented activities for mobility (Vipperman & Rager, 1980).

School age children can be helped to cope by determining what the child knows, clarifying, and using diagrams, models, and equipment; encouraging the child to verbalize feelings; preparing the child for stressful events; encouraging continuation of schoolwork; allowing decision making about care whenever possible; setting limits (e.g., it is okay to scream but not to move); providing books and games; allowing the child to handle equipment; being a good listener (to their jokes, etc.); being a good sport (play jokes); sharing cartoons and anecdotes; encouraging optimum activity; encouraging parents to keep the child informed about home activities; and encouraging participation in their own care (Vipperman & Rager, 1980).

To help adolescents cope with their chronic condition, nurses can determine what the youngster knows and clarify misconceptions (remember that intellectualization and big words do not necessarily mean understanding); use diagrams, models, equipment; encourage verbalization of feelings; prepare for stressful events; encourage continuation of schoolwork; allow the adolescent to make decisions about care; help interpret normal body changes from abnormal; anticipate future changes; encourage self-expression (e.g., keep diary, write poetry); respect need to conform to peers; encourage socialization with peers; arrange contact with role models (e.g., famous people with same problem); encourage participation in own care; set reasonable limits but be flexible; and provide for optimal activity (Vipperman & Rager, 1980).

Therapeutic Play

Play is a vehicle for teaching and clarifying misconceptions. Therapeutic play is used when there is some problem or concern causing emotional stress or anxiety (Walker, 1989). Therapeutic play, conducted by a professional (e.g., nurse, child-life worker) knowledgeable about child growth and development differs from play therapy, conducted by a professional therapist. Therapeutic play allows children to release tension (anger, hostility, aggression), make sense of painful experiences, enjoy a temporary escape, and provide a link to their life outside the hospital. Thus, play can be either diversional or tension reducing. Nurses should encourage and participate in therapeutic play. Make sure the hospitalized child has play materials available for diversion as well as opportunities (time, materials) for hospital play. Being involved in the child's play is one way

Table 12–6 Therapeutic Techniques for Children

Body tracings	An art technique to promote better understanding of body image. Child lies on floor or stands against wall while body is traced, then fills in details with crayons; can also be made into marionettes by means of fasteners at joints of limbs and adding strings.
Clown make-up and hats	Need full length mirror. Children should feel in control and make decisions whether to wear hats, use makeup, or look at self.
Videotape	Can be distressing to some of the children, may begin by watching others. By seeing self can observe appearances (e.g., in traction, with bandages)
Books and art	Allow distancing, denial, projection, or symbolic handling of stressful issues
Fantasy play	For children with death anxieties (e.g., drawing, story telling), without stressing or reinforcing death themes

Source: Cameron, Juszczak, & Wallace, 1984.

nurses can identify troublesome issues for children and help them to deal with them.

Creative arts have been used to help children cope with altered body image (Cameron, Juszczak, & Wallace, 1984). Art therapy is a treatment that requires highly specialized training; however, using art to help hospitalized children express their feelings and concerns is appropriate. Some creative approaches used by child-life specialists for therapeutic purposes are described in Table 12–6.

Summary

Assessment of individual stressors and coping strategies involves internal resources, including health and energy, knowledge, feelings, and sexuality. External resource assessment of individual and family includes relationships, communication and external support. While information regarding general coping strategies is useful, specific strategies used for current stressors are particularly important in planning care.

Effective nursing interventions are based on the specific needs and strengths of family members and the family unit. Clients and families are more likely to adhere to the regimen of care and be equal partners with health care professionals when nurses take time to explain the patient's regimens, learn how they fit into family life-style and goals, discuss variations and alternatives, and arrive at mutually agreeable methods of treatment. Intervention strategies to help clients and families understand the situations they face and, when possible, preparing them for anticipated stressor events may facilitate an adequate level of functioning. Assisting them to develop a repertoire of coping strategies with which to handle these stressors is also valuable.

Stress can be reduced through various interventions, including stress inoculation training, a cognitive-behavioral approach; stress management techniques, such as relaxation, problem solving, reality testing, or assertiveness; and cognitive strategies, such as cognitive restructuring, problem solving, and guided self-dialogue. The focus of cognitive intervention is to change thoughts as well as feelings and actions, whereas relaxation training is offered to alter perceptions of bodily experiences. Contingency management, another useful intervention strategy, involves goal setting, contracting, reinforcement, and response-cost condition. Mutually derived contracts can be effective strategies for promoting positive health outcomes. Crisis intervention is used to focus on rapid mobilization of the client's emotional resources to resolve an immediate stressful situation.

References

Angell, J. (1982, Jan 14). The quality of mercy. *N Engl J Med, 306,* 98–99.

Annon, J. (1976). The PLISSIT model: A proposed conceptual scheme for the behavioral treatment of sexual problems. *J Sex Educators Therapists, 2,* 1–15.

Aquilera, D.G., & Messick, J.M. (1982). *Crisis intervention: Theory and methodology* (4th ed.). St. Louis: Mosby.

Barofsky, I. (1981). Issues and approaches to the psychosocial assessment of the cancer patient. In K. Proktop

& L.A. Bradley (Eds.), *Medical psychology: Contributions to behavioral medicine.* (pp. 55–65). New York: Academic Press.

Beck, D.E., Fennell, R.S., Yost, R.J., et al. (1979). Evaluation of an educational program on compliance with medication regimens in pediatric patients with renal transplants. *J Pediatr, 96,* 1094–1097.

Brykczynski, K. (1982). Health contracting. *Nurse Pract, 7*(5), 27–31.

Burish, T.G., & Bradley, L.A. (1983). Coping with chronic disease: Definitions and issues. In T.G. Burish & L.A. Bradley (Eds.), *Coping with chronic disease* (pp. 3–12). New York: Academic Press.

Burns, D.D. (1980). *Feeling good: The new mood therapy.* New York: William Morrow.

Butler, R.N. (1974). Mental health and aging. *Geriatrics, 29,* 53–54.

Butler, R.N. (1963). The life review. *Psychiatry, 26,* 65–76.

Cameron, C.O., Juszczak, L., & Wallace, N. (1984). Using creative arts to help children cope with altered body image. *Child Health Care, 12*(3), 108–112.

Capone, M.A., Westie, K.S., Chitwood, J.S., et al. (1979). A functional model for hospitalized cancer patients. *Am J Orthopsychiatry, 49,* 598–607.

Chewning, B. (1982). *Strategies to promote self management of chronic illness.* AHA/CDC Health Education Project. Chicago: American Hospital Association.

Childress, A.R., & Burns, D.D. (1981). The basics of cognitive therapy. *Psychosomatics, 22*(12), 1017–1027.

Cohen, J.A. (1986). Sexual counseling of the patient following myocardial infarction. *Critical Care Nurse, 6*(6), 18–27.

Cromer, B.A., & Tarnowski, K.J. (1989). Noncompliance in adolescents: A review. *J Dev Behav Pediatr, 10*(4), 207–215.

Cunningham, A.J., & Tocco, E.K. (1989). A randomized trial of group psychoeducational therapy for cancer patients. *Patient Educ Counseling, 14,* 101–114.

Damrosch, S.P., & Perry, L.A. (1989). Self-reported adjustment, chronic sorrow, and coping of parents of children with Down syndrome. *Nurs Res, 38*(1), 25–30.

deRaymon, P.B. (1983). The final task: Life review for the dying patient. *Nursing 83, 13*(2), 43–47.

Douglas, D., & Anisman, H. (1975). Helplessness or expectation incongruency: Effects of aversive consequence on subsequent performance. *J Exp Psychol [Hum Percept], 1,* 411–417.

Dunst, C.J., Trivette, C.M., & Deal, A.G. (1988). *Enabling and empowering families: Principles and guidelines for practice.* Cambridge, MA: Brookline Books.

Ertzwiler, D.D. (1974). Why not put your patients under contract? *Prism, 2,* 26–28.

Faust, J., & Melamed, B.G. (1984). Influence of arousal, previous experience, and age on surgery preparation of same day of surgery and in-hospital pediatric patients. *J Consult Clin Psychol, 52,* 359–365.

Flodberg, S.O. (1990). Sexuality. In I.M. Lubkin (Ed.), *Chronic illness: Impact and interventions* (2nd. ed.). (pp. 232–260). Boston: Jones and Bartlett.

Folkman, S., & Lazarus, R.S. (1980). An analysis of coping in a middle-aged community sample. *J Health Soc Behav, 21,* 219–239.

Gatchel, R.J., & Baum, A. (1983). *An introduction to health psychology.* Reading, MA: Addison-Wesley.

Hamilton, D.B. (1985). Reminiscence therapy. In G.M. Bulecheck, & J.C. McCloskey (Eds.), *Nursing interventions: Treatments for nursing diagnoses.* Philadelphia: W.B. Saunders.

Heinrich, R.L., & Schag, C.C. (1984). A behavioral medicine approach to coping with cancer: A case report. *Cancer Nurs, 7*(3), 243–247.

Herje, P.A. (1980). Hows and whys of patient contracting. *Nurse Educator, 5*(1), 30–34.

Horowitz, M.J., & Wilner, N. (1980). Life events, stress and coping. In L. Poon (Ed.), *Aging in the 1980s: Selected contemporary issues.* Washington, DC: American Psychological Association.

Hull, M.M. (1980). Family needs and supportive nursing behaviors during terminal cancer: A review. *Oncol Nurs Forum, 16*(6), 787–792.

Hyman, R.B., Feldman, H.R., Harris, R.B., et al. (1989). The effects of relaxation training on clinical symptoms: A meta-analysis. *Nurs Res, 38*(4), 216–220.

Hymovich, D.P. (1981, May 13). Chronic childhood illness: Family impact and parent coping. Association for the Care of Children's Health, Toronto, Canada.

Hymovich, D.P. (1984). Development of the chronicity impact and coping instrument: Parent questionnaire (CICI:PQ). *Nurs Res, 33*(4), 218–222.

Hymovich, D.P. (1989, unpublished). The parent perception inventories: Guidelines for administration and scoring.

Hymovich, D.P., (1990). Measuring parental coping when a child is chronically ill. In O.L. Strickland & C.F. Waltz (Eds.), *Measurement of nursing outcomes vol. 4. Measuring client self-care and coping skills* (pp. 96–117). New York: Springer.

Jalowiec, A., Murphy, S.P., & Powers, M.J. (1984). Psychometric assessment of the Jalowiec Coping Scale. *Nursing Research, 33*(3), 157–161.

Johnson, J.E., Kirchhoff, K., & Endress, M.P. (1975). Altering children's distress behavior during orthopedic cast removal. *Nurs Res. 24,* 404–410.

Johnson, S.B., Silverstein, J., Rosenbloom, A., et al. (1986). Assessing daily management in childhood diabetes. *Health Psychol, 5*(6), 545–564.

Katzin, L. (1990). Chronic illness and sexuality. *Am J Nurs, 90*(1), 55–59.

Kendall, P.C., & Watson, D. (1981). Psychological preparation for stressful medical procedures. In C.E. Prokop & L.A. Bradley (Eds.), *Medical psychology* (pp. 197–221). New York: Academic Press.

Kerfoot, K.M., & Buckwalter, K.C. (1985). In G.M. Bulechek & J.C. McCloskey (Eds.), *Nursing interventions: Treatments for nursing diagnoses.* Philadelphia: W.B. Saunders.

Kikuchi, J. (1975). How the leukemic child chooses his confidant. *Can Nurse, 71*(5), 22–23.

Klorman, R., Hilpert, P.L., Michael, R., et al. (1980). Effects of coping and mastery modeling on experienced and inexperienced pedodontics patient's disruptiveness. *Behav Ther, 11,* 156–168.

Lazarus, R. (1984). The costs and benefits of denial. In S. Breznitz (Ed.), *Denial of stress.* New York: International Universities Press.

Leiber, D. (1986). Laughter and humor in critical care. *Dimens Crit Care Nurs, 5*(3), 163–170.

McCaffrey, M., & Bebee, A. (1989). *Pain: Clinical manual for nursing practice.* St. Louis: Mosby.

McCann, M.E. (1989). Sexual healing after heart attack. *Am J Nurs, 89*(9), 1133–1138.

McCubbin, H.I., & Comeau, J.K. (1987). FIRM: Family Inventory of Resources Management. In H.I. McCubbin & A.L. Thompson (Eds.), *Family assessment inventories for research and practice* (pp. 143–159). Madison, WI: University of Wisconsin-Madison.

McCubbin, H.I., Patterson, J.M., Cauble, A.E., et al. (1981). *Systematic assessment of family stress, resources, and coping: Tools for research, education and clinical investigation.* St. Paul, MN: University of Minnesota.

McCubbin, H.I., & Thompson, A.L. (Eds.). (1987). *Family assessment inventories for research and practice.* Madison, WI: University of Wisconsin-Madison.

Meichenbaum, D. (1985). *Stress inoculation training.* New York: Pergamon.

Meichenbaum, D., & Novaco, R. (1978). Stress inoculation: A preventative approach. In C.D. Spielberger, & I.G. Sarason (Eds.), *Stress and anxiety* (Vol 5). New York: Halstead.

Meichenbaum, D., & Turk, D.C. (1987). *Facilitating treatment adherence: A practitioner's guidebook.* New York: Plenum.

Melamed, B.G., Dearborn, M., & Hermecz, D. (1983) Necessary considerations for surgery preparation: Age and previous experience. *Psychosom Med, 45,* 517–525.

Melzak, R. (1983). *The puzzle of pain.* New York: Basic Books.

Miller, J.F. (1983). *Coping with chronic illness: Overcoming powerlessness.* Philadelphia: F.A. Davis.

Mishel, M.H., & Braden, C.J. (1988). Finding meaning: Antecedents of uncertainty in illness. *Nurs Res, 37*(2), 98–103, 127.

Mogtader, E.M., & Leff, P.T. (1986). "Young healers": Chronically ill adolescents as child life assistants. *Child Health Care, 14*(3), 174–177.

Molleman, E., Krabbendam, P.J., Annyas, A.A., et al. (1984). The significance of the doctor-patient relationship in coping with cancer. *Soc Sci Med, 18,* 475–480.

Moos, R.H. (1974). Psychological techniques in the assessment of adaptive behavior. In G.V. Coelho, D.A. Hamburg & J.E. Adams (Eds.). *Coping and adaptation.* New York: Basic Books.

Munro, B.H., Creamer, A.M., Haggerty, M.R., & Cooper, F.S. (1988). Effect of relaxation therapy on post-myocardial infarction patients' rehabilitation. *Nurs Res, 37*(4), 231–235.

Osterweis, M. (1987). Illness behavior and experience in chronic pain. In M. Osterweis, A. Kleinman, & D. Mechanic (Eds.), *Pain and disability: Clinical behavior and public policy perspectives.* Washington, DC: National Academy Press.

Patel, C., Marmot, M.G., Terry, D.J., et al. (1985). Trial of relaxation in reducing coronary risk: Four year follow up. *Br Med J, 290,* 1103–1106.

Pender, N.J. (1985). Effects of progressive muscle relaxation training in anxiety and health locus of control among hypertensive adults. *Nurs Res Health, 8,* 67–72.

Pruyser, P.N. (1987). Maintaining hope in adversity. *Bull Menninger Clin, 51*(5), 463–474.

Robinson, V. (1977). *Humor and the health professions.* New York: SLACK.

Rolland, J.S. (1987). Family systems and chronic illness: A typological model. *J Psychother Fam, 3*(3), 143–168.

Rosomoff, H., & Steele-Rosomoff, R. (1988, March). Pain management programs for low back disorders. *Miami Med, 59,* 25–26.

Savedra, M.K. (1977). The severely burned child: Moving from hospital to home. *Matern Child Nurs, 1,* 220–222.

Schneider, J.S. (1980). Hopelessness and helplessness. *J Psychiatr Nurs Ment Health Serv, 18*(3), 12–21.

Seligman, M. (1975). *Helplessness: On depression, development, and death.* San Francisco: W.H. Freeman.

Shipley, R.H., Butt, J.H., & Horowitz, E.A. (1979). Preparation to reexperience a stressful medical examination: Effect of repetitious videotape exposure and coping style. *J Consult Clin Psychol, 47,* 485–492.

Simon, J.M. (1989). Humor techniques for oncology nurses. *Oncol Nurs Forum, 16*(5), 667–670.

Simons, R.D., Morris, J.L., Frank, H.A., et al. (1979). Pain medication contracts for problem patients. *Psychosomatics, 20*(2), 122–123, 127.

Skipper, J.K., & Leonard, R.C. (1968). Children, stress and hospitalization: A field experiment. *J Health Hum Behav, 9,* 275–287.

Spirito, A.A., Russo, D.C., & Masek, B.J. (1984). Behavioral interventions and stress management training for hospitalized adolescents and young adults with cystic fibrosis. *Gen Hosp Psychiatry, 6,* 211–218.

Steckel, S.B., & Swain, M.A. (1977). Contracting with patients to improve compliance. *Hospitals, 51,* 81–84.

Stein, R.E.K., & Jessop, D.H. (1984). Does pediatric home care make a difference for children with chronic illness? Findings from the pediatric ambulatory care treatment study. *Pediatrics, 73,* 845–853.

Snyder, M. (1986). Stressor inventory for persons with epilepsy. *J Neurosci Nurs, 18*(2), 71–73.

Swain, M.A., & Steckel, S.B. (1981). Influencing adherence among hypertensive. *Res Nurs Health, 4,* 213–222.

Taylor, C., Lieberman, R.P., Agras, W.S., et al. (1982). Treatment evaluation and behavior therapy. J.M. Lewis & G. Usdin (Eds.), *Treatment planning in psychiatry.* Washington, DC: American Psychiatric Association Press.

Thoresen, C.E., Friedman, M., Powell, L.H., et al. (1985). Altering type A behavior pattern in postinfarction patients. *J Cardiopulmonary Rehabil, 5,* 258–266.

Tobin, D.L., Reynolds, R.V.C., Holroyd, K.A. & Creer, T.L. (1986). Self-management and social learning theory. In K.A. Holroyd, & T.L. Creer (Eds.), *Self management of chronic disease* (pp. 29–55). Orlando, FL: Academic Press.

Turner, J.A., & Clancy, S. (1986). Strategies for coping with chronic low back pain: Relationship to pain and disability. *Pain, 24,* 355–364.

Ureda, J.R. (1980). The effect of contract witnessing on motivation and weight loss in a weight control program. *Health Educ Q, 7,* 163–185.

Vaillot, S.M.C. (1970). Living and dying: Part I. Hope, the restoration of being. *Am J Nurs, 70,* 268–272.

Vipperman, J.F., & Rager, P.M. (1980). Childhood coping: How nurses can help. *Pediatr Nurs, 6,* 11–17.

Walker, D.K., Epstein, S.G., Taylor, A.B., et al. (1989). Perceived needs of families with children who have chronic health conditions. *Child Health Care, 18*(4), 196–201.

Wasik, B. (1984). *Teaching parents effective problem-solving: A handbook for professionals.* Unpublished manuscript. University of North Carolina, Chapel Hill.

Weinert, C. (1987). A social support measure: PRQ85. *Nurs Res, 36*(5), 273–277.

Wickler, L., Wascow, N., & Hatfield, E. (1981). Chronic sorrow revisited: Parent vs. professional depiction of the adjustment of parents of mentally retarded children. *Am J Orthopsychiatry, 51,* 63–67.

Worden, J.W., & Sobel, H.J. (1978). Ego strength and psychosocial adaptation to cancer. *Psychosom Med, 40,* 585–592.

Zangari, M.E., & Duffy, P. (1980). Contracting with patients in day-to-day practice. *Am J Nurs, 80*(3), 451–455.

Zola, I.K. (1982). Denial of emotional needs in people with handicaps. *Arch Phys Med Rehabil, 63,* 63–67.

SECTION V
Level of Functioning

This section contains two chapters, Strengths and Needs and Level of Functioning. System strengths and needs arise from developmental and situational stressors and strategies used to cope with them. These strengths and needs have a direct bearing on the system's level of functioning. Nursing interventions arise from assessment of strengths, needs, and level of functioning. They are provided to foster strengths and facilitate need reduction.

Chapter 13, Strengths and Needs, defines **strengths** as system resources, assets, and abilities; and **needs** as motivating forces initiating behavior to maintain internal consistency and harmony with the external environment. When needs are met, they may become strengths. Potential individual and family strengths and needs include positive self-esteem, knowledge, coping resources, autonomy, independence, and support. Also included in this chapter are guidelines for assessing strengths and needs. Intervention strategies include (1) establishing and maintaining trust, (2) providing support and guidance, (3) providing information based on principles of teaching and learning, and (4) providing anticipatory guidance.

Chapter 14, Level of Functioning, discusses individual and system level of functioning, or current state of adaptation to the chronic condition. Variables influencing functioning, such as the condition itself, environmental characteristics, and achievement of developmental and situational tasks are discussed. Nursing intervention strategies to foster independence and to facilitate control, adherence to regimen, and access to resources are discussed. The nurse's collaborative role is also included in this chapter.

13 Strengths and Needs

All human beings are unique, with diverse strengths and needs. Although system strengths and needs are partially contingent upon identified stressors and coping strategies, they also play a role in determining perceptions of stressors (primary appraisals) and one's ability to cope with stressors (secondary appraisals). Strengths reflect system abilities and assets, whereas needs reflect potential system weaknesses or limitations in coping with stressors. Nursing assessment and intervention focus on determining system assets and capabilities to foster growth and use in meeting identified needs.

This chapter provides an overview of the concepts of strengths and needs, followed by selected potential strengths and needs of individuals and families. The relationship of strengths and needs to other variables in the Contingency Model of Long-Term Care is depicted in Figure 13-1. It can be seen from the figure that although strengths and needs arise from stressors and coping strategies, they also play a role in determining whether something becomes a strength or a need. For example, a family with many resources is more likely to identify resources as a strength rather than as a need. However, if they are lacking financial resources, then financial resources will be identified as a need. If this need is satisfied, it will no longer be a stressor and may become a strength.

Characteristics perceived as strengths in one situation may become needs or stressors in another situation. A person needing money to purchase a new home may have a strong work orientation (strength) enabling her or him to work overtime to obtain the needed money. However, if that person becomes chronically ill or disabled and can work only a limited amount of time, this strong work orientation can become a stressor.

Strengths

Strengths are system resources, assets, and capabilities. They may be identified subjectively by the individual or objectively by others. Strengths form the foundation for individual and family system level of functioning and potential for growth. **Capable individuals and families** are those able to use their assets and strengths to cope with stressors throughout the life cycle.

Strengths can be classified on the basis of who perceives them. **Self-assessed strengths** are the system's (e.g., individual, family, community) assessment of it's own capabilities, whereas **other-assessed strengths** are capabilities perceived by someone outside the system. Although similarities may exist, it is unlikely that other-assessed strengths would be identical to those that are self-assessed. Discrepancies in self-assessed and nurse-assessed perceptions of strengths are likely to affect the appropriateness of interventions and their eventual outcome.

Systems have both internal and external strengths. Internal strengths include health; high energy level; self-esteem and self-respect; autonomy

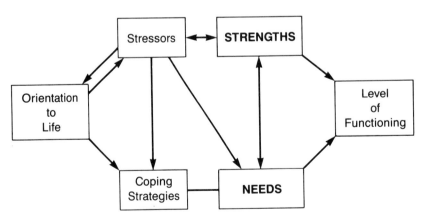

FIGURE 13–1 Relationship of Strengths and Needs to Orientation to Life, Stressors, Coping Strategies, and Level of Functioning

Table 13–1 Family Strengths

- Ability to provide for family physical, emotional, and spiritual needs

- Clear set of family rules, values, and beliefs

- Open and honest communication that emphasizes positive interactions

- Ability to provide support, security, and encouragement

- Maintain and build relationships within the family

- Maintain and build relationships within the community

- Balance between use of internal and external family resources

- Ability to help oneself and to accept help when needed

- Flexibility in family functions and roles

- Mutual respect and appreciation for individuality

- Ability to use crisis as a means for growth

- Family unity, loyalty, and intrafamily cooperation

- Growing through and with children

- Varied repertoire of coping strategies, including problem-solving abilities

- Child-rearing practices implemented by both parents, mutual respect for each parent's views, and self-discipline fostered in children

- Commitment toward promoting family well-being

- Concentrated effort to spend time together as a family

Sources: Adapted from Dunst, Trivette, & Deal (1988) and Otto (1973).

and independence; ability to communicate with others; and feelings of love, belongingness, acceptance, security, protection, faith, and self-control.

Family strengths are capabilities and resources that enable a family to meet each member's needs as well as those of the family unit. Family resources differ from individual resources because they are a combination of individual characteristics that reflect the interdependence among family members (Walker, 1988). Family strengths are influenced by forces inside and outside the family. They are

. . . those relationship patterns, interpersonal skills and competencies, and social and psychological characteristics which create a sense of positive family identity, promote satisfying and fulfilling family interaction among family members, encourage the development of the potential of the family group and individual family members, and contribute to the family's ability to deal effectively with stress and crisis (Williams, Lindgren, Rowe, et al, 1975, preface)

Otto (1973) defined family strengths as "those factors or forces that contribute to family unity and solidarity and that foster the development of potentials within the family" (p. 88). This research has been a major force in encouraging professionals to focus on capabilities rather than just on weaknesses or limitations. Recent work by Dunst and colleagues (1988) has led to a reformulation of Otto's family strengths. Family strengths are listed in Table 13–1 and examples of comments regarding family strengths are in Box 13–1.

Needs

A **need** is a motivating force that initiates behavior to maintain internal consistency and harmony with the external environment. It "is something (e.g., a resource) that is desired or lacking but wanted or required to achieve a goal or attain a particular end" (Dunst, Trivette, & Deal, 1988, p. 13). In other words, there is a discrepancy between what is present and what one desires. It is felt as a tension that can be reduced by a specific source of satisfaction. As a need increases, so does the tension. Individual and family needs are fundamental to family systems theory (Hartman & Laird, 1983).

Illness alters perceptions of strengths and needs by shifting their priorities (Maslow, 1968). Changes in perceptions are influenced by the nature of the condition and the system's identifying characteris-

Box 13–1 *Statements of Family Strengths*

Statements by Adults

"The nurse asked me if anyone had helped me through this. I said my son had been wonderful, but I realized that I had never told him. So I went home and told him how helpful he had been. He said 'Mom, any son would have done the same.' He's going to take me out to lunch on my last day of treatment."

"My daughters have been terrific. They each take turns to bring me in. They all have families and have jobs, but they arranged their schedules for me. I feel so guilty."

"I don't know how I would have managed without my husband. He comes with me to all of my doctor's appointments."

"I didn't want to tell anyone, but I'm glad I did. Everyone is so thoughtful. They send cards. It's nice to know that someone cares and is thinking about you."

Statements by Children

"My sister teases me, but I know she really cares."

"Dad says we'll make it because we stick together. Even if Mom gets worse, he said we'd be okay. . . . Yeah, I believe him."

tics. The degree of need for any individual or family may vary widely at any given time, and family members may disagree over the relative priority among needs. Similarly, individual and family perceptions of strengths will vary.

Needs can be classified on the basis of who perceives them (Magi & Allander, 1981). **Self-assessed needs** are the system's (e.g., individual, family, community) assessment of it's own situation, whereas **other-assessed needs** are the situation as perceived by someone outside the system. Because self-assessed needs are unique and subjective, complete congruence with other-assessed needs is rare. Differences between clients and health professionals, such as social and educational background, influence perceptions of need. Differences in perceptions and

values regarding the client's present and future may affect the suitability of interventions and their eventual outcome. "The less agreement there is on the factual contents of the need situation, the greater the possibility for disagreement on a value basis" (Magi & Allander, 1981, p. 54).

Generally, the medical approach to those with chronic conditions has focused on the practical possibilities of people's limitations rather than on their potentialities and strengths (Zola, 1982). While medical focus is on the disease and its treatment, the accompanying disability and handicap are of greater consequence in daily functioning of the individual. Nurses have a crucial role in helping the client and family achieve a balance of their medically defined disease needs and their self-defined illness needs and strengths. In part, client satisfaction with nursing care depends upon the extent of agreement between clients' perceptions of needs and need priorities and those of nurses (Williamson, 1978). If clients and nurses can identify needs and set mutually agreeable goals, the goals more likely will be met.

Individuals and families need to accomplish their developmental and situational tasks to function effectively within the constraints of the chronic condition. People differ in ability to accomplish tasks and, consequently, in the extent of their strengths and needs. Systems function adequately as long as their basic needs are being satisfied. Maslow states a need is "basic or instinctoid" if,

1. its absence breeds illness,
2. its presence prevents illness,
3. its restoration cures illness,
4. under certain (very complex) free choice situations, it is preferred by the deprived person over other satisfactions,
5. it is found to be inactive, at a low ebb or functionally absent in the healthy person.
(Maslow, 1968, p. 22)

There is, also, a subjective "conscious or unconscious yearning or desire, and a feeling of lack or deficiency" when the need is present (Maslow, 1968, p. 22).

Hierarchy of Needs

Maslow (1968) suggested a hierarchy of needs, with basic or lower-level needs having to be satisfied before moving to more complex ones. His hierarchy consists of five basic needs, each having higher level priority than the one preceding it. In ascending order, these needs are (1) physiological, (2) safety and security, (3) belonging and love, (4) social esteem, and finally (5) self-actualization. Needs are related in a hierarchical and developmental way in order of strength and priority. All needs are steps toward self-actualization. Needs overlap and higher-level needs may emerge before lower-level ones are totally satisfied.

Physiological needs predominate in the motivation of human behavior and are essential for life. They include regulation of respiratory, nutritive, and excretory functions and water and electrolyte balance; body temperature maintenance, rest and sleep, and avoidance of pain. If these basic physiological needs are not met, they dominate the conscious mind. Thus, a person with a chronic condition interfering with any of these physiological needs may spend a considerable amount of time and energy in meeting them. For example, it may take a long time to feed oneself or to complete a recommended elimination program.

Safety and security needs include psychological as well as physical factors. One must feel protected and safe in all aspects of life. Illness threatens one's safety and security. When safety is assured, higher needs and impulses can emerge; when it is endangered, regression to the more basic needs occurs. Consider Jenny, an adolescent with cystic fibrosis. When she developed pneumonia, treatment of her physical illness took priority over her school performance. When Mr. Feltzer was placed on home oxygen because of his COPD, he would tell his friends, "You can't smoke here anymore, I have my oxygen. Be careful with those matches."

Belonging and love includes the need for affection. If physiological and safety needs are satisfied, one will then seek companionship, friendship, and recognition of others. Once Jenny's pneumonia was over, she began to worry about when her friends would visit and whether she would fit in with the group when she returned to school. Initially, Mr. Feltzer had to spend so much energy and time controlling his disease that he had little time or energy left to spend on friends or companions. However, when his symptoms were under control, he again became interested in companionship.

The need for esteem includes both self-esteem and social esteem. A person needs to be recognized as an individual with a distinct personality. According to Maslow (1968), needs for social esteem and self-actualization are rarely satisfied completely. If these needs are rarely met for healthy persons, consider how much more difficult they will be for those with chronic conditions who are faced with social stigma.

Self-actualization is an episode in which one's powers come together in an efficient and enjoyable way: One becomes open for experience, more idiosyncratic, more expressive or spontaneous, fully functioning, more creative and more independent of lower needs. Maslow describes the self-actualizing person as more truly himself or herself, closer to the core of his or her being, and more fully human. Maslow estimated that only about 1% of the population reaches self-actualization; some may be too economically deprived, whereas others are satisfied with meeting lower-level needs. For most it is a hope, a yearning, a drive, a something wished for but not yet achieved.

Systems have both internal and external needs. Internal needs are related to health status, energy level, self-esteem, and autonomy and independence. Family systems have basic physical needs for food, shelter, clothing, medications, care of health problems, and cleanliness. Psychological needs include information concerning self, therapy, communication with others, respect for self, recognition for accomplishments, and entertainment. Children, whether chronically ill or healthy, have the following basic needs: love, acceptance, security, protection, independence, faith, guidance, and control (National Association for Mental Health, 1954). Adults have a need for personal achievement in both personal and spiritual matters (Hymovich & Chamberlin, 1980). Categories of needs identified by Dunst et al (1988) include financial adequacy, food and shelter, health and protection, communication and mobility, vocational opportunities, availability of time; education, enrichment, and growth; and cultural/social involvement.

Dunst and colleagues (1988) report that need hierarchies are highly personalized and unique to individual families. For example, a family whose basic needs for food, shelter, and so forth are met will be more likely to focus its hierarchy on the higher-level needs than will a family just scraping by with barely enough food. The latter family invests emotional and physical energy and time meeting these needs.

Potential Strengths and Needs

Potential psychosocial strengths or needs of individuals with chronic conditions include positive self-esteem, self-control, knowledge, coping resources, autonomy, independence, and support. Based on Hymovich's (1976) earlier work, we have identified the following potential needs of individuals who are chronically ill, disabled, or handicapped, and their families. These are related to trust, self-efficacy, spirituality, self-esteem, orientation to life, self-expression and understanding, and independence.

Internal Strengths and Needs

In his classic study with healthy adults, Otto (1965) developed a framework of personal strengths or assets. He noted that strengths are present in a latent or unused form in all people, but that healthy persons function at only 10% to 15% of their potential. He identified a number of areas related to self-concept and self-esteem that can aid people in coping with stressors. A modified list that includes these and other strengths is presented in Table 13–2. An absence of many of these strengths may indicate a need for intervention.

Trust　Interpersonal trust is defined as the "expectancy held by an individual that the communication behaviors of another individual or other individuals can be relied on" (Northouse, 1979, p. 366). Trust has been conceptualized and measured as two independent constructs. The first construct, general trust, indicates a person's trust in people in general. The second construct, specific trust, refers to trust in a particular person. People who are generally trusting do not necessarily trust a particular person; e.g., a family may trust nurses in general, but not the nurse caring for their family member now.

To use their strengths to manage the condition effectively, chronically ill individuals and their families must be able to trust in themselves and each other to manage their feelings and the daily requirements of their illness and its treatment. In addition, they need to trust the health care professionals with whom they come in contact.

Self-efficacy　**Self-efficacy** or control is the real or perceived belief that one has the power to determine the outcome of an event (Gatchel & Baum, 1983). People who feel a sense of control are better able to cope with focal stressor events than are those who do not believe they can be effective in determining what happens to themselves or their families. Generally, people who feel they have the ability to affect their own lives are, or want to be, active participants in decision making and self-care. Ability and flexibility are other aspects of self-efficacy or control that enable the person or family to function within the constraints of the condition. Self-efficacious individuals can regulate their time to fit into schedules, or modify schedules to fit the demands of their condition.

People need to feel they can control their own life and destiny. They need opportunities for taking action, exercising judgment, and making decisions to the degree allowed by the nature of the condition (Germain, 1977). They also need the freedom to

Table 13–2　Individual Strengths

- Trust and confidence in self and others
- Positive self-concept and self-esteem
- Hope
- Spectator sports and similar activities
- Sports and activities
- Hobbies and crafts
- Expressive arts
- Strengths through family and others
- Imaginative and creative strengths
- Other strengths (e.g., humor, perseverance)
- Large repertoire of coping skills
- Education, training, and related areas
- Work, vocation, job, or position
- Special aptitudes or resources
- Intellectual strengths
- Aesthetic strengths
- Organizational strengths
- Relationship strengths
- Spiritual strengths
- Emotional strengths
- Knowledge and understanding of illness, treatment
- Skills
- Temperament
- Genetic factors
- Health status

Sources: Adapted from Elliott & Eisdorfer (1982) and Otto (1965).

make choices and to have some control over their situation.

Spiritual   Spiritual needs are factors necessary to establish and/or maintain a person's personal relationship with their God and to experience forgiveness, love, hope, trust, and meaning and purpose in life (Stallwood & Stoll, 1975). Spiritual beliefs are covered more fully in Chapter 9, Orientation to Life.

During crisis situations, people have indicated that prayer is a strategy that helps them deal with the immediate situation. In fact, one woman with osteoarthritis indicated she had not prayed in years, but when admitted to the hospital for hip replacement surgery, the first thing she did was stop in the chapel to pray.

Positive self-esteem   Positive self-esteem includes feeling worthwhile, positive about oneself, and confident in oneself and one's capabilities. Self-esteem is enhanced in many ways for persons with chronic conditions as well as for their care givers. For example, learning to care for the child's disability made mothers ($n = 27$) of children with long-term tracheostomies feel better about themselves (Singer & Farkas, 1989). This strong sense of mastery of the necessary skills enhanced the self-concept and self-esteem of the mothers.

Hope and a positive orientation to life   **Hope** is a feeling or belief that something desired will occur. It is something that sustains a system through stressful periods (Skolny & Riehl, 1974). Although hope has been defined in many ways, it is generally considered to be a positive personal attribute. Erikson (1963) described hope as a virtue formed in early childhood as a result of having a favorable ratio of trust over mistrust. Hope helps one to deal with a situation when needs and goals have not been met (Korner, 1970). Miller and Powers (1988) describe three levels or intensities of hope: The first level consists of superficial wishes, such as for a nice day or basic material goods. The second level includes hoping for self-improvement, self-accomplishments, and relationships. The third level is hoping for relief from some form of personal suffering.

Rideout and Montemuro (1986) noted the influence a positive outlook can have on adaptation. They found that hopeful patients maintained their involvement in life regardless of the physical limita-tions imposed by their chronic heart failure. They suggested that more hopeful individuals with chronic illness may be able to ignore or suppress certain realities of their illness. Similarly, Stoner and Keampfer (1985) found that patients terminally ill with cancer had just as much hope as patients in other stages of the disease. Cassileth and colleagues (1980) found that patients who were actively involved in their own care were more hopeful than those who did not participate in their care. People who wanted information, either good or bad, were significantly more hopeful than those who wanted only minimal information or only good news.

Understanding and expression of feelings   All individuals need to feel they are understood. For example, all parents in a study of hospitalized children with cancer indicated a need to feel someone understood what it was like for them to have a hospitalized child, to understand the everyday events, losses, and fears associated with hospitalization (Hayes & Knox, 1984).

Mattsson (1972) found that children able to express their feelings of hope and despair were better adjusted to their chronic conditions than were children who could not. Zola (1982), who is disabled, points out the need for those who are disabled to express their feelings of anger. However, he notes that they often are denied this opportunity for fear they may not receive needed help or will be considered ungrateful by their care givers. In addition, they may be physically unable to express anger because they cannot kick or hit. Under the stress of illness, personal animosities, angers, and disappointments may not be expressed. Energy and attention are focused on the immediate situation. Once the crisis has passed and remission is achieved, the old problems resurface. Following the crisis, family members may feel they should be able to meet their own deferred personal needs and gain restitution for their previous sacrifices. "A flexible family structure can allow for conflict and the expression of anger as well as the redevelopment of positive, but appropriate affect toward the patient in remission" (Mailick, 1984, p. 92).

Independence   People need to be able to function autonomously. When this is not possible, they need people who are willing to assist them maintain as high a degree of autonomy as possible. Each system (individual and family) needs to have the maximum physical, cognitive, emotional, social, and spiritual independence possible within the limits imposed by the chronic condition.

Chronic conditions make coping difficult because they may alter strengths. Instead of feeling safe and secure, clients may feel vulnerable and threatened. Just when they need to feel in charge and capable, they may be feeling less coherent and in control, not more. To control the environment and lessen anxiety, people may become rigid and inflexible.

Vulnerability.

Vulnerability is defined as an inadequacy of psychologic and social resources needed to deal with demands in something that matters to the person (Murphy & Moriarty, 1976). If there is a deficit in these resources, functioning is impaired, leaving the individual vulnerable. To be vulnerable means to be susceptible to being wounded or hurt; open to attack or assault. When people are vulnerable, they are weak and defenseless. The degree of vulnerability is determined by the deficit and the relationship between one's pattern of commitment and resources for warding off threats to those commitments. Persons with chronic illnesses are potentially vulnerable at all times. Vulnerability is a potential threat that becomes active when something valued is put in jeopardy (Lazarus, 1984). For example, the personal vulnerability of people with cancer was described by Pelligrino (1981) as a state of being in pain, anxious, dependent, and "unable to pursue other activities until he or she becomes well again."

Information and skills

Adequate knowledge about the condition and its management is a prerequisite to effective functioning. Specific information needed by patients or their family members is listed in Table 13–3. These information needs come from many sources and include topics that have been identified by patients, family members, and health care personnel. Although some needs may be basic for all patients or their family care givers, others will vary with the focal stressors and other contingency variables.

Nurses can anticipate that information is needed by newly diagnosed persons and their family members. They need not only disease-related information but also information related to themselves (physical and psychological well-being, future goals), their family, and social situation (job, leisure, special

Table 13–3 Potential Information and Skill Needs

Disease process	Financial planning
Change in treatment protocols	Financial aid
	Insurance plans
Options for alternative treatment protocols	Social and recreational opportunities
Community resources available	Support groups
When to call physician	Transportation
Nutrition and feeding	Bathing, grooming
Medications	Treatments,
Administration	procedures
Side effects	

Sources: Bartholomew et al, 1988; Ferraro & Longo, 1985; Walker et al, 1989.

interests) (Derdiarian, 1986). Although these needs were identified for adults with cancer, all persons should have the opportunity to obtain such information.

Parents of children hospitalized with long-term disabilities identified the need to understand the illness experience, become familiar with the hospital environment, adapt to their changing relationship with the child and other family members, and negotiate with the health professionals about their child's care (Hayes & Knox, 1984). A study by Hull (1989) identified the needs of family members of a dying patient by analyzing the content of 13 studies focused on family needs. A common finding was that family members wanted clear and honest information about the patient's condition, prognosis, and signs of impending death.

While some studies report similarities and differences in nurse and patient perceptions of learning needs (Casey, O'Connell, & Price, 1984), other studies report only differences in perceptions. Educational needs following myocardial infarction agreed upon by nurses ($n = 33$), physicians ($n = 12$), and patients ($n = 30$) were signs and symptoms of heart attack, ways to modify or change personal risk factors, medication dosage and side effects, and personal risk factors (Casey, O'Connell, & Price, 1984). Studies of patients requiring hemodialysis (Goddard & Powers, 1982) and cancer (Lauer, Murphy, & Powers, 1982) report significant differences between the two groups.

The response of a 16-year-old boy with cystic fibrosis to the question "What should patients know

Box 13–2 *What Adolescents Want to Know About Their Illness*

"They should know EVERYTHING. They should know how they are doing compared to other cystic fibrosis kids. They should know who is doing research, how many people are working on a cure, and where they are working. I'm not interested in the heredity part. I'm just interested in what is going to happen to me. They should know what the pulmonary function test tells the doctor. They should know what the x-rays tell the doctor. Just hearing that "you are doing OK" isn't good enough, because I always get told that. They should know if there is any decline, because ever since I've been little I've been told that I'm OK, but I know that I'm not as well as I was 10 years ago . . . I want to know about other people my age and older with CF. I want to know if they have girlfriends, if they quit school and why, how many get married, if they work, what kind of work they are doing."

Source: Nolan et al, 1986, p. 235.

about CF?" is in Box 13–2. This youngster believed patients should be able to read their hospital records to know that doctors were not hiding anything from them.

People with chronic conditions and those caring for them need to learn what they **should** do to manage the condition as well as what they **should not** do because it may have a harmful outcome. Burckhardt (1987) describes difficulties patients may have when they need to inhibit their actions. She states that patients may have to engage in certain activities before they are able to give them up. For example, a woman with arthritis may be able to garden one day but not for several days afterwards because of the pain the activity caused. In some cases, there may be a fine line between inhibiting and permitting activities to maintain one's self-esteem. Patients and care givers need instructions **and** practice in doing procedures. This helps to reassure the patient and the care giver that they are capable of meeting special needs.

Parents of children with chronic conditions need information about child and family growth and development (Hymovich, 1979; Singer & Farkas, 1989). Children need information about the nature of their condition, and as they get older, more information. They need to know the self-care strategies

they can use to monitor and manage the condition. As they develop, they need to know how to take medicines, do treatments, and help to recognize the small ways they can take control over their health.

Several kinds of skills are generally needed by the person who is ill, disabled, or handicapped, as well as by significant others. Among them are skills that enable clients to manage their own condition, such as performing procedures and preparing appropriate diets. Also needed are skills to enable clients and their families to negotiate with health care providers and others about their care.

Health and energy Physical health, energy, and strength are needed to cope with stressors impinging on family life. **Health status** refers to the person's or the health professional's appraisal of physical and/or mental well-being. For example, siblings of chronically ill children report preoccupation with their own health (Cairns et al, 1979). Some individuals with chronic conditions report they feel healthy in spite of having a diagnosed disease, while others, such as elderly persons with urinary incontinence, tend to rate their health as fair or poor (Harris, 1986).

Energy is the capacity to do work needed to meet the demands of the chronic condition and other family and individual demands. According to Ferraro and Longo (1985), family strength is determined by the physical strength and reserve of each member, the strength of the marital dyad and sibling support, and the health of the family members. Parents of chronically ill children and care givers of chronically ill adults often report fatigue and lack of energy.

Role flexibility Role flexibility and resiliency are strengths often needed by families of chronically ill or disabled persons. As mentioned previously, roles shift as the patient's condition changes and with admission to and discharge from the hospital. As a father remarked about his children, "I was amazed at how helpful they were while she [wife] was in the hospital. They pitched right in without my even having to tell them."

Social support The presence of a social support system can buffer the effects of stress and crisis (Boyce, 1985; Friedland & McColl, 1987; Gatchel & Baum, 1983). Although definitions of social support differ, they generally have one or more of the following components: (1) giving emotional support (nurturance, empathy, encouragement), (2) conveying a sense of belonging, (3) providing tangible help (material assistance) when needed, (4) suggesting information about how to cope, and (5) expressions of sharedness (Elliott & Eisdorfer, 1982; Mechanic, 1986). Kahn and Antonucci (1980) defined it as "interpersonal transactions that include one or more of the following key elements: Affect, affirmation, and aid" (p. 267). Affective transactions involve expressions of liking, admiration, respect, or love; affirmation transactions are expressions of agreement or acknowledgement that some act or statement of another person is right or appropriate; and direct aid or assistance involves giving such things as information, money, or time. To Cobb (1976), support is information that leads people to believe they are loved, cared for, esteemed, and belong to "a network with mutual obligations" (p. 300). On the other hand, instrumental support such as adequate finances may be protective during a major life event like the presence of a long-term condition.

For optimal development to occur, some primary attachment relationship needs to be formed during the first year of life. Later life experiences contribute to the continuity or discontinuity and stability or change of the relationship. Relationships between care giver and infant are reciprocal. For serious chronic conditions at any age, the reciprocity may change considerably when the care giver provides care and the patient has limited or no opportunity to reciprocate. Reciprocity refers to the perception of bidirectional exchange of valued resources (Tilden & Gaylen, 1987). Bidirectional support over time may prevent feelings of indebtedness and dependency.

The concept of adult social support is derived from the concept of attachment based on Bowlby's (1969) work with infants. Bowlby defined attachment as "seeking proximity to the primary caretaker (usually the mother) in times of stress or danger." The concept was later expanded, and others began to apply it to interpersonal activities throughout the life span, suggesting it is equivalent to adult social support (Kahn & Antonucci, 1980).

Social support has been beneficial in mediating the effects of acute and chronic stress and buffering the potentially negative effects of crisis events. Increasing evidence suggests that, for adults, social supports contribute to longer life, lower incidence of physical disease, better morale, more positive mental health, and quicker recovery from illnesses such as congestive heart failure, heart attacks, and asthma. Natural support systems can be effective in buffering stressful events (Ayers, 1989; Boyce, 1985; Hamburg, 1982; Vachon, 1986), influencing use of health services, and maintaining adherence to medical regimens.

Social networks are made up of the people with whom a person communicates and the links between these relationships. Important features of support networks include their structural properties (size, stability, availability, number of people in the network who know each other, heterogeneity among types of contacts) and the nature of the links within the group (reciprocity of relationships, intensity, and frequency of interactions)´ (Elliott & Eisdorfer, 1982; Kahn & Antonucci, 1980). The characteristics of a person's support groups are likely to change as losses occur through death and gains or losses occur through changes in location, school, and jobs.

The need for social support may increase when any of a person's major life roles undergo changes, especially if these changes are not wanted or expected. Under such circumstances the buffering effect of social support may also be increased. An instance of this occurs when the family breadwinner, diagnosed with severe COPD, is required to consider early retirement. The help and support of family and friends during this period are likely to facilitate the change. As one man said, "I don't think I could have done it without their help. It wasn't easy, but I could never have done it alone."

Quality of support may be more important than frequency of interaction (Kahn & Antonucci, 1980). The number of people in the support network appears crucial if the difference is between zero (no support) and one (supportive person). A person with at least one close supportive relationship is able to tolerate a stressful event better than someone with no support.

Social support can be viewed objectively (properties and links) or subjectively (perceptions). People evaluate the actions of others as either supportive (assets) or not supportive (stressors). Actions experienced as threatening one's need for control or interfering with one's ability to make choices are not likely to be perceived as supportive. The majority of nurse-developed social support measures emphasize the receipt of support rather than its provision or reciprocal nature (Stewart, 1989). Equity and reciprocity may be important components of effective relationships. Even when actions are perceived accurately, they may not necessarily be supportive: If people believe they are receiving more support than they think is necessary or can be repaid, its effects may be negative (Kahn & Antonucci, 1980). Other examples of stressful relationships within one's support system were discussed in Chapter 10, Stressors.

Part of the family's support system can be the health care system, yet generally greater support is offered to patients rather than their healthy spouses or other family members. Northouse (1988) reports that husbands of women post-mastectomy perceived significantly less support from health professionals than did patients throughout the course of the illness. A study by Hymovich (1990) indicates that some spouses and children of parents with cancer perceive little or no supportive contact with members of the health care system.

"The kind of support appropriate for a given situation is influenced at least in part by the nature of the stressful situation, the timing of support and the resources of the affected person" (Dimond & Jones, 1983, p. 241). The types of support provided may be instrumental, emotional, appraising, or informational.

Siblings of chronically ill children and children of parents with chronic conditions need to be involved and informed from the beginning of the illness to avoid some of their feelings of isolation and support feelings of belonging and contributing. Children who are not included are likely to feel lonely and guilty about expressing their own feelings (Sargent, 1984). It is important to remember, however, that children differ in the extent to which they want to be involved in their ill sibling's care (Fine & Friedman, 1984), and probably in their parent's care as well. Their desired involvement needs to be determined and honored. Sibling needs are listed in Table 13–4.

Table 13–4 Potential Needs of Children with a Chronically Ill Sibling or Parent

- Social support
- Psychosocial preparation
- Anticipatory guidance
- Assistance in processing information
- Knowledge and information about disease, treatment, and person's condition
- Open and honest communication within the family
- Involvement in the sick person's care to the extent they feel comfortable

Care-giver needs.

Findings concerning care-giver burden and care-giver stress and satisfaction remain equivocal. Variables like the amount of care required, level of impairment, and mental condition of the patient have been identified as important in some studies but not in others (Baille, Norbeck, & Barnes, 1988). Medical problems and physical-care needs were usually found to be less important than mental impairment or psychologic problems of the elderly person. Care givers of elderly persons who indicated the need for social support were significantly lower on dimensions of well-being than were those who reported having sufficient social support (George & Gwyther, 1986), reduced burden, and coping effectiveness (Scott, Roberto, & Hutton, 1986). Zarit et al (1980) also found that frequency of family visits to the elderly person was significantly related to care-giver burden.

Home care of children and adults with complex medical problems is on the rise. Families need a great deal of support beyond the hospital's normal boundaries of care, not only for their medical needs but also for their social and financial needs.

External Resources

Families unable to meet their needs within the family system may require supporting services. They may need assistance with home help, laundry, housing, aids to living (e.g., wheelchairs), and day-care facilities (Pless & Perrin, 1985). Organizational procedures and policies that respect life-styles, cultural values, and social supports are needed to foster trust between the health care system and clients (Germain, 1977). Need for health services refers to the diagnostic, therapeutic, rehabilitative, or compensatory regimen for supporting or restoring well-being once it is compromised (Soldo & Manton, 1985). External resources are discussed more fully in Chapters 7 and 10.

Financial resources Some families may have resources to meet financial obligations imposed by the chronic condition, but a substantial number have limited resources. They may need financial aid in the form of assistance for medical and related services or free or partial-pay clinics and social and counseling services (Pless & Perrin, 1985). Other forms of financial assistance include food stamps, vocational rehabilitation, disability income, and financial benefits to discharged veterans. Assistance with medications can be had through agencies (e.g., American Cancer Society, Leukemia Society), drug companies, Social Security, or Medicare benefits.

Occupation.

Many persons can continue their usual work roles despite their chronic condition, but there may be times when the condition or its therapy necessitates a change in occupation. If ability to work is permanently interfered with, vocational counseling and rehabilitation may be needed. Physical rehabilitation or occupational therapy may alleviate the physical problem and result in improved strength and coordination. Persons who need to change occupations may be eligible for job retraining through the Vocational Rehabilitation Act of 1973. Counseling may facilitate return to work for those unable to deal with the emotional impact of the disability.

It is possible that other family members may have to adjust their work schedules. For example, a spouse may need to curtail working hours to provide care in the home. On the other hand, a family member may have to take on a new or additional job to lessen the family's financial burden.

Youngsters who have grown up with a chronic condition or acquire one sometime in their youth also need counseling. Chronic conditions may limit career options, but discussion with a guidance counselor as early as possible may prevent later disappointments. Since work is significant in the formation of a good self-image, it is important that a realistic and satisfying career choice be made.

Community resources A variety of community resources may be needed by families of those with chronic conditions. Strengths exist when these services are available and the family is able to make use of them. These resources are discussed in Chapters 6 and 7. Adequate resources can help families maintain independence, relieve certain demands, and maintain quality of life. It is helpful if the family has the name of a contact person and clear directions for getting to an agency. In addition, they need to know what to expect regarding admission criteria, services, policies, and fees.

Anticipatory Needs

Persons with chronic conditions and their families need to anticipate what will be happening to them in the future. The anticipatory needs include preparation for experiences like procedures and hospitaliza-

tions, as well as the feelings likely to accompany their experiences. They may also need to anticipate changes in skills, capacities, and personal or family needs over the life cycle.

Parents facing long-term implications of their child's disability or illness may need to grieve and deal with their anger once the acute life-threatening aspects of an illness are resolved (Heisler & Friedman, 1981). Often, this process occurs when earlier supports are no longer available. Acute care workers need to recognize this need and plan for follow-up. Parents need to plan for the future when they are no longer available to provide care for their adult children. Likewise, elderly adults may need to make contingency plans for the time the care giver can no longer care for a spouse.

Hospitalized patients need preparation for expectations following discharge, whether it be a rehabilitation center, nursing home, or their own home. When the hospital stay is relatively brief and the person is going home, little time is needed for psychologic preparation prior to discharge. More time is needed for those whose stay has been lengthy, especially when life has been in danger and the person has been dependent on others for every aspect of care.

Assessment

Assessment of individual and family strengths and needs involves interviewing and observation. Nurses assess each area previously discussed and come to mutual agreement with family members regarding their self-assessed needs and strengths and those assessed by the nurse and others on the health care team. General guidelines for assessing strengths appear in Table 13–5 and instruments for assessing strengths and needs appear in Table 13–6.

Nursing Intervention Strategies

The nursing interventions discussed in this section are establishing, and maintaining trust, providing support and guidance, providing information, and providing anticipatory guidance.

Establish and Maintain Trust

Trust Trust involves understanding the values, attitudes, and beliefs of one's clients as well as the psy-

Table 13–5 General Areas to Assess Individual and Family Strengths and Needs

STRENGTHS	
Individual and family	Ability to accomplish tasks
	Use of effective coping strategies
	Satisfaction with task accomplishment
	Use of family strengths
NEEDS	
Individual and family	Trust
	Support
	Guidance and counseling
	Information
	Skill Training
	Resource identification
	Health
	Housing
	Financial assistance
	Vocational
	Food
	Clothing

Strengths	Needs

Table 13–6 Instruments for Assessment of Individual and Family Strengths and Needs

Help Scale of the Parent Perception Inventory: Concerns (PPICONC) (Hymovich, 1990).
16 items measuring desire for information related to child development (social, emotional, physical, intellectual), child care (e.g., sleep, nutrition, managing behavior), and health care of child (e.g., dental, minor illnesses)

Sibhelp Scale of the Parent Perception Inventory: Siblings (PPISIB) (Hymovich, 1990).
7 items measuring desire for information about siblings of index (chronically ill) child, including child development (social, emotional, physical, intellectual), and managing child behavior

Family Needs Scale (Dunst, Trivette, & Deal, 1988).
41 items measuring 9 categories of needs: basic resources (e.g., health care, child care, transportation), specialized child care (e.g., respite, dental, medical), personal and family growth (e.g., travel, vacation, educational opportunities), financial and medical resources, child education, future child care, financial and budgeting, household support

Family Resource Scale (Dunst, Trivette, & Deal, 1988).
31 items measuring growth, financial support, health, necessities, nutrition, communication, employment, child care, and time

Family Functioning Style Scale (Experimental Instrument) (Dunst, Trivette, & Deal, 1988).
26 items measuring 12 qualities of family strengths: commitment, appreciation, allocation of time, sense of purpose, congruence, communication, rules and values, coping strategies, problem solving, positivism, flexibility and adaptability, and balance

chosocial variables that impact on that person's perceptions of the current situation. A trusting relationship is a two-way process in which the health care provider learns to trust the client and vice versa. A warm trusting relationship needs to be established to facilitate an ongoing relationship. Such a relationship does not develop overnight, and once established it is constantly tested. Characteristics of the nurse that engender a trusting relationship include warmth and a desire to cooperate with clients and to accurately understand their perspectives. The law of reciprocity seems to operate in this area of trust; that is, people tend to respond in the way they are treated (Thorne & Robinson, 1988). If a person is treated with acceptance and trust by the nurse, the person is likely to respond by accepting and trusting in return.

Trust can be fostered in a variety of ways as nurses, clients, and family members interact. The nurse's accessibility; communication; and providing of individualized information, telephone numbers, and other ways clients and families can contact you or another member of the team contribute to clients' sense of security. Taking time to explain regimens, learning how they fit into the patient's life-style and goals, discussing variations and alterations, and arriving at mutually agreeable methods of treatment also facilitate trust. Clients are more likely to adhere to the regimen if there is a coalition between the health care provider and client. When appropriate, physical contact through *touch* may facilitate development of a trusting relationship with chronically ill patients (Larkin, 1987).

When a child or adult is hospitalized, trust can be established by learning enough about the person so that unique strengths and needs can be respected. Among the stressors encountered by clients who have chronic conditions is the lack of recognition for the care they have been providing for themselves at home. People who have medicated themselves for years, or parents who know the best way to feed and comfort their youngster, can become frustrated when entering the hospital without the opportunity to continue these activities themselves or share their knowledge with the nursing staff.

When working with ethnic groups who use folk remedies, it is important to respect and accept their practices. "The blending of folk remedies with scientific cures can help bridge the communication gap between nurse, client, and family, thereby increasing trust. Once trust is established, the individual and his family will be much more open to the re-

placement of a potentially harmful folk practice by a medically validated one." (McKenzie & Chrisman, 1977, p. 329).

Communication   Communication skills are important in developing a mutually trusting relationship. Some nurses have been observed avoiding communication and purposefully distancing themselves from their patients (Flaskerud, 1979). Such behavior can be especially difficult for persons with chronic conditions. Health professionals are apt to avoid specific kinds of patients, such as those with cancer and those nearing death, at a time when they most need someone to be with them (Larkin, 1987).

No communication is totally independent of context, and all meaning has an important contextual component. Few people realize how dependent the meaning of even the simplest statement is on the context in which it is made. For example, two people who have lived together for years know much of what the other is expressing nonverbally. They do not always have to spell things out; they can tell from such things as tone of voice. When one moves from these personal relationships (e.g. being admitted to the hospital, seeing an unfamiliar nurse) everything must be spelled out. The unfamiliar language used by health personnel and the idiosyncratic language of families, coupled with the anxiety of client and family, can lead to lack of understanding on both sides. We often comment on "how long" it took before someone understood what we were trying to tell him. Conversely, clients are likely to complain that we have not "taken enough time" to help them understand, or that health professionals do not have a lot of time, so they do not want to bother them with their concerns and questions.

Early studies by Korsch and Negrete (1972, 1980), Davis (1968), and Svarstadt (1976) indicate that the health care provider's manner significantly influences patient satisfaction and adherence to suggested regimens. Physician affect, such as words used, tone of voice, and body language were found to influence client outcome (Davis, 1968). Svarstadt (1976) reinforced this by finding that 78% of the clients who received both high friendliness and high instruction from their providers followed their medication regimens, compared with only 42% who received only high instruction. Korsch and Negrete (1980) found lowered trust in the medical profession to be a variable predicting high risk for noncompliance with immunosuppressive therapy for children following renal transplant. In a retrospective study, patients with cancer indicated that most of the information and advice they received from doctors and nurses was not helpful (Thorne, 1988). In addition, most of the unhelpful instances were associated with a communication style characterized by lack of concern.

An atmosphere in which clients feel free to express their feelings needs to be created by listening without condemnation or annoyance; showing respect for individuals with unique characteristics, beliefs, and feelings; and using empathy when talking with them. It is possible to recognize and accept the problem from their perspective while gently guiding them to see alternatives. Meichenbaum (1985) suggested that when something unfavorable is mentioned, the nurse might say, "It's understandable that you might feel this way about yourself at times and want to change." When something favorable is mentioned, an appropriate response might be, "It's obvious you have a lot going for you." If clients believe their opinions are valued and worthwhile, this may enhance their sense of self and sense of trust.

Physicians and patients tend to view health status in fundamentally different ways. Physicians are trained to differentiate discrete illnesses to the extent possible, and have no adequate measures of holistic functioning, vitality, or well-being. Patients tend to view health more globally and experientially. They may be concerned with specific symptoms but tend to view their health in terms of an overall sense of well-being and the extent to which the symptoms disrupt ability to function or interfere in some significant fashion with life activities (Mechanic, 1986, p. 100). Nurses are educated to have a more holistic approach to health and illness and consequently have the background to perceive different points of view. This background plus an understanding of patient theories of illness, family systems, and contingency variables offers nurses the potential for improved communication and effective therapeutic interactions with patients and families.

Provide Support and Guidance

Support refers to the help available that has the potential to enhance a person's coping with stressors. Chronically ill people need long-term and sometimes continuous support when coping with the stressors of their chronic conditions. Support may be informal, like that offered by family and friends, or formal, as provided by nurses and other health care professionals. Dyer (1973) reports a study conducted on a chronic illness ward of a large hospital. Patients were asked whom they talk to concerning their illness. Patients mentioned everyone from friends and other patients to aides, orderlies, and other nonmedical personnel. No patient mentioned nurses, doctors, or other professional personnel. Northouse (1988) found that patients with breast cancer perceived significantly more support from health professionals than did their husbands, even though the husbands perceived as much distress over the course of the illness.

Nurses can be a valuable support to clients who come to the health care setting. The goal of providing support and guidance is to facilitate growth and independence in clients and families as they are able to cope with the stressors they face. To give emotional support, nurses or other health care professionals can show concern and caring, indicate that the person is valued, and provide a sympathetic ear. By conveying a sense of belonging, we are participating in a reciprocal network of shared obligations (Elliott & Eisdorfer, 1982). Other ways to support include providing tangible help when needed and suggesting alternative coping strategies. However, Meichenbaum (1985) cautions us to be careful in proposing any specific coping technique, to discuss honestly with clients what is known and not known about coping, and to have clients collaborate in determining useful strategies. He also stresses the importance of being flexible in tailoring the coping training to the individual's specific situation and strengths. Health professionals need to understand the patient's and family's tensions and struggles to control their emotions and to reduce fear and anxiety.

Recognizing and enhancing family strengths can be supportive because it projects a sense of concern, involvement, and personal interest on the part of the nurse. However, health care professionals need to take care not to project the feeling that one must always be strong and capable, lest the patient or family member be afraid to share uncertainties and vulnerabilities that could benefit from intervention. For example, the mother of a boy with spina bifida always appeared confident, strong, and supportive of her son and was constantly praised for her behaviors. Whenever he was hospitalized she would be at his bedside, usually around the clock. The youngster was scheduled for surgery, and the mother was encouraged to remain with the boy. When the nurse asked her whether she felt she always had to appear strong and invulnerable, she burst into tears, talked about how overwhelmed she felt, how she was always praised for her strength, and how she wished she could just have a few hours for herself. Plans were made to give her some relief during the child's hospitalization, and she felt she did not have to be there 24 hours a day "because that's what everybody expects of me."

While the actual techniques of providing support and guidance vary with the individuals involved and the particular situation, there are certain commonalities including (1) helping people verbalize unexpressed fears (fantasies are often more frightening than reality); (2) helping them sort out real issues from unreal ones; (3) recognizing the validity of the patient's and the family's fears; (4) reassuring when appropriate, without giving false assurances; and (5) discouraging self-blame (e.g., "If only I came for help sooner, things would be different"), and (6) acknowledging their need for control.

Psychologic support is a means of providing reassurance and support to facilitate individual and family adjustment. Its many diverse methods include individual psychotherapy, group discussions to voice fears and anxieties, and puppet play with children (Watson & Kendall, 1983). Inherent in the nurse's ability to provide psychologic support is the formation of a trusting and good relationship with the person or persons to be supported. Techniques include listening, reflecting feelings, and providing reassurance when fears and anxieties are normal. The nurse also reinforces the person's strengths to cope successfully with the situation and, when appropriate, encourages the individual or family to increase its part in decision making.

Kendall and Watson (1981) reviewed the research literature regarding psychologic support for both children and adults, all of whom were hospitalized. They concluded that studies with both adult medical patients and with children produced some evidence of the effectiveness of this intervention but that the results are equivocal. They recommend that the approach is probably best used in conjunction with other methods that have established efficacy. Several studies show that children demonstrate less distress during medical procedures when their parents are present than when they are absent (Gross et al, 1984; Shaw & Routh, 1982). Hull (1989) recently reported that, contrary to the importance attached to emotional support by family members of dying patients, the least supportive nursing interventions for them were behaviors designed to encourage ventilation of their own feelings. During the terminal phase of the illness they wanted the nurses to focus on the patient, especially when the nurse had limited time.

Interventions with parents of adolescents should address the struggles for control that may interfere with the youngster's health (e.g., decision making, consent, confidentiality), encouraging the adolescent to accomplish developmental tasks, promoting the adolescent to be an active participant in care, and specifying a safe time or place for releasing anger surrounding the condition (Buhlmann & Fitzpatrick, 1987).

Instead of being judgmental or authoritarian, health professionals need to take stock of a family's ways of adapting to different situations. "The true test is not whether the family is doing something in the way we personally feel is best, but whether it works for them. . ." and whether the person is receiving adequate care (Boch, 1984, p. 29)

Many times our primary role is to facilitate communication among the family members. Acceptance of roles and of the family hierarchy is important. That hierarchy often changes when the child comes home. One person may play dominant role while the child is in the hospital and another when the child is home.

Support groups　Support groups can be constructive in providing necessary information, encouragement, and tangible assistance to people with chronic conditions and their families. However, little is known about their long-term effectiveness because there has been no follow-up of those who drop out of the groups. Support groups can facilitate an understanding of problems, assessment of their meaning, and making realistic and comforting comparisons. Self-help support groups have the capacity to be effective or potentially ineffective at different times and for different people (Mechanic, 1986).

People tend to seek help from these groups when the help they need is not available from family, friends, or professional helping networks (Borkman, 1976). Support groups can be useful in promoting understanding and mastery of distressing feelings related to one's own or a family member's chronic condition, thereby helping to improve relationships. Such support can only come from peers. Groups can provide avenues for clients to learn from others about the daily aspects of care, as people often share how they manage common problems. Sometimes they may find it easier to accept helpful suggestions and criticism from others with a similar problem than from a professional. People learn they are not alone, and they may gain insight, comfort, and support from each other, as well as increase their self-awareness of both strengths and limitations. Some members are positive role models for others. However, support groups are not a substitute for professional care and cannot fill the gap when professional services are inadequate (Silverman, 1978; Singer & Farkas, 1989).

There are also hazards in support groups. Highly disturbed and manipulative individuals may preclude group cohesiveness and identification. Groups that are inappropriate or poorly timed for the individual may create additional stress, rather than alleviate it (Ayers, 1989). Initially, groups may be difficult for newly diagnosed patients or family members who may become overwhelmed and anxious as they listen to others. Much of this can be avoided if the group leader is alert to their anxiety and can muster some reassuring and constructive resources in the group.

Support groups may be ineffective as a continuing resource for some people because they are likely to give undue emphasis to the disability as a crucial part of the patient's identity. Although some people may require this continuing support (shared need), others do not, and may even resent it. Dixon (1981) cautions us to examine the relationships between a person's self-concept and the attitudes toward chronic illness and disability in a self-help group before we recommend the group. For example, if the person has a poor self-concept and the self-help group emphasizes the condition as central to one's self-concept, this factor could increase the negative self-concept. Patients and families should be given guidelines for the types of things they might want to consider when selecting a group for themselves.

Timing of attendance at support group meetings is an issue that needs to be considered in discussing such groups with clients. Other factors include the purpose of the group (information, support, fund raising), membership, and leadership (lay, professional). The leadership role is crucial in providing a balance between giving information and allowing for individual expressions of feelings. The most effective leadership style for these groups tends to be a nondirective approach. Mechanic (1986) believes that support groups are almost always helpful during the acute phases of a chronic illness, especially when they include people who have coped successfully (role models) with the realistic problems and frustrations of the situation. Explanations and information

---

Box 13-3 *Example of Potential Stressors in a Support Group*

New parents attended their first parent meeting about 2 weeks after their infant was born with osteogenesis imperfecta (brittle bone disease). This was the parents' first baby, and everyone was anxious to provide them with information about the care their baby would need. One thing they stressed was the importance of protecting the infant's fontanel (soft spot) because they "could hurt the baby's brain real bad." These parents rarely invited health professionals to their meeting, but on this particular week, a nurse was there as a visitor. She recognized the increasing anxiety of the new parents and the misinformation they were receiving. The nurse was able to intervene by (1) correcting the misinformation, (2) helping to put the number of problems presented into perspective in view of the infant's age, (3) guiding the discussion onto a more positive note by asking the parents to share some of their positive experiences, and (4) talking with the new parents after the meeting about the experience and realistic expectations for their child.

---

are given in response to questions as they arise, rather than presented in a didactic form. The example in Box 13-3 describes some potential stressors associated with the timing and nature of a support group.

Provide Information

The nurse's role in providing information to patients who have chronic conditions and their families is vital. In fact, evidence indicates that patient education can improve the quality of care, reduce future hospitalizations, and have other benefits (Blue Cross, 1980). Studies have shown that patient education contributes to shortening the length of hospital stays, reducing complications, and more effective use of services (Schwartz, 1982). Greater utilization includes improved patterns of utilization, greater number of appointments kept, and enhanced self-care and clinic use rather than emergency room use (Green et al, 1980).

In general, the literature on patient education indicates that teaching produces better outcomes than not teaching, and teaching efforts that tend to be personalized and include emotional support are better than only providing facts (Mazzuca, 1982, Mumford, Schlesinger, & Glass, 1982). Mumford et al (1982), using meta-analysis techniques, reported that interventions aimed at relieving anxiety and providing emotional support were more effective than those that provided information only, while a combination of psychologic support and information was superior to either alone. Mazzuca (1982) found that personalizing teaching was more effective in improving compliance and health outcomes than general patient education. Personalized teaching was accomplished by using the patient's own daily routine and bolstering social support, in addition to medication and telephone monitoring.

Much of the research on prescription drugs and compliance has implications for teaching. Problems of compliance arise when multiple drugs are prescribed for patients. Noncompliance can be manifested in ways such as failing to take the proper dose, failing to take the drug at the proper times, forgetting to take the drug, and sharing drugs with others. Darnell and colleagues (1986) reported that for each diagnosed illness, most patients have two drugs to consume. Sands and Holman (1983) found no relationship between compliance of elderly individuals with hypertension and their knowledge of hypertension. Only a small majority of the subjects scored above average on the knowledge scale. In addition, although patients were highly compliant in other areas that were measured, 33% of these patients forgot to take their medications. Second, compliance was related to education, and those with at least a high school education were more compliant than those who had not graduated from high school. This study again reinforces the importance of a thorough assessment. It also implies that nurses must find ways to help patients remember when to take their medications, suggesting that knowledge alone may be an insufficient basis for self-care.

Three meta-analytic studies have been done looking at the effects of patient teaching in chronic illness. Two of these studies (Mullen, Green, & Persinger, 1985; Posovac, 1980) included chronic conditions, and one (Brown, 1988) concerned only diabetes. The conclusion from these studies was that patient education interventions increase patient knowledge. Brown (1988) also reports enhanced self-care behaviors and metabolic control as a result of patient education. Of note is the finding in a study of diabetic education (Surwut, Scovern, & Feinglos, 1982) that over 50% of the patients made errors in insulin administration and failed to comply with diet and foot care, although all could demonstrate or describe the correct techniques. In clinical practice, the most successful patient teaching occurs with longitudinal programs involving frequent contact and reinforcement. Unfortunately, attrition rates from these programs is high (Brown, 1988). Patient satisfaction was found to be greater as a result of increased educational efforts by care givers (Bartlett, 1984).

Redmond and Thomas (1985) express concern about the state of patient education. Some tools used for assessment and intervention lack vital information, consistency, and structure. Although much has been achieved, the findings suggest that rigor needs to be applied in practice and research in patient education. Ways of standardizing the patient education process, diffusion of information about superior patient education models, careful definition of measurement of components of educational interventions, and development of comprehensive educational services need to be addressed.

Teaching and learning   Knowledge of the principles of teaching and learning is essential to providing information that will be readily learned by patients and their families. Teaching is the process of passing facts and ideas to others. It involves the transmission of knowledge in a manner likely to stimulate interest and retention on the part of the learner. **Instruction** is the process whereby one individual intentionally influences the learning of another by structuring the environment so that the latter will learn a desired behavior. **Learning** is a relatively permanent change in behavior due to practice or experience.

Several learning theorists have contributed to our understanding of teaching and learning. Thorndike, a stimulus-response theorist, contributed the "law of exercise," which stated that connections are strengthened with use and weakened with disuse (Van Hoozer, Bratton, Ostmoe et al, 1987). For example, the family member who has to give injections daily will become increasingly skilled in the procedure, while someone who only gives an occasional injection will be less skillful. Skinner (1971), another stimulus-response theorist, concluded that learning is the result of reinforcement of desired responses. His ideas of teaching in small steps and giving immediate positive reinforcement were a major contribution. Praising or rewarding patients for their progress or giving information in small increments illustrates how this theory is applied in practice.

The cognitive field theorists were basically concerned with cognitive processes and contributed many ideas about the importance of perception and the activity of the learner. An individual's need will determine what he or she will learn and how he or she will act. Brunner (1966) proposed "discovery learning," whereby the learner is more likely to acquire a better understanding by discovering information by himself or herself, rather than by being told what we think should be known. The "whole-part-whole principle" is an effective strategy in which the teacher presents an overlying framework and then breaks the information into its components, discusses each part, and concludes with putting everything back together again in the whole framework. These and other theories form the basis of the principles of learning that can guide educational interventions.

Principles of teaching and learning   Hymovich and Hagopian (1989) summarized principles of teaching and learning that can guide nurses in their educational interventions. These principles are listed in Table 13–7.

Evaluation of teaching effectiveness can be done through periodic assessments of progress and accomplishments. Evaluation should be based on behavioral objectives. Knowledge obtained from the evaluation gives direction for future learning needs.

It is often assumed that once patients learn the basics about a health problem, they generally require little or no additional information. Most educational programs are aimed at assisting people with initial information, because the need is obvious and the information can be standardized. However, the need for reteaching is essential, especially for people who are chronically ill. Anxiety may interfere with initial learning, forgetting occurs, motivation declines, and there may be a need to provide new skills for dealing with changes in situational and developmental stressors and changes in self-concept (Hymovich & Hagopian, 1989). Patient knowledge needs to be reassessed periodicaly. Rapid advances

Table 13–7   Principles of Teaching and Learning

1. The characteristics of the individual will influence learning. Factors such as heredity, environment, goals, aspirations, and desires impact on learning. Personalized intervention based on this information is more likely to be effective than general instruction.
2. A comfortable, quiet environment without distractions will enhance learning.
3. Motivation will influence learning. People are more likely to learn things that interest them rather than those not of interest or those that they consider unimportant.
4. Effective communication is essential. When teaching, do not make assumptions, define all terms, be succinct, and present information as simply as possible.
5. It is essential to set aside time for teaching. The telephone can be an important tool for teaching purposes (Hagopian & Rubenstein, 1990). A short telephone call can allow the nurse to verify, give, repeat, and/or reinforce information.
6. Teach new information in short sessions and make information meaningful. Fatigue and boredom may interfere with learning. Make important points early, reinforce frequently, and summarize at the end of the session. It is better to teach a little thoroughly than a lot superficially.
7. Keep the learner active. An active person learns more effectively than a passive one. Strategies to keep the learner active include frequent practice, discovery learning (letting the patient learn information on his or her own), or drawing up a written contract with the patient.
8. Try to build new information on what the patient already knows and capitalize on the patient's past experience. Teach from the simple to the complex, and from the known to the unknown, to enhance the learning process.
9. Provide for practice when teaching skills. In teaching a skill, 10% of the time should be devoted to explanation, 25% to demonstration, and 65% to practice. Practice actively involves the learner.
10. Provide positive reinforcement to increase the likelihood that the behavior will be repeated.
11. Evaluate the person's learning periodically. Learning will be enhanced by frequent feedback about progress, mistakes, and successes.

Source: Hymovich & Hagopian (1989).

mean potential changes in patient therapy, and new information needs to be shared with patients.

Promoting learning readiness.

Patients who are ready to learn do so more efficiently and effectively than those who are not ready. It is important for the nurse to assess readiness to learn by recalling factors that can influence readiness:

- *Comfort.* Patients must be comfortable both physically and psychologically.
- *Energy.* Patients who do not have enough energy may have a decreased ability to learn.
- *Motivation.* People who are motivated are more likely to learn than those not motivated.
- *Capacity.* People with severe physical and mental handicaps may not be able to learn as readily as those who are not handicapped (Hymovich & Hagopian, 1989).

Although readiness is the responsibility of the learner, the nurse can try to stimulate readiness. The strategies that can stimulate readiness include (Hymovich & Hagopian, 1989):

- Help the patient identify the need for learning. Pose a problem to the patient and ask how he or she would solve it.
- Start teaching with information that the patient wants to know to maintain patient interest.
- Make the information easy, concrete, short, meaningful, and manageable.
- Put the patient in control. Allow the patient to make decisions about what is to be learned and when, if at all possible.
- Provide rewards. This might include improving the patient's support system or drawing up a written contract that includes meaningful rewards when certain goals are accomplished.

Establishing objectives and priorities.

Once learning needs have been identified and the patient is ready to learn, the content and priorities for teaching should be established. This step can be accomplished by using behavioral objectives that are learner centered, realistic, individual, observable, and measurable. Once written, the objectives should be prioritized by determining the informa-

tion the patient must know, should know, and could know.

- *Must know.* This is essential information that people must know for their own survival, protection, safety, and well-being.
- *Should know.* This information is valuable and interesting and can be taught if there is time or information that patients should know about in order to manage their health problems.
- *Could know.* This information consists of "trimmings or frills." If patients are interested and motivated and have learned what they must and should know, teaching information in this category is appropriate.

There are clinical benefits to be expected from providing problem-focused educational interventions. Once given the information they need, patients and families should feel in control of the situation. This may lead to reduced fear and anxiety, enhanced coping, a better self-image, and optimal quality of life (Hagopian, 1987).

Special considerations   In addition to the general principles of teaching and learning, there are special considerations for specific clients.

Children.

Of particular importance for nurses working with children and their parents is ensuring the children receive adequate information. Children need information that is developmentally appropriate and relevant to their beliefs about health, illness, and their bodies (Clark et al, 1988). Children who are chronically ill, their siblings, and children of chronically ill parents should not be shielded from the realities of what is happening to the family. When attention is given to an ill child or parent, the children need to know why parents are spending more time with the ill person.

Children acquire most behaviors through simple conditioning, discovery learning, trial and error, practice, imitation, and association. To ensure that the child receives adequate information, the nurse may work with the child directly and/or indirectly through the parents. Direct intervention with the child involves providing information at a cognitively appropriate level, clarifying misunderstandings, and providing new or similar knowledge as the child develops. Indirect intervention includes educating parents about children's thought processes, being certain parents understand the necessary information, and encouraging updates as the child matures (Hymovich, 1986).

Educating Adults.

When working with chronically ill adults or with parents of chronically ill children, remember that adults have special learning needs. Knowles (1973) makes the following assumptions about adult learners:

1. The adult self-concept is that of a self-directed person. Adults need to be perceived by others as self-directed. Tension develops when adults are put in a situation in which they cannot be self-directed.
2. The adult has an accumulated reservoir of experience that is a valuable learning resource. The mature person has rich experience that provides a broad base upon which to relate new learning. It is important to recognize each person as unique and possessing wide experience.
3. The adult is ready to learn those things that are viewed as important. This motivation to learn is usually oriented toward the tasks of the social role the adult plays.
4. The adult has a problem-centered orientation to learning. An adult who experiences some inadequacy in dealing with current life problems usually seeks education to solve the problem and wants to apply this knowledge immediately.

Older adult.

The older adult usually requires more time to learn new knowledge and skills. Although intelligence and ability to learn remain, reaction time tends to decrease. In addition, lack of use of information leads to forgetting. The saying "If you don't use it, you lose it" applies to the older adult and refers to the law of exercise.

Reading comprehension.

It is helpful to keep in mind that 23 million Americans read at fifth grade level or below, and that 1.5 million people are functionally illiterate. In addition, a person reads, hears, and comprehends at an equivalent of two grades below the highest grade level completed.

Providing information about resources

The patient and family managing the chronic condition on their own may not need or want help. Others may need assistance but not know it, or they may not realize it is available. They are afraid or embarrassed to ask, or they may not think they can afford assistance. Many organizations are available to assist clients with chronic conditions and their families. Among the services these organizations offer are home-health care, medical equipment, transportation, nutritional services, family service or counseling, senior citizen services, financial assistance, hospice, support groups, and vocational and physical rehabilitation. By using health and other support services, people with chronic conditions are able to spend less time in the hospital, maintain independence, and deal more effectively with health-related problems.

Usually the health care worker can put the patient and family in touch with the appropriate resource. There are books for nurses, patients, and families to identify needed assistance. These books may include resources at national or local levels. Some books list agencies and services and are useful in locating the appropriate agency. One such book is *Handicapping Conditions and Services Directory* (Clearinghouse, 1981). This directory provides a list of organizations throughout the country, along with the address, telephone number, and the handicapping condition served. Information is also provided about the organization and its services. *Voluntary Health Organizations: A Guide to Patient Services* (Scheinberg & Schneider, 1987) is another comprehensive, easy-to-use reference. Diseases or disorders are listed and described, followed by a list of national organizations, addresses and telephone numbers. This guide lists information on local chapters and indicates the name of a contact person. The services provided are described in detail. Norback and Weitz's (1983) *Sourcebook of Aid for the Mentally and Physically Handicapped* covers topics such as careers and training, sources of legal information, affirmative action, telecommunications for the deaf, and rehabilitation information and facilities. They also include information on the Architectural Barriers Act, highway rest areas for the handicapped, and national parks accessible to the handicapped.

Other books describe how to take care of a family member in the home. One useful title is *Home Care: Patient and Family Instruction* (Zastocki & Rovinski, 1989), a compilation of instruction guides for patients. This book consists of many simple instructions for procedures, information on diseases, common symptoms, medications, diet, and exercise. General information is provided, along with guidelines for care, needed equipment, detailed steps of procedures, important points, and under what circumstances to call the doctor. Also included are useful logs, diagrams, forms for record keeping, checklists and flow sheets. The pages of the book may be reproduced to distribute to patients. A similar book for the care of the child is *Home Care for the Chronically Ill or Disabled Child* (Jones, 1985). This book, written by a parent, discusses meeting the child's medical, physical, educational, and social needs, as well as family needs.

"Family Caregiving for the Elderly: An Overview of Resources," an article by Blieszner and Alley (1990), provides a short review of literature on family care givers and a long list of resources available for the family caring for an elderly member. The resource list for care givers includes articles, reports, books, curriculum guides, hotlines, newsletters, organizations, programs, videotapes, and films. This article should prove valuable to health care workers.

Provide Anticipatory Guidance

Much coping activity is anticipatory, that is, the person prepares to overcome or avoid the danger. Such anticipation changes the nature of the ultimate transaction along with its associated emotions. Hamburg and Inoff (1982) suggest that preparation for major stressful transitions may be valuable in preventing human suffering. Anticipatory guidance enables a person to make a potentially unfamiliar event more familiar and predictable, thus facilitating adaptation. Intervention strategies to help individual and family systems understand the situations they face and, when possible, prepare them for anticipated stressful events may facilitate their ability to function. Helping clients and families develop a repertoire of coping strategies for handling these stressors is also valuable.

Summary

Persons with chronic conditions and their families have a variety of internal and external strengths. A reciprocal relationship exists between strengths and needs, whereby strengths may become needs, and needs, once met, may lead to new strengths. Internal strengths and needs are related to trust, self-efficacy, spirituality, self-esteem, orientation to life, self-expression and understanding, and independence. External strengths and needs include community and financial resources.

Assessing and reinforcing system strengths and coping abilities are an important nursing role. Guidelines for assessment and intervention were provided in this chapter. Once an effective working relationship based on trust and good communication is established, nursing intervention strategies based on needs include providing support and guidance, information based on principles of teaching and learning, and anticipatory guidance. If nursing intervention strategies are effective, needs will be met and new strengths may emerge.

References

Ayers, T.D. (1989). Dimensions and characteristics of lay helping. *Am J Orthopsychiatry, 59*(2), 215–225.

Baille, V., Norbeck, J.J., & Barnes, L.E.A. (1988). Stress, social support, and psychological distress of family caregivers of the elderly. *Nurs Res, 37*(4), 217–222.

Bartholomew, L.K., Seilheimer, D.K., Parcel, G.S., et al. (1988). Planning patient education for cystic fibrosis: Application of a diagnostic framework. *Patient Educ Counseling, 13*(1), 57–68.

Bartlett, E.E. (1984). The medical and educational models of health care under prospective pricing. *Patient Educ Counseling, 6*(2), 57–60.

Blieszner, R., & Alley, J.M. (1990). Family caregiving for the elderly: An overview of resources. *Fam Relat, 39*(1), 97–102.

Blue Cross and Blue Shield Associations. (1980). *Financing for health education services in the United States.* Atlanta: Centers for Disease Control.

Boch, R. (1984). Strategies for building expertise within report on a conference held May 27, 1984, Houston, Texas. Association for the Care of Children's Health.

Borkman, T. (1976). Experimental knowledge: A new concept for the analysis of self-help groups. *Soc Serv Rev, 50,* 445–456.

Bowlby, J. (1969). *Attachment and loss* (Vol. 1). New York: Basic Books.

Boyce, W.T. (1985). Stress and child health: An overview. *Pediatr Ann, 14*(8), 531–542.

Brown, S.A. (1988). Effects of educational interventions in diabetes care: A meta-analysis of findings. *Nurs Res 37*(4), 223–230.

Brunner, J. (1966). *Toward a theory of instruction.* Cambridge, MA: Harvard University Press.

Buhlmann, U., & Fitzpatrick, S.B. (1987). Caring for an adolescent with a chronic illness. *Primary Care, 14*(1), 57–68.

Burckhardt, C.S. (1987). Coping strategies of the chronically ill. *Nurs Clin North Am, 22*(3), 543–550.

Cairns, N.U., Clark, G.M., Smith, S.D., & Lansky, S.B. (1979). Adaptation of siblings to childhood malignancy. *J Pediatr, 95*, 484–487.

Casey, E., O'Connell, J.K., & Price, J.H. (1984). Perceptions of educational needs for patients after myocardial infarction. *Patient Educ Counseling, 6*(4), 77–82.

Cassileth, B.R., Zupkis, R.V., Sutton-Smith, K., & March, V. (1980). Information and participation preferences among cancer patients. *Ann Intern Med, 92*, 832–836.

Clark, N.M., Rosenstock, I.M., Hassan, H., et al. (1988). The effects of health beliefs and feelings of self efficacy on self management behavior of children with a chronic disease. *Patient Educ Counseling, 11*(2), 131–139.

Clearinghouse on the Handicapped. (1981). *Handicapping conditions and services directory.* Detroit: Grand River.

Cobb, S. (1976). Social support as a moderator of life stress. *Psychosom Med 38*, 300–314.

Darnell, J.C., et al. (1986). Medication use by ambulatory elderly: An in-home survey. *J Am Geriatr Soc, 34*(1), 1–4.

Davis, M.S. (1968). Variations in patients' compliance with doctors' advice: An empirical analysis of patterns of communication. *Am J Public Health, 58*, 274–288.

Derdiarian, A.K. (1986). Informational needs of recently diagnosed cancer patients. *Nurs Res, 35*(5), 276–281.

Dimond, M., & Jones, S. (1983). *Chronic illness across the life span.* Norwalk, CT: Appleton-Century-Crofts.

Dixon, J.K. (1981). Group-self identification and physical handicap: Implication for patient support groups. *Res Nurs Health, 4*, 299–308.

Dunst, C.J., Trivette, C.M., & Deal, A.G. (1988). *Enabling and empowering families: Principles and guidelines for practice.* Cambridge, MA: Brookline.

Dyer, W.G. (1973). The nurse-patient system relationship. In A. Reinhardt & M. Quinn (Eds.), *Family centered community nursing* (pp. 87–94). St. Louis: Mosby.

Elliott, G.R., & Eisdorfer, C. (Eds.). (1982). *Stress and human health.* New York: Springer.

Erikson, E.H. (1963). *Childhood and society* (2nd ed.). New York: Norton.

Ferraro, A.R., & Longo, D.C. (1985). Nursing care of the family with a chronically ill, hospitalized child: An alternative approach. *Image, 17*(3), 77–81.

Fine, L.L., & Friedman, M.S. (1984). The sibling experience: Developmental considerations. *Children are different: Behavioral development monograph series: Number 11.* Columbus, OH: Ross Laboratories.

Flaskerud, J.H., Halloran, E.J., Janken, J., et al. (1979). Avoidance and distancing: A descriptive view of nursing. *Nurs Forum, 18*, 158–174.

Friedland, J., & McColl, M. (1987). Social support and psychosocial dysfunction after stroke: Buffering effects in a community sample. *Arch Phys Med Rehabil, 68*, 475–480.

Gatchel, R.J., & Baum, A. (1983). *An introduction to health psychology.* Reading, MA: Addison-Wesley.

George, L.K., & Gwyther, L.P. (1986). Caregiver well-being: A multidimensional examination of family caregivers of demented adults. *Gerontologist, 26*, 253–259.

Germain, C.B. (1977). An ecological perspective on social work practice in health care. *Soc Work Health Care, 3*(1), 67–76.

Goddard, H.A., & Powers, M.J. (1982) Emotional needs of patients undergoing hemodialysis: A comparison of patient and nurse perception. *Dial Transplant, 11*, 578–583.

Green, L., Squiers, W.D., D'Altroy, L.H., & Herbert, B. (1980). What do recent evaluations of patient education tell us? In W. Squiers (Ed.), *Patient education: An inquiry into the state of the art* (pp. 11–38). New York: Springer.

Gross, A.M., Stern, R.M., Levin, R.B., et al. (1984). The effect of mother-child separation on the behavior of children experiencing a diagnostic medical procedure. *J Consult Clin Psychol, 51*, 738–785.

Hagopian, G.A. (1987). Teaching adults in a hospice setting. *Hospice J, 3*(1), 59–65.

Hagopian, G.A., & Rubenstein, J.H. (1990). The effects of telephone call interventions in a radiation therapy department. *Cancer Nurs, 13*(6), 339–349.

Hamburg, D.A. (1982). Forward: An outlook on stress research and health. In G.R. Elliott & C. Eisdorfer (Eds.), *Stress and human health* (pp. ix–xxii). New York: Springer.

Hamburg, B.A., & Inoff, G.E. (1982). Relationships between behavioral factors and diabetic control in children and adolescents: A camp study. *Psychosom Med, 44*, 321–339.

Harris, T. (1986). Aging in the eighties, prevalence and impact of urinary problems in individuals age 65 years and over. *Advancedata*, No. 121, August 27, 1986. USDHHS.

Harman, A., & Laird, J. (1983). *Family-centered social work practice.* New York: Free Press.

Hayes, V.E., & Knox, J.E. (1984). The experience of stress in parents of children hospitalized with long-term disabilities. *J Adv Nurs, 9*, 333–341.

Heisler, A., & Friedman, S. (1981). Social and psychological considerations in chronic disease with particular reference to seizure disorders. *J Pediatr Psychol, 6,* 231–248.

Hull, M.M. (1989). Family needs and supportive nursing behaviors during terminal cancer: A review. *Oncol Nurs Forum, 16*(6), 787–792.

Hymovich, D.P. (1976). Parents of sick children: Their needs and tasks. *Pediatr Nurs, 2,* 13–22.

Hymovich, D.P. (1979). Assessment of the chronically ill child and family. In D.P. Hymovich & M.U. Barnard (Eds.), *Family health care: Vol. 1. General perspectives* (pp. 280–293). New York: McGraw-Hill.

Hymovich, D.P. (1990, January). The impact of cancer in a parent on family functioning. Presentation. University of Pennsylvania.

Hymovich, D.P. (1986). Child and family teaching: Special needs and approaches. *Hospice J, 2*(1), 103–120.

Hymovich, D.P. & Chamberlin, R.W. (1980). *Child and family development: Implications for care.* New York: McGraw-Hill.

Hymovich, D.P., & Hagopian, G.A. (1989). The teaching role of the office nurse. *Office Nurse, 2*(5), 30–32.

Jones, M.L. (1985). *Home care for the chronically ill or disabled child.* New York: Harper & Row.

Kahn, R.L., & Antonucci, T.C. (1980). Convoys over the life course: Attachment, roles and social support. In P.B. Baltes & O.G. Brim (Eds.), *Life-span development and behavior* (pp. 253–286). New York: Academic.

Kendall, P.C., & Watson, D. (1981). Psychological preparation for stressful medical procedures. In C.E. Prokop & L.A. Bradley (Eds.), *Medical psychology* (pp. 197–221). New York: Academic.

Knowles, M. (1973). *The adult learner: A neglected species.* Houston: Gulf.

Korner, I.N. (1970). Hope as a method of coping. *J Consult Clin Psychol, 34*(2), 134–139.

Korsch, B., & Negrete, V. (1972). Doctor-patient communication. *Sci Am, 227,* 66–74.

Korsch, B.M., & Negrete, V.F. (1980). Counseling patients and their families in a chronic renal disease program. *Patient Educ and Counseling, 2*(2), 87–91.

Larkin, J. (1987). Factors identifying one's ability to adapt to chronic illness. *Nurs Clin North Am, 22*(3), 535–542.

Lauer, P., Murphy, S.P., & Powers, M.J. (1982). Learning needs of cancer patients: A comparison of nurse and patient perceptions. *Nurs Res, 31,* 11–16.

Lazarus, R. (1984). The costs and benefits of denial. In S. Breznitz (Ed.), *Denial of stress.* New York: International Universities Press.

McKenzie, J.L., & Chrisman, N.J. (1977). Healing herbs, gods, and magic. *Nurs Outlook, 25*(5), 326–329.

Magi, M., & Allander, E. (1981). Towards a theory of perceived and medically defined need. *Sociol Health Illness, 3*(1), 49–71.

Mailick, M. (1984). The impact of severe illness on the individual and family: An overview. In E. Aronwitz, & E.M. Bromberg (Eds.), *Mental health and long-term physical illness* (pp. 83–94). Canton, MA: Prodist. Reprinted from *Soc Work Health Care, 5*(2) 1980.

Maslow, A.H. (1968). *Toward a psychology of being* (2nd. ed.). New York: Van Nostrand Reinhold.

Mattsson, A. (1972). Long term illness in childhood: A challenge to psychosocial adaptation. *Pediatrics, 50,* 801–805.

Mazzuca, S.A. (1982). Does patient education in chronic disease have therapeutic value? *J Chronic Dis, 35,* 521–529.

Mechanic, D. (1986). *From advocacy to allocation: The evolving American health care system.* New York: Macmillan.

Meichenbaum, D. (1985). *Stress inoculation training.* New York: Pergamon.

Miller, J.F., & Powers, M.J. (1988). Development of an instrument to measure hope. *Nurs Res, 37*(1), 6–10.

Mullen, P.D., Green, L.W., & Persinger, G.S. (1985). Clinical trials of patient education for chronic conditions: A comparative meta-analysis of intervention types. *Prev Med, 14,* 753–781.

Mumford, E., Schlesinger, H.J., & Glass, G.V. (1982). The effects of psychological intervention in recovery from surgery and heart attacks: An analysis of the literature. *Am J Pub Health, 72,* 141–151.

Murphy, L. (1962). *The widening world of childhood.* New York: Basic Books.

Murphy, L.B. & Moriarty, A.E. (1976). Vulnerability, coping, and growth. New Haven: Yale University Press.

National Association for Mental Health. (1954). *What every child needs.* New York: National Association for Mental Health.

Nolan, T., Desmond, K., Herlich, R., & Hardy, R. (1986). Knowledge of cystic fibrosis in patients and their parents. *Pediatrics, 77,* 221–235.

Norback, J., & Weitz, P. (1983). *Sourcebook of aid for the mentally and physically handicapped.* New York: Van Nostrand Reinhold.

Northouse, P.G. (1979). Interpersonal trust and empathy in nurse-nurse relationships. *Nurs Res, 28*(6), 365–368.

Northouse, L.L. (1988). Social support in patients' and husbands' adjustment to breast cancer. *Nurs Res, 37*(2), 91–95.

Otto, H.A. (1965). The human potentialities of nurses and patients. *Nurs Outlook, 12*(8), 32–35.

Otto, H.A. (1973). A framework for assessing family strengths. In A. Reinhardt & M. Quinn (Eds), *Family centered community nursing* (pp. 87–94). St Louis: Mosby.

Pellegrino, E. (1976). Lecture delivered to the International Institute of Health Care, Ethics, and Human Values, Mt. St. Joseph College, Mt. St. Joseph, Ohio, July. Cited in L. Curtain, (1977). Human values in nursing. *Journal of New York State Nurses Association, 8*(4), 31–40.

Pless, I.B., & Perrin, J.M. (1985). Issues common to a variety of illnesses. In N. Hobbs & J.M. Perrin (Eds.), *Issues in the care of children with chronic illness* (pp. 41–60). San Francisco: Jossey-Bass.

Posovac, E.J. (1980). Evaluation of patient education programs. *Eval Health Professions, 3*, 47–62.

Redmond, B.K., & Thomas, S.K. (1985). In G.M. Bulechek & J.C. McCloskey, (Eds.) *Nursing interventions: Treatments for nursing diagnoses.* Philadelphia: W.B. Saunders.

Rideout, E., & Montemuro, M. (1986). Hope, morale and adaptation in patients with chronic heart failure. *J Adv Nurs, 11*, 429–438.

Sands, D., & Holman, E. (1983). Does knowledge enhance patient compliance. *J Gerontol Nurs, 11*(4), 23–29.

Sargent, J. (1984) Assessing and building family coping skills and confidence. *Home care for children with serious handicapping conditions* pp. 44–53. A report on a conference held May 27, 1984, Houston, Texas. Association for the Care of Children's Health.

Scheinberg, L., & Schneider, D.M. (1987). *Voluntary health organizations: A guide to patient services.* New York: Demos.

Schwartz, B. (1982). The friction of time: Access and delay in the context of medical care. In E.H. Mizruchi, B. Glassner, & T. Pasorello (Eds.), *Time and aging: Conceptualization and application in sociological and gerontological research* (pp. 75–111). Bayside, NY: General Hall.

Scott, J.P., Roberto, K.A., & Hutton, J.T. (1986). Families of Alzheimer's victims: Family support to the caregivers. *J Am Geriatr Soc, 34*, 348–354.

Shaw, E.G., & Routh, D.K. (1982). Effect of mother presence on children's reactions to aversive procedures. *J Pediatr Psychol, 7*, 33–42.

Silverman, P. (1978). *Mutual help groups: A guide for mental health workers* (NIMH Monograph, DHEW No. ADM 78–646). Washington, DC: U.S. Government Printing Office.

Singer, L., & Farkas, K.J. (1989). The impact of infant disability on maternal perception of stress. *Fam Relat, 38*, 444–449.

Skinner, B.F. (1971). *Beyond freedom and dignity.* New York: Knopf.

Skolny, M.A., & Riehl, J.P. (1974). Hope: Solving patient and family problems by using a theoretical framework. In J.P. Riehl & C. Roy (Eds.), *Conceptual models for nursing practice* (pp. 206–218). New York: Appleton-Century-Crofts.

Soldo, B.J., & Manton, K.G. (1985). Health status and service needs of the oldest old: Current patterns and future trends. *Memorial Fund Q/Health Soc, 63*(2), 286–319.

Stallwood, J., & Stoll, R. (1975). Spiritual dimension of nursing practice. In I.L. Beland & J.Y. Passos (Eds.) *Clinical nursing.* 3rd ed. New York: Macmillan.

Stewart, M.J. (1989). Social support instruments created by nurse investigators. *Nurs Res, 38*(5), 268–275.

Stoner, M.H., & Keampfer, S.H. (1985). Recalled life expectancy information, phase of illness and hope in cancer patients. *Res Nurs Health, 8*, 264–274.

Surwut, R.S., Scovern, A.W., & Feinglos, M.N. (1982). The role of behavior in diabetes care. *Diabetes Care, 5*, 337–342.

Svarstadt, B. (1976). Physician-patient communication and patient conformity with medical advice. In D. Mechanic (Ed.), *The growth of bureaucratic medicine* (pp. 220–238). New York: Wiley.

Thorne, S.E. (1988). Helpful and unhelpful communications in cancer care: The patient perspective. *Oncol Nurs Forum, 15*(2), 167–172.

Thorne, S.E., & Robinson, C.A. (1988). Reciprocal thrust in health care relationships. *Journal of Advanced Nursing, 13*, 782–789.

Tilden, V.P., & Gaylen, R.D. (1987). Cost and conflict: The darker side of social support. *West J Nurs Res, 9*(1), 13–18.

Vachon, M.L. (1986). A comparison of the impact of breast cancer and bereavement: Personality, social support and adaptation. In S. Hobfoll (Ed.), *Stress, social support and women* (pp. 187–204). New York: Hemisphere.

Van Hoozer, H.L., Bratton, B.B., Ostmoe, P.M. et al. (1987). *The teaching process: Theory and practice in nursing.* Norwalk, CT: Appleton-Century-Crofts.

Walker, A.J. (1985). Reconceptualizing family stress. *J Marr Fam, 47*, 827–837.

Walker, C.L. (1988). Stress and coping in siblings of childhood cancer patients. *Nurs Res, 37*(4), 208–212.

Wakker, D.K., Epstein, S.G., Taylor, A.B., et al. (1989). Perceived needs of families with children who have chronic health conditions. *Children's Health Care, 18*(4), 196–201.

Watson, D., & Kendall, P.C. (1983). Methodological issues in research on coping with chronic disease. In T.G. Burish & L.A. Bradley (Eds.), *Coping with chronic disease* (pp. 313–81). New York: Academic.

Williams, R., Lindgren, H., Rowe, G., et al. (Eds.). (1975). *Family strengths: Enhancement of interaction* (Preface). Lincoln, NE: Department of Human Development and the Family, Center for Family Strengths, University of Nebraska.

Williamson, Y.M. (1978). Methodological dilemmas in tapping the concept of patient needs. *Nurs Res, 27*(3), 172–177.

Zarit, S.H., Reever, K.E., & Bach-Peterson, S. (1980). Relatives of impaired elderly: Correlated feelings of burden. *Gerontologist, 20*, 649–655.

Zastocki, D.Z., & Rovinski, C.A. (1989). *Home care: Patient and family instructions.* Philadelphia: W.B. Saunders.

Zola, I.K. (1982). Denial of emotional needs in people with handicaps. *Arch Phys Med Rehabil, 63*, 63–67.

14 Level of Functioning

This chapter focuses on the individual and family systems level of functioning. **Level of functioning** refers to the system's current state of adaptation and is determined by the extent to which the system is able to accomplish its developmental and situational tasks. The system's ability to function may change over time as the individual and family develop, the chronic condition progresses, or new focal stressors occur. Included in this chapter are several variables, not mentioned elsewhere, that have an important bearing on individual and family functioning. These variables are related to the characteristics of the chronic condition and the environment. Also included is an overview of situational tasks to be accomplished by individuals and their families. Evidence indicating their successful or unsuccessful adaptation is discussed. The relationship between level of functioning and the other variables in the Contingency Model of Long-Term Care is depicted in Figure 14–1.

Variables Mediating Level of Functioning

Characteristics of the Condition

A number of illness-related factors may mediate the impact of a chronic condition on all systems, and hence the level of functioning at any point in time. Rolland's typology of illness provides a framework for understanding many of these factors (Rolland, 1987, 1988). The typology consists of four categories (onset, course, outcome, and degree of incapacitation) related to the time phases of the illness (crisis, chronic, terminal) that are linked by periods of transition. These time phases were discussed in Chapter 8.

Sudden onset of an illness, such as a spinal cord injury, creates a crisis with which the family must cope immediately, whereas a condition with a more

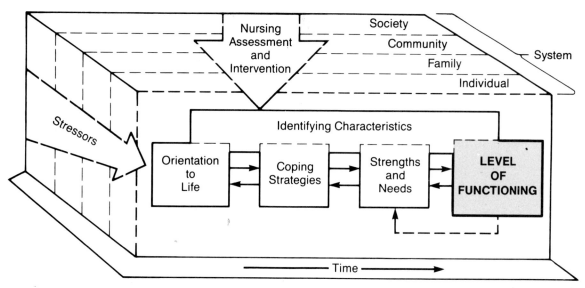

FIGURE 14—1 The Relationship of Level of Functioning to Other Variables in the Contingency Model of Long-Term Care

gradual onset, such as arthritis, provides family members with a longer period of adjustment. The course, or trajectory, of a chronic condition may be either progressive, with gradual increase in severity of symptoms (e.g., COPD); constant, with a fairly stable and predictable course (e.g., paralysis); or episodic, with periods of exacerbations and remissions characterized by uncertainty as to when the next crisis will occur (e.g., asthma). The outcome of illness is related to the family's initial expectation of the disease's effect on the person's life span (no effect, shorten, death). This potential impact on the life span influences the degree to which families experience anticipatory grief. The types of incapacitation (mobility, sensation, cognition, energy production, disfigurement) also influence adjustments the family must make. For example, a person with asthma may be minimally or severely incapacitated, or at times, not incapacitated at all.

Other variables related to the condition are its complexity, frequency of occurrence, symptoms (frequency, intensity), genetic transmission, severity, and the efficacy of treatment available for it. Still other mediators include place of treatment (home, hospital, institution, community agency, school), amount of time involved in management, and the people needed to manage the illness (patient, parent, outsider).

Environmental Characteristics

Three elements related to the environment can affect the individual: (1) Something in the environment becomes the activator, (2) the individual reacts to the activator, and (3) the reaction leads to consequences (Elliott & Eisdorfer, 1982). A single event may produce many reactions, and responses to environmental situations or conditions vary from individual to individual and from time to time within the same individual. Reactions may vary in intensity, effectiveness, or appropriateness. For example, a person falling down a few steps may react by crying if in pain or laughing if in front of others and not hurt. Those observing the event may respond by showing concern, laughing, or turning away. If the person is on crutches, it is unlikely that laughter would be a response, at least not by those observing the incident. The child who is teased by playmates because he has lost his hair from chemotherapy for his leukemia may respond by running away, wearing a cap, or explaining why he has no hair (see Figure 14–2).

Physical environment Physical environment includes geographic location, climate, nutritional substances, natural resources, shelter, and harmful or dangerous substances. People who are chronically ill, disabled, or under stress are more likely to be

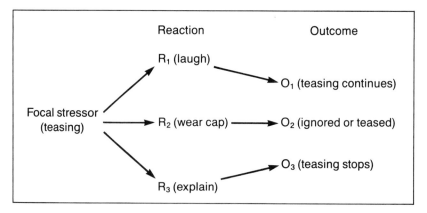

FIGURE 14–2 Relationship Among a Focal Stressor, Possible Reactions, and Possible Outcomes

influenced by these environmental conditions than are those persons not facing these stressors.

The weather is likely to influence the activities of people with certain chronic conditions. People with chronic respiratory problems and those with limited mobility may be restricted at various times because they cannot go out of doors. People with arthritis report increased pain as "stormlike pressure and humidity" increase (Moos, 1979). Increased mortality has been associated with heat waves and extreme cold weather, especially for the poor, elderly, physically handicapped, and those with circulatory problems. Climate has been found to be related to suicide, homicide, accident rates, and physical symptoms.

Level of Functioning as a Coping Outcome

Coping outcome refers to the effect a coping strategy has in relieving the stressor. Because people perceive their chronic conditions subjectively and cope in different ways, the outcome of coping is likely to be variable. The goal of health care professionals should be to facilitate coping so that children and adults with chronic conditions and their families are able to accomplish their developmental and situational tasks while balancing the stressors of the condition. A task should be accomplished "according to standards that are tolerable to both the individual and the group in which he lives" (Hamburg & Adams, 1967, p. 280). The expected level of functioning outcomes for persons living with chronic conditions and their families are listed in Table 14–1.

An important issue to be addressed involves how the coping behavior is determined to be effective or adaptive (Barofsky, 1981; Singer, 1984). This is partially a question of judging the intent or purpose of the behavior. It requires making a judgment between different domains of the individual (physical, psychological, social), over different periods of time (short term, long term), as a function of different situations (e.g., diagnosis, hospitalization). For example, in studies of adults, Hackett and Weisman (1964) found that denial was psychologically beneficial for patients with myocardial infarction at one

Table 14–1 Level of Function Outcomes

- The individual and family are able to accomplish their developmental tasks to the extent that is possible, given the limitations of the chronic condition.
- The individual and family are able to effectively accomplish their situational tasks.
- The psychosocial and financial costs to the individual and family are minimal.
- Rewarding interpersonal relationships are maintained.
- Disability is limited and function is maximized.
- Patients and families are satisfied with their quality of life.
- Parents understand the coping behaviors of their child(ren).
- Parents are able to facilitate their children's coping.
- The terminally ill person dies with dignity.

stage of their illness but not for patients with terminal cancer. Determining the outcome of coping also means imposing a set of value judgments that may vary across individuals and cultures, making it likely that different outcomes will be attributed to the coping strategies. Little attention has been given to predicting those who are likely to cope poorly or are most likely to benefit from professional or self-help interventions (Bradley & Burish, 1983).

Adaptation has been defined as "coming to terms existentially with the reality of chronic illness as a state of being, discarding both false hope and destructive hopelessness, and restructuring the environment in which one must now function . . . so that there is meaning and purpose in living that transcends the limitations imposed by the illness" (Feldman, 1974, p. 290). Successful adaptation depends on a continuing willingness to remain engaged in everyday social activities and concerns (Mechanic, 1986). However, this is often difficult to do because there is natural tendency to withdraw in response to a chronic condition. White (1974) views adaptation as striving toward a compromise between triumph over and surrender to the environment. Consequently, the individual and family systems are interacting with the environment as they come to terms with the chronic condition. Within the context of the Contingency Model of Long-Term Care, **adaptation** refers to the extent to which the individual or family system is accomplishing its developmental and situational tasks.

Adaptation to a chronic condition is a complex, dynamic coping process that occurs over time. Because it is a dynamic process, the stages of adaption may overlap at times. They may also be reexperienced as the disease progresses or new stressors arise; in fact, at times a person may need to adapt on a daily basis (Shocken & Carson, 1987).

Characteristics of successful adaptation or adjustment of coping include (1) keeping one's distress within reasonable limits; (2) maintaining a realistic appraisal of the situation, positive outlook, and positive self-concept; and (3) being able to function or carry out socially desired goals (Silver & Wortman, 1980). Although clients may appear to have adjusted well to the chronic condition, it is possible for them to have setbacks.

> Adoption of the chronic sick role constitutes a form of adaptation and is viewed as a meaningful alternative to full recovery or complete dependence. Characteristic traits of adaptation include reduction or alteration in work activity, diet control, changes in personal health habits such as smoking, and adjustments in family relationships. (Smith, 1975, p. 153)

Some people cope by using measures that may be harmful to themselves or to others. Coping strategies that are abusive to oneself may include self-destructive behaviors such as substance abuse or physical and verbal abusive behaviors directed at others (Gray-Price & Szczesny, 1985).

An unfortunate outcome of coping with a chronic condition may be maltreatment of the ill or handicapped individual. For analytic clarity, maltreatment is generally divided into abuse and neglect. Abuse is usually defined as an intentional act of commission, whereas neglect is an act of omission of needed care. Although there have been reports of both child and elderly abuse, more research is needed in this area. In a recent review of the literature regarding childhood physical disabilities and child maltreatment, White and colleagues (1986) conclude that linkages do exist between disabilities and maltreatment, but the nature of these linkages remains unclear. Although there is some indication that children with preexisting disabilities and chronic illness are abused, it is not known whether they are at increased risk for such abuse. Studies by Glaser and Bentovim (1979) and Dimond and Jones (1983) suggest that children with preexisting illness are more likely to be maltreated through neglect than through abuse. Some studies suggest that the presence of a child with a physical disability may be most stressful if the parents are already vulnerable because of low socioeconomic status. Other variables, such as parental age, race, and family structure, have been investigated but do not consistently differentiate families who maltreat their youngsters, from other families. Families who maltreat their children may have poor general coping and parenting skills, may suffer from social isolation, or be highly responsive to negative behavior (Garbarino, 1983).

Elderly abuse can take many forms, such as withholding food, money, medications for services, in addition to inflicting pain and injury. Also, it could involve threats, insults, being sworn at, confinement, or management of the elderly person's finances (Eliopoulos, 1984). The groups most prone to abuse are those who are very old, female, disabled, living with a relative, and physically, socially, or financially dependent (Select Committee on Aging, 1987).

Pillemer and Finkelhor (1989) recently questioned the widely accepted proposition that elderly abuse results from stress and burden placed on the care giver by sick and dependent elderly. Until now, much literature focused on strains of caring for the elderly. Because of "generational inversion" (elderly dependence on offspring), costs for the care giver increase while the rewards diminish, leading to abuse by the care giver. Evidence suggests that the abusive care giver is financially dependent on the elderly victim resulting in perceived powerlessness. In addition, care givers often depend on the elderly for social support. In a study of 61 identified abuse victims and a comparison group of elderly persons who were not abused, Pillemer and Finkelhor (1989) found that abuse appears to be a reflection of the abusers' problems rather than of the elderly victims' characteristics. Spouses rather than adult children were more likely to be the abusers. The abusers were more likely to have some socioeconomic maladjustment than the care givers in the comparison group.

Developmental Tasks

Individuals and family units have to accomplish both developmental and situational tasks. Developmental tasks are growth responsibilities that arise at a critical time in the person's or family's life that must be accomplished in order for them to accomplish tasks that follow (Duvall, 1977). Developmental tasks serve as guidelines that enable individuals and families to know society's expectations of them at any given stage of development. Developmental tasks of the individual were discussed in Chapter 4 and family developmental tasks in Chapter 5. Although it is beyond the scope of this book to discuss the developmental tasks for each level, nurses need to be aware of these expectations. Unfortunately, the expectations for individuals with chronic conditions and their families are not as clearcut as they are for those who are healthy. Overall individual and family developmental tasks are listed in Table 14–2.

Situational Tasks

Situational tasks arise as a result of stressors caused by the chronic condition. These tasks are responsibilities that must be accomplished in order to successfully cope with and adapt to the chronic condition. Situational tasks need to be accomplished by

Table 14–2 Individual and Family Developmental Tasks

INDIVIDUAL DEVELOPMENTAL TASKS

1. Develop and maintain healthy growth and nutrition patterns
2. Learn to manage one's body satisfactorily
3. Learn to understand and relate to the physical world
4. Develop self-awareness and a satisfying sense of self
5. Learn to relate to others

FAMILY DEVELOPMENTAL TASKS

1. Meet the basic physical needs of the family (e.g., food, health care, shelter, and money)
2. Assist all family members develop their own potential
3. Meet the emotional needs of all family members
4. Maintain and adapt family organization and management to meet family needs
5. Function in the community

Source: Hymovich & Chamberlin, 1980.

the child or adult who is chronically ill, by their care givers, and by other members of their families.

When a family member dies, remaining family members are faced with accomplishing certain tasks in order to return to an effective level of functioning. Lindemann (1965) described the grief work of the normal individual, delineating the intrapsychic tasks of "working through" the loss. Goldberg (1973) outlined family tasks of grieving as (1) facilitating the process of mourning for all members, (2) assigning the proper role to the memory of the deceased, (3) reassigning roles and expectations among the remaining members, and (4) establishing new or altered relationships outside the family.

Children with chronic conditions The majority of children with chronic disorders of varying degrees of severity cope successfully and adapt well to their situation (Stein, 1989). Recent studies show that, although seriously ill children and their families are more likely to have mental health problems than are families with healthy children, severe psychopathology is rare. Children with chronic conditions may experience difficulty completing their developmental tasks and achieving independence from their parents as they mature. They may also have difficulty finding and maintaining employment and forming social and sexual relationships.

Situational tasks to be completed by chronically ill children are listed in Table 14–3. The extent to which children are able to accomplish these tasks influences their level of functioning with the chronic condition.

Evidence of satisfactory adaptation includes (1) ability to function effectively in school and at home, (2) good understanding of the disorder and realistic understanding of one's limitations, (3) social competence, (4) good self-concept, (5) belief in one's ability to control one's own health status, (6) age-appropriate dependence on parents and other family members, and (7) participation in medical management (Mattsson, 1972; Simmons et al, 1985). In addition, the children have little need for secondary gains and have a sense of self-preservation. Their

Table 14–3 Situational Tasks of Children and Adults with Chronic Conditions

- Master, within limits of the condition, age-appropriate developmental tasks
- Develop an age-appropriate understanding of the condition and its management
- Develop and preserve a sense of control over the situation
- Adjust to potential role changes
- Maintain control of symptoms (e.g., pain, incapacitation, decreased control of bodily functions)
- Deal with the uncertainty of the condition and prepare for an uncertain future
- Develop or refine one's value system
- Develop or preserve relationships with family and friends
- Understand and cope with emotional impact of the condition
- Master the ability to provide care for self, within the limits of the condition and one's developmental level
- Make age-appropriate decisions regarding one's care
- Develop trust in oneself and one's care givers
- Develop and maintain a positive self-concept and sense of self-esteem

patterns of social interactions, although sometimes modified, are adequate. Compensatory activities, such as intellectual or physical pursuits, are developed and give the children satisfaction. Children who have adapted successfully can express sad and angry feelings when they are frustrated and feelings of confidence and guarded optimism as appropriate. The use of denial as an adaptive mechanism has also been noted. Denial enabled children to deal with uncertainty about their future and to maintain hope. Some children became altruistic by wishing to become nurses or doctors and help others with the same problem they had. Others identified with children who had similar problems and wished for cures for anybody who was sick (Mattsson, 1972).

Following a study of chronically ill adolescents, Zeltzer and colleagues (1980) concluded that the adolescents were psychologically healthy and that the group differences reflected the realities of the various diseases and treatments. This finding suggests that intrapsychic explorations may not be as useful as psychosocial rehabilitation aimed at alleviating disease- and treatment-related problems.

Children who fail to adapt successfully fall along a continuum (Prugh, 1983). At one end are the children who remain overly dependent on their families, especially their mothers. They tend to be fearful and overly anxious and are passive or withdrawn, lack outside interests, and often have strong needs for secondary gains from their illness. These children are likely to become overly dependent or inhibited. Although there is no direct correlation between parent behavior and behavior of these withdrawn children, their parents tend to be overprotective, over-anxious, and, sometimes, overindulgent.

At the other end of the continuum are the overly independent children who tend to deny their limitations. They may act as if they are not sick, push themselves unrealistically, or become risk takers. While there was no significant correlation between parent behavior and child adaptation, the parents, usually the mother, tend to be oversolicitous. Predictors of poor adaptation of children one year following renal transplant were low family income, absence of father in the home, sense of being less happy than other families, poor understanding of the medical condition, and lowered trust in the medical profession. Items in the child's personality tests most predictive of poor psychosocial adjustment were anxiety, poor sense of personal worth, low popularity, and antisocial tendencies (Korsch & Negrete, 1980).

Considerable evidence indicates that children with mild disabilities are more likely to have emotional problems than are those with severe disabilities (Stein, 1989). Stein and Jessop (1984) reported increased negative consequences for both child and parents when the child's chronic condition was not visible. These negative effects included dissatisfaction with medical care, psychiatric symptoms in the mothers, and mother reports of poor functional status in the child. On the positive side, normal appearance was associated with increased involvement in the community and reduced dependency in the child, reduced numbers of days hospitalized, and improved health care maintenance. Children with mild conditions are more likely to conceal their problem and try to pass for normal, resulting in psychosocial adjustment problems. For example, adolescents whose seizures were under good control were less likely to communicate with family and friends and had poorer self-images and poorer expectations for the future than those who were not under good control (Hodgman et al, 1979).

Adults with chronic conditions Adults with chronic conditions are faced with many tasks and potential psychosocial adjustment difficulties that may interfere with their level of functioning. As with children, adults have to accomplish certain situational tasks that are superimposed on their normal developmental tasks. Table 14–3 lists some of these situational tasks.

Although many people can function very well when they have a chronic condition, others may not function well. For example, recent studies show that survivors of strokes are affected by psychosocial dysfunction. Leisure activities are considerably decreased, as are social activities, even for people who achieve complete physical restoration. Weisman & Worden (1975) found that when patients maintained active and mutually responsive relationships with those persons responsible for their experience, they had longer periods of survival.

Meenan and colleagues (1981) studied the psychosocial outcome of 245 adults with rheumatoid arthritis. Changes in marital and employment status and leisure activities were explored. Work disability was the major impact of the illness, with the group earning an average of 50% of the income predicted for them if they had not had arthritis. In this study, 18% of the sample, compared with national average of 11%, were never married; 59% stopped working completely, and the majority of the others reduced their hours or changed occupations. In addition, 85% reported changing their leisure activities, 18% changed residence because of the rheumatoid arthritis, and 6% of the family members changed employment status to compensate for the impact of the condition. Only 15% had been referred to a social worker. Major losses in the area of work, finances, and family structure were reported.

Studies indicate that family reactions following sudden physical disability such as stroke are formed within the first month following the diagnosis and that initial family coping patterns are not as rigid as they may become over time (Evans et al, 1987). Hospital time was reduced for patients following stroke by positive family support and responsiveness. Problem solving, communication skills, self-care scores, and baseline patient adjustment were predictors of patient adjustment at 6 and 12 months poststroke. Pollack (1986) found sex and social status were significantly related to physiologic and psychosocial adaptation in adults with rheumatoid arthritis, diabetes mellitus, and hypertension. In this study, age, health improvement regimens, length of time the illness was present, days lost from work, and marital status were not significantly related to adaptation. The presence of hardiness was significantly related to adaptive behavior only in the persons with diabetes.

Families of children with chronic conditions Situational tasks for families of chronically ill children arise as a result of the child's condition and are superimposed on individual and family developmental tasks. A number of important situational tasks of parents and siblings are pertinent to nursing care. Parent situational tasks are listed in Table 14–4.

Parents.
Mattsson (1972) noted that the parents of children who adapted successfully were usually able to understand and accept their children's limitations. They could permit appropriate dependence and were able to make good use of the children's capacities and strengths.

Contrary to previous reports, current data provide no evidence that divorce rates are higher in families of chronically ill children than they are for control groups (Buhlmann & Fitzpatrick, 1987). However, marital distress is higher in these families than in control groups. Positive outcomes, such as increased family closeness, have also been noted (Hymovich & Baker, 1985). For example, mothers

Table 14—4 Situational Tasks of Parents of Chronically Ill Children

- Obtain adequate health care
- Meet financial burden of the condition
- Maintain health of all family members
- Understand and manage the condition
- Meet the developmental needs of each family member
- Learn areas in which child's life and function are not affected by the condition and develop plan to assure as much normalcy as possible (Sargent, 1983)
- Maintain their own health
- Maintain the individual integrity of each family member
- Establish and maintain support system
- Establish a philosophy of life to cope with the condition
- Help child(ren) understand and cope with the condition
- Assign condition management tasks to child appropriate for age and developmental status
- Understand and cope with the emotional impact of the condition on family
- Adjust family organization to accommodate person with the chronic condition
- Adjust to changes in lifestyle
- Become an advocate for self and family
- Seek and use appropriate health and community resources

Sources: Hymovich, 1979; Sargent, 1983.

of children with long-term tracheostomies reported that their child's condition had brought the family closer together. In addition, the mothers thought that learning to care for the children made them feel better about themselves (Singer & Farkas, 1989).

Adjustment to living with a child who has a chronic condition is an ongoing task. There may be frequent medical crises as a result of the nature of the illness (e.g., asthma). Parents are required to be constantly alert to potential changes in the child's condition, and changes in occupational status may be required, especially by the mother. At the same time, parents are expected to provide as normal a life as possible for the child and siblings. Many of

these conflicting tasks are faced by parents of children receiving continuous ambulatory peritoneal dialysis (CAPD) at home:

> Parents are asked to monitor the child's physical state intensely. They are also told not to allow the child's medical problems to become the main family focus. Parents are instructed that an error in the sterile technique could result in their child's serious illness, yet staff is also concerned that parents should not experience excessive anxiety. Parents are asked to function as both medic and parent, and yet it is also expected that the child will be able to progress through normal stages of separation and individuation. Parents are encouraged to allow their adolescents the usual opportunities to test out independence and self-care skills in their own medical management. Nevertheless, they must also closely support a youth who is often rejected by peers and who acts out self-rejection in the form of medical non-compliance. (LePontois, Moel, & Cohen, 1987, p. 53)

Siblings of children with chronic conditions and children of parents with chronic conditions.
As with the parents, there is a wide range of functioning levels of well children in families of children or parents with chronic conditions. It is reasonable to assume that any member of the family system is at risk for potential psychosocial adjustment difficulties and should be considered when planning nursing care.

Some siblings may be well adjusted, while others may have adjustment problems (Breslau & Prabucki, 1987; Simeonsson & McHale, 1981). Evidence suggests that siblings of children with mild chronic conditions have more psychosocial adjustment problems than those with more severe handicaps. Sibling adaptation may be mediated by the quality of the family's reaction.

Although there has been relatively little research with children whose parents are chronically ill, it appears they may have potential difficulties adjusting to the condition and changes within the family. Situational tasks that siblings must accomplish also need to be mastered by children whose parent has a chronic condition. These situational tasks are listed in Table 14–5.

Spouses and care givers of chronically ill adults.
When a spouse or parent is chronically ill, adult care givers may find themselves adapting to new re-

Table 14—5 Situational Tasks of the Siblings
of Chronically Ill Children and
Children of Chronically Ill Parents

- Master age-specific development tasks
- Understand the condition and its associated care
- Master the feelings that accompany the stressors associated with the condition (e.g., jealousy)
- Communicate openly with those who can handle it and practice mutual pretense with those who cannot (Bluebond-Langner, 1988)
- Understand and master changes in parents and family life

sponsibilities. They must learn about the condition, its course, and treatment; what to expect; what to report; how to perform special procedures; and understand medications and their side effects. These and other situational tasks of care givers are listed in Table 14–6. Brody (1981) refers to the burden of women care givers as "women-in-the-middle," who must care for their own children and their aging parents. These added responsibilities cause increasing stress as the aging parent becomes more frail. The care givers will often suffer from psychological and

Table 14—6 Situational Tasks of Care Givers
of Chronically Ill Adults

- Establish and maintain a support system
- Establish a philosophy of life to cope with the condition
- Master the feelings that accompany the stressors associated with the chronic condition
- Understand the condition and its associated care
- Maintain one's own health
- Adjust to changes in life-style
- Adjust family organization to accommodate person with the chronic condition
- Develop and preserve a sense of control over the situation
- Adjust to potential role changes
- Deal with the uncertainty of the condition and prepare for an uncertain future
- Develop or refine one's value system

somatic symptoms. Social support has been found to be an important factor in the adjustment of spouses of women with breast cancer (Northouse, 1988; Vachon, 1986) as well as the adjustment of others.

Assessment and Intervention

Assessment

Individuals and families are assessed according to their stage in the life cycle. The extent to which they are accomplishing their developmental and situational tasks is an important consideration in the nurse's assessment and intervention. Guidelines for assessing individual and family developmental tasks are included in Table 14–7 and situational tasks are in Table 14–8.

Intervention

This section includes nursing interventions to facilitate individual and family functioning that were not covered in previous chapters. The goal of intervention is to enhance the system's ability to function at its highest possible level. Interventions in this chapter and in preceding chapters are related to facilitating level of functioning.

Foster independence through self-care Effective management of a chronic condition depends upon the person's ability to actively regulate the condition and to slow or prevent deterioration. The role of health care providers is to support and encourage patient management of the condition so that the patient feels comfortable enough to return for additional help as management problems arise or new stressors emerge (Chewning, 1982). To provide such care, an ongoing relationship between client and provider is necessary so that modifications can be made in response to changes in the client's self-awareness, condition, or circumstances.

"Self care is the practice of activities that individuals personally initiate and perform on their own behalf in maintaining life, health, and well-being" (Orem, 1991, p. 17). Adults normally take care of their own health needs, and self-care contributes to one's health. During illness, self-care demands may exceed the person's ability to meet them, and nursing care may be required to help the person regain a steady state.

Table 14—7 Assessment of Individual and Family Coping Strategies

Area	Useful Information
Usual way of coping	Satisfaction with previous coping
Ability to cope with this event	Beliefs about ability to manage
Management of condition	Seek information Use information Use of skills Seek resources Use of resources Monitor self or other Adhere to regimen
Incorporate illness into life style	Manage time Maintain normalcy Modify roles Modify environment
Cope with feelings	Search for meaning Attribute causes and outcome Make comparisons Maintain hope Use defense mechanisms

Strengths	Needs

Nursing is based on the values of self-help and help to others. **Self-care** is the practice of activities that people initiate and perform on their own behalf. To engage in self-care activities, the individual must have the ability and skills to initiate and sustain self-care practices. When there is a self-care deficit, the patient needs assistance in learning and performing self-care activities (Orem, 1991); the role of the nurse is to provide the necessary assistance.

To facilitate self-care, the regimen should be tailored to the individual. Whenever possible, the regimen should not be intrusive and should be planned to minimize inconvenience. For example, treatment and medication schedules should be planned to fit the person's daily schedule. Scheduling medications around regular habits (mealtime, bedtime) may facilitate adhering to them because they are tied to specific activities. Preserving things perceived as special in the client's schedule or habits sustains quality of life and makes life worth living.

Patients need meaningful activities they can do despite the presence of disease. "Assisting the individual with a meaningful contribution to society is as important an activity for nursing as assuring adherence to a regimen of exercise, diet, or medication" (Larkin, 1987, p. 539). This letter from a 75-year-old woman during rehabilitation following hip surgery indicates her perception of prescribed activities:

It could be an amusing story—like to keep patients occupied, I had to attend a cooking class!! I don't intend to start cooking! Also an exercise group for strengthening muscles from the waist up—we are all in wheelchairs. Plus, an arts and crafts class, can you believe? Like camp, where I made a ceramic trivet, a work of *art*—The cost of this is probably about $20,000 of hospitalization there.

Table 14—8   Assessment of Individual and Family Developmental Tasks

Area	Useful Information
Individual (depends upon age)	Extent to which accomplishing tasks assess each member, using appropriate individual tasks Establish and maintain healthy growth and nutrition patterns Develop and maintain control over body Understand and relate to the physical world Develop and maintain self-awareness and satisfying sense of self Establish and maintain effective relationships with others

Family	Meet basic physical needs
	  (e.g., food, health care, shelter, money)
	Assist each member develop individual potential (appropriate for age, condition)
	Meet needs for emotional support
	  Communicate effectively
	Understand needs
	Adapt organization and management (perform roles)
	Function in community

Strengths	Needs

Optimal daily self care makes considerable demands on a person's knowledge, skill, motivation, time, energy, and social supports. In a recent survey of 73 persons with diabetes, 43 (59%) were able to complete all required care themselves, while 23 (32%) needed occasional help, 5 (7%) did nothing special for their diabetic care, and 2 (5%) needed care by someone else (e.g., insulin injections, managing hypoglycemia) all the time (Germain & Nemchik, 1988).

The relationship between client variables and successful self-management are relatively unexplored. Social support may have a strong relationship to success in managing one's chronic condition. For example, disorganized or dysfunctional family processes can undermine a person's efforts (Gurman, 1981). Especially problematic for successful self-management are family (or societal) promotion of secondary gain for illness behavior or active constraints on self-care activities in the family or work

environment (Turk, Meichenbaum, & Genest, 1983). As mentioned in Chapter 11 (Coping Strategies), self-monitoring is a method for coping and is, in fact, necessary for self-care. Therefore, patients and their families need to know what should be monitored, based on the nature of the chronic condition and its treatment.

Self-management depends on the patient's awareness of activities and treatments that alleviate the symptoms or make them worse (Shekleton, 1987). Patients can be encouraged to keep a log or diary of daily routines, feeling states, and associated symptoms of disease. The log can be reviewed to determine causes of exacerbations.

Studies of the effectiveness of self-management training on adherence to medical regimens are still limited. Most investigations focus on such strategies as the value of individual versus group instruction, the value of sequencing learning skills, and patient versus professional educational group leaders. More investigations on the techniques of teaching and the loss of skills over time are needed.

One potentially useful strategy is self-talk, whereby a person verbally praises herself or himself. Self-talk might involve changing negative thoughts to positive ones. For example, "I hate to test my urine—it's such a bother, so I'll just skip it this morning" could be changed to "Testing my urine gives me feedback on how I'm doing today, so I will do it before breakfast."

Facilitate control Fuchs (1987) notes that teaching promotes behavioral control. To facilitate cognitive control, nurses can give patients information about such things as their laboratory values or blood pressure and their relationship to the disease. Decisional control can be fostered by providing information about available options. See Chapter 12 for specific teaching guidelines.

Facilitate adherence to regimen Generally, it is more difficult for people to follow complex regimens than fairly simple ones (Sackett, 1986). Because client success is the key to shaping behavior, regimens should focus on tasks the client believes he or she can perform successfully (Steckel & Swain, 1977). Implied is the importance of considering client priorities in helping plan a regimen. Unfortunately, meeting this objective may not always be possible, as some conditions require tasks clients may be unable to accomplish successfully. In these cases, helping them determine an appropriate support system would be necessary.

Education about the medical regimen has two components: information needed to make informed decisions and behavioral skills needed to act on the information. Kirscht and Rosenstock note that

> . . . the only serious ethical question arises in the case of clients whose motives are such that they do not wish to modify a particular behavior. It is our view that in such cases it is inappropriate to attempt to change motives (even if it were possible). Any informed person who wishes to engage in any personal practices that are not conducive to good health, should, if those practices do not constitute danger to others, be free to do so. (Kirscht & Rosenstock, 1979, p. 214)

As noted previously, admissions of noncompliance are usually accurate and interventions performed with this group of patients have been found to show the greatest improvement (Cromer & Tarnowski, 1989; Epstein & Cluss, 1982).

Parrish (1986) compiled a list of the methods commonly used to strengthen child and adult compliance. These approaches involve education, combination of education and behavioral management, self-management (self-monitoring, goal setting, and reinforcement), environmental rearrangement, contingent reinforcement, adjustment to regimen (reduce complexity of treatment), and organizational strategies within the health care system to facilitate appropriate behaviors. Organizational strategies include helping the patient to problem solve or facilitating transportation to clinic. Strategies to reduce complexity of treatment include the use of timed-release medications, anticipating major side effects and prescribing appropriate medications for them, and the use of individual prompting strategies (e.g., use pocket alarm, take pills with meals).

Cromer and Tarnowski (1989) identified several trends in intervention to improve compliance. These included increased emphasis on quality of health care provider and patient relationships, increased use of combined interventions (e.g., education and behavioral approaches), and individually tailored interventions. We recommend including family members in these individual plans to facilitate patient support in adhering to the therapeutic regimen. Southam and Dunbar (1986) note that the combination of several approaches to compliance are more effective than a single strategy.

Two examples of studies to foster adherence are presented here. In one study (Nessman et al, 1980), two training methods were compared for patients with hypertension. The first was a patient-operated group supervised by a nurse and a psychologist and the other was a group who listened to audiotaped information on hypertension and were managed in a nurse-operated clinic. Although both programs increased patient adherence, the patient-operated group had greater reductions in systolic and diastolic pressures. Fireman et al (1981) investigated the effect of a program to teach self-management skills to children with asthma and to their parents. The experimental group of children and parents received training in self-management skills by a nurse using individual and group instruction, plus telephone monitoring. The comparison group was instructed in the data collection format and the management of asthma but received the usual physician's care. Children in the experimental group had fewer and less severe asthmatic attacks, and fewer hospitalizations and emergency room visits than did the comparison group.

Facilitate access to resources Providing economic resources that enable the patient to obtain needed services and modify the environment is a tangible approach to facilitating access to resources. Although health care professionals cannot provide the needed finances, they can put people in contact with the appropriate agencies, facilitate the use of their available support system, and advocate for legislation and policy changes that address this area.

Collaboration with others Although there is much the nurse can do to facilitate family functioning when chronic illness or disability is present, many family needs extend beyond the scope of nursing, and in fact beyond the scope of the health care system. A multidisciplinary team is necessary to ensure comprehensive care for these patients and their families. Nurses play a pivotal role as members of these teams.

There are rigid traditional functions of health professionals, such as territoriality, that still interfere with collaboration, although it is clear that we can no longer independently fulfill all the needs of clients. Each team member has both unique contributions and shared responsibilities. Teams need to clarify their functions. They need to decide who should coordinate the team efforts, establish goals, and show mutual respect for the abilities and contributions of others. Flexibility of roles within the team is often useful in meeting patient and family needs.

Summary

Individual and family level of functioning was discussed as it relates to adaptation to chronic conditions. Effective functioning implies the ability to accomplish, within the constraints of the chronic condition, developmental tasks. In addition to developmental tasks, certain situational tasks must also be accomplished. **Level of functioning** refers to the system's current state of adaptation. It is determined by the extent to which the system is able to accomplish its developmental and situational tasks. Ability to function may change over time as the individual and family develop, the chronic condition progresses, or as new focal stressors occur. Two variables relevant to level of functioning were explored: characteristics of the chronic condition and characteristics of the environment.

This chapter included an overview of situational tasks to be accomplished by adults and children with chronic conditions. Situational tasks of other family members, primarily siblings of the chronically ill child, children of parents with chronic conditions, spouses and care givers were also discussed. Nursing interventions included fostering independence through self-care, facilitating control, facilitating adherence to regimen, facilitating access to resources, and the nurse's role in collaborating with others.

References

Barofsky, I. (1981). Issues and approaches to the psychosocial assessment of the cancer patient. In K. Proktop & L.A. Bradley (Eds.), *Medical psychology: Contributions to behavioral medicine* (pp. 55–65). New York: Academic.

Bluebond-Langner, M. (1978). *The private worlds of dying children.* Princeton, NJ: Princeton Univ. Press.

Bradley, L.A., & Burish, T.G. (1983). Coping with chronic disease: Current status and future direction. In T.G. Burish & L.A. Bradley (Eds.), *Coping with chronic disease* (pp. 475–482). New York: Academic.

Breslau, N., & Prabucki, K. (1987). Siblings of disabled children. *Arch Gen Psychiatry, 44,* 1040–1046.

Brody, E. (1981). Women in the middle and family help to older people. *Gerontologist, 21,* 471–480.

Buhlmann, U., & Fitzpatrick, S.B. (1987). Caring for an adolescent with a chronic illness. *Primary Care, 14*(1), 57–68.

Chewning, B. (1982). *Strategies to promote self management of chronic illness.* AHA/CDC Health Education Project. Chicago: American Hospital Association.

Cromer, B.A., & Tarnowski, K.J. (1989). Noncompliance in adolescents: A review. *J Dev Behav Pediatr, 10*(4), 207–215.

Dimond, M., & Jones, S. (1983). *Chronic illness across the life span.* Norwalk, CT: Appleton-Century-Crofts.

Duvall, E.M. (1977). *Marriage and family development.* Philadelphia: Lippincott.

Eliopoulos, C. (1984). Assessment of the family system. In C. Eliopoulos (Ed.), *Health assessment of the older adult* (pp. 37–46). Reading, MA: Addison-Wesley.

Elliott, G.R., & Eisdorfer, C. (Eds.). (1982). *Stress and human health.* New York: Springer.

Epstein, L.H., & Cluss, P.A. (1982). A behavioral medicine perspective on adherence to long-term medical regimens. *J Consult Clin Psychol, 50,* 950–971.

Evans, R.L., Bishop, D.S., Matlock, A., et al. (1987). Family interaction and treatment adherence after stroke. *Arch Phys Med Rehabil, 68,* 513–517.

Feldman, D.J. (1974). Chronic disabling illness: A holistic view. *J Chronic Dis, 27,* 287–291.

Fireman, P., Friday, G.A., Gira, C., et al. (1981). Teaching self-management skills to asthmatic children and their parents in an ambulatory care setting. *Pediatrics, 68,* 341–348.

Fuchs, J. (1987). Use of decisional control to combat powerlessness. *ANNA Am Nephrol Nurses Assoc J, 14*(1), 11–13, 56.

Garbarino, J. (1983). What we know about child maltreatment. *Child Youth Serv Rev, 5,* 3–5.

Germain, C.P., & Nemchik, R.M. (1988). Diabetes self management and hospitalization. *Image, 20*(2), 74–78.

Glaser, D. & Bentovim, A. (1979). Abuse and risk to handicapped and chronically ill children. *Child Abuse Negl, 3,* 565–575.

Goldberg, S. (1973). Family tasks and reactions in the crisis of death. *Soc Casework, 54,* 398–405.

Gray-Price, H., & Szczesny, S. (1985). Crisis intervention with families of cancer patients: A developmental approach. *Top Clin Nurs, 7*(1), 58–70.

Gurman, A.S. (1981). Integrative marital therapy: Toward the development of an interpersonal approach. In S.H. Budman (Ed.), *Forms of brief therapy.* New York: Guilford.

Hackett, T.P., & Weisman, A.D. (1964). Reactions to the imminence of death. In G.H. Grosser, H. Wechsler, & M. Greenblatt (Eds.), *The threat of impending death.* Cambridge, MA: M.I.T. Press.

Hamburg, D., & Adams, J. (1967). A perspective on coping behavior: Seeking and utilizing information in major transitions. *Arch Gen Psychiatry, 17,* 227–284.

Hodgman, C.H., McArarney, E.R., Meyers, G.H., Iker, H. (1979). Emotional complications of adolescent grand mal epilepsy. *J. Pediatr 95,* 309–312.

Hymovich, D.P. (1979). Assessment of the chronically ill child and family. In D.P. Hymovich & M.U. Barnard (Eds.), *Family health care: Vol. 1. General perspectives* (pp. 280–293). New York: McGraw-Hill.

Hymovich, D.P., & Baker, C. (1985). The needs, concerns and coping of parents of children with cystic fibrosis. *Fam Relat, 34,* 91–97.

Hymovich, D.P., & Chamberlin, R.W. (1980). *Child and family development: Implications for care.* New York: McGraw-Hill.

Kirscht, J.P., & Rosenstock, I.M. (1979). Patients' problems in following recommendations of health experts. In G.C. Stone, F. Cohen, & N.E. Adler (Eds.), *Health psychology—A handbook* (pp. 189–215). San Francisco: Jossey-Bass.

Korsch, B.M., & Negrete, V.F. (1980). Counseling patients and their families in a chronic renal disease program. *Patient Counseling Educ, 2*(2), 87–91.

Larkin, J. (1987). Factors identifying one's ability to adapt to chronic illness. *Nurs Clin North Am, 22*(3), 535–542.

LePontois, J., Moel, D.I., & Cohen, R.A. (1987). Family adjustment to pediatric ambulatory dialysis. *Am J Orthopsychiatry, 57*(1), 78–83.

Lindemann, E. (1965). Symptomatology and management in acute grief. *Crisis intervention.* New York: Family Service Association of America.

Mattsson, A. (1972). Long term illness in childhood: A challenge to psychosocial adaptation. *Pediatrics, 50,* 801–805.

Mechanic, D. (1986). *From advocacy to allocation: The evolving American health care system.* New York: Macmillan.

Meenan, R.F., Yelin, E.H., Nevitt, M., & Epstein, W.V. (1981). The impact of chronic disease: A sociomedical profile of rheumatoid arthritis. *Arthritis Rheum, 24*(3), 544–549.

Moos, R.H. (1979). Social-ecological perspectives on health. In G.C. Stone, F. Cohen, & N.E. Adler (Eds.), *Health psychology—A handbook* (pp. 523–547). San Francisco: Jossey-Bass.

Nessman, D.G., Carnahan, J.E., & Nugent, C.A. (1980). Increasing compliance: Patient-oriented hypertension groups. *Arch Int Med, 140,* 1427–1430.

Northouse, L.L. (1988). Social support in patients' and husbands' adjustment to breast cancer. *Nurs Res, 37*(2), 91–95.

Orem, D.E. (1991). *Nursing: Concepts of practice.* New York: McGraw-Hill.

Parrish, J.M. (1986). Pediatric compliance with medical and behavioral recommendations. In N.A. Krasnegor, J.D. Arasteh, & M.F. Cataldo (Eds.), *A behavioral pediatrics perspective.* New York: Wiley.

Pillemer, K., & Finkelhor, D. (1989). Causes of elder abuse: Caregiver stress versus problem relatives. *Am J Orthopsychiatry, 59*(2), 179–187.

Pollack, S.E. (1986). Human responses to chronic illness: Physiologic and psychosocial adaptation. *Nurs Res, 35,* 90–95.

Prugh, D.G. (1983). *The psychosocial aspects of pediatrics.* Philadelphia: Lea & Febiger.

Rolland, J.S. (1987). Family systems and chronic illness: A typological model. *J Psychother Fam, 3*(3), 143–168.

Rolland, J.S. (1988). A conceptual model of chronic and life-threatening illness and its impact on families. In C.S. Chilman, E.W. Nunnally, & F.M. Cox (Eds.), *Chronic illness and disability* (pp. 17–68). Newbury Park, CA: Sage.

Sackett, D. (1986). The magnitude of compliance and noncompliance. In D.L. Sackett & B.B. Haynes (Eds.), *Compliance with therapeutic regimens* (pp. 9–25). Baltimore: Johns Hopkins Press.

Sargent, A.J. (1983). The sick child and the family. *J Pediatr, 102*(6), 982–987.

Select Committee on Aging. (1984). U.S. House of Representatives 97th Congress. April 3, 1981. *Elder abuse:*

An examination of a hidden problem. Committee Publication #97-277.

Shekleton, M.E. Coping with chronic respiratory difficulty. (1987). *Nurs Clin North Am, 22*(3), 569–581.

Shocken, K.L., & Carson, V.J. (1987). Responding to the spiritual needs of the chronically ill. *Nurs Clin North Am, 22*(3), 603–611.

Silver, R.L., & Wortman, C.B. (1980). Coping with undesirable life events. In J. Garber & M.E.P. Seligman (Eds.), *Human helplessness* (pp. 279–340). New York: Academic.

Simmons, R.J., Corey, M., Cowen, L., et al. (1985). Emotional adjustment of early adolescents with cystic fibrosis. *Psychosom Med, 47*(2), 111–122.

Simeonsson, R.J., & McHale, S.M. (1981). Review: Research on handicapped children: Sibling relationships. *Child Care Health Dev, 7*, 153–171.

Singer, J.E. (1984). Some issues in the study of coping. *Cancer, 53*(Supplement), 2303–2315.

Singer, L., & Farkas, K.J. (1989). The impact of infant disability on maternal perception of stress. *Fam Relat, 38*, 444–449.

Smith, R.T. (1975). Societal reaction and physical disability: Contrasting perspectives. In W.R. Gove (Ed.), *The labelling of deviance: Evaluating a perspective* (pp. 147–156). New York: Wiley.

Southam, M.A., & Dunbar, J. (1986). Facilitating patient compliance with medical interventions. In K.A. Holroyd, & T.L. Creer (Eds.), *Self management of chronic disease* (pp. 163–187). Orlando, FL: Academic.

Steckel, S.B., & Swain, M.A. (1977). Contracting with patients to improve compliance. *Hospitals, 51*, 81–84.

Stein, R.E.K. (Ed.). (1989). Caring for children with chronic illness: Issues and strategies. New York: Springer.

Stein, R.E.K., & Jessop, D.J. (1984). General issues in the care of children with chronic physical conditions. *Pediatr Clin North Am, 31*, 189–198.

Turk, D.C., Meichenbaum, D., & Genest, M. (1983). *Pain and behavioral medicine.* New York: Guilford.

Vachon, M.L. (1986). A comparison of the impact of breast cancer and bereavement: Personality, social support and adaptation. In S. Hobfoll (Ed.), *Stress, social support and women* (pp. 187–204). New York: Hemisphere.

Weisman, A.D., & Worden, J.W. (1975). Psychological analysis of cancer deaths. *Omega, 6*, 71–75.

White, R. (1974). Strategies of adaptation: An attempt at systematic description. In G. Coelho, D. Hamburg, & J. Adams (Eds.), *Coping and adaptation* (pp. 47–68). New York: Basic Books.

White, R., Benedict, M.I., Wulff, L., & Kelley, M. (1986). Physical disabilities as risk factors for child maltreatment: A selected review. *Am J Orthopsychiatry, 57*(1) 93–101.

Zeltzer, L., Kellerman, J., Ellenberg, L., et al. (1980). Psychological effects of illness in adolescence. II. Impact of illness in adolescents—crucial issues and coping styles. *J Pediatr, 97*(1), 132–138.

15 Case Examples Using the Contingency Model of Long-Term Care

Introduction

Long-term conditions affect all aspects of a person's being and family and other associated systems. In-depth assessment is critical in developing a plan of care, identifying short- and long-term goals, and fostering appropriate coping skills. Hymovich's Contingency Model of Long-Term Care provides a viable framework for assessing patients with disabling conditions. The following case studies are actual examples using Hymovich's contingency model and assessment guidelines. Several people were asked to use the model and guidelines as they were being developed to assess their use with a variety of patients. The nurses using the guidelines and framework found them to be appropriate for families with children and adults having chronic conditions.

This chapter contains three case examples based on Hymovich's Contingency Model of Long-Term Care. The first concerns early intervention with a 13-year-old boy newly diagnosed with insulin dependent diabetes mellitus. The individual and family data are presented according to the guidelines for interview assessment presented in the Appendix. The second study presents a 49-year-old man with a disc herniation and compression fracture. The third case informs about a 36-year-old woman diagnosed with cancer 7 years prior to the assessment. Because these cases were assessed during stages of development of the guidelines, their formats may differ slightly from one another and from the guidelines in the Appendix.

Hymovich's Contingency Model of Long-Term Care Clinical Assessment Guide

by: Terri H. Lipman, PhD., R.N.

DATE: _____

PERSON(S) INTERVIEWED: _____ **Mother** _____

GENERAL INFORMATION: **13-year-old white male with 2-week history of polyuria and polydypsia; 10-pound weight loss in 2–3 weeks. Presented with blood glucose of 700 ng/dl.**

Diagnosis **New onset type 1 diabetes mellitus**

I. IDENTIFYING CHARACTERISTICS

Name	**Ethan**
Age	**13 years**
Sex	**male**
Education	**9th grade**
Occupation	**student**
Race	**white**
Ethnicity	
Religion	**Jewish**

Personality characteristics (e.g., introspection, hardiness, locus of control, dispositional optimism, temperament)

Developmental level (Emotional, cognitive, social)
 very mature for age

Family (Other members of household)

Name	Age	Sex	Education	Occupation	Roles (e.g., wage earner)
Sharon	**34**	**F**	**college**	**dancer**	**child care giver, wage earner**
Donald	**36**	**M**	**college**	**college prof**	**child care giver, wage earner**
Thomas	**15**	**M**	**HS**		
James	**14**	**M**	**Jr. high**		
					roles fairly traditional

Income	middle class
Sources	both parents employed
Insurance	HMO
Recreation	baseball, ballet

GENOGRAM

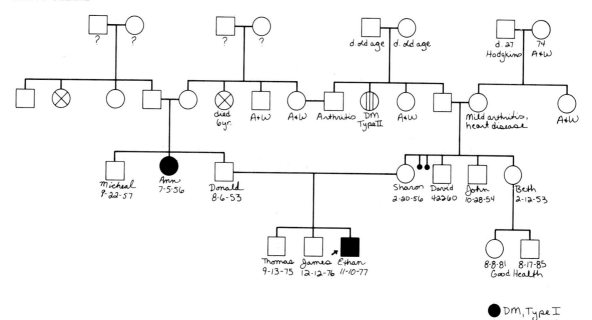

● DM, Type I
◍ DM, Type II

II. TIME AND TIME MANAGEMENT

Past (Relevant past health history and experiences)
history of nephrotic syndrome age 9 years

Development prior to illness
normal

Present
Onset of illness
2 week history polyuria, polydypsia

Stage of illness
new onset IDDM, not very ill

Stage of reaction to illness (shock, anger, denial, despair, guilt, depression)
parents: shock, acceptance
Ethan: denial

Future (Goals and plans)
law school

TIME MANAGEMENT: Daily routine (Describe)
need for blood glucose monitoring sometimes interferes with after-school activities

Treatments (Schedule, how often able to do treatments, how interfere with usual schedule)
both parents work, children in school—only minor changes since illness

Available help (Would client use help?)
would probably use help

How labor is divided for situational and developmental tasks
give children much responsibility

PASSAGE OF TIME: (Usually slow or rapid; when pressured more slowly or rapidly)

III. ORIENTATION TO LIFE

Health (Values placed on health, beliefs about health, illness, death, hospitalization)
"If we all work together, we'll be fine."
very positive about hospitalization

Health system (Beliefs about health system)

Satisfaction with past experiences with health system (Doctors, nurses, hospitals)
satisfied with previous hospitalization and management of nephrotic syndrome

Treatment (Expectations about type of treatment needed and outcome)
expected medical treatment for diabetes (insulin, monitoring, etc.)

Religious beliefs (Importance of religion, God, prayer; amount of reliance on religion when stressed)
Jewish, moderately religious

Spirituality (Source of strength and hope, if ever asks why this is happening, if a God or deity functions in daily life)
unknown

IV. INDIVIDUAL AND FAMILY STRESSORS

Internal Resources

Focal stressor event(s) Developmental and situational (Onset, manifestations, duration, intensity)
2 week hx polydypsia, polyuria

Health & energy (Current health status, rest & sleep patterns, available energy, current difficulties (new, chronic)
good health—no sleep disturbances

Knowledge & information
Disease (General knowledge about disease, name of present illness, what caused it, onset of symptoms, initial thoughts, what illness is doing to self, course of disease, severity, expectations re course [short, long])
Ethan and parents have excellent knowledge about disease

Treatment (Purpose, possible side effects, complications, skills needed, unanswered questions about treatment)
same as above

Resources (What is available, how to use)
Received information from American Diabetes Association & Juvenile Diabetes Foundation. Know how to utilize available resources.

Feelings (Self-efficacy or control, hopefulness, uncertainty)
initially appeared in control; with follow-up, apparent he was utilizing denial

FAMILY
Health and energy
everyone in good health

Knowledge of disease and treatment
Ethan and parents learned quickly

Relationships (Supportive)
strong, close
children especially close to father

How labor is divided
children given much responsibility

Changes in responsibilities (For care of ill person, other)
most of responsibility is Ethan's

Role changes and flexibility
flexible—family work together

Communication (open, closed)
open, except Ethan, who keeps feelings to self

Boundary permeability   **open**

Tolerance for difference   **?**

Necessity for respite care   **none**

External Resources

Informal support
People who provide help when needed

Feelings about support (Comfort in asking or accepting it)

Satisfaction with support

  __X__ Yes   ___ No   Explain

Types of help (Check type of support currently receiving or needed and explain.)

Type of help	Receive	Need	Explanation
Listen	X		ask many questions
Information	X		
Problem solving	X		elicit help with problem solving
Tangible: food, money			
Child care			
Household tasks			
Errands			
Transportation			
Social support outside family	X		Ethan's friends; Mother's, father's friends & coworkers

Formal support (Check type of support currently receiving or needed and explain)

Type of help	Receive	Need	Explanation
Educational	X		
Occupational	X		both parents employed
Financial			
Housing			
Child care			
Respite care			
Recreational			

V. INDIVIDUAL AND FAMILY COPING STRATEGIES

Usual way of coping (Satisfaction with previous coping)
   Ethan: internalizes, then gets angry
   Mother & other children express and share feelings

Ability to cope with this event
   very quiet, accepting
   pulled together, very determined

Beliefs about ability to manage   **confident in ability to manage**

Management of illness

Seek information
    Use information—**met with all team members**
    Use of skills
    Seek resources
      sought community assistance

    Use of resources

    Monitor self or other
      Ethan performed self-monitoring
    Adhere to regimen
      Ethan initially adhered to regimen; then appeared that blood sugar results were fabricated

Incorporate illness into life-style (Manage time, maintain normalcy modify roles, modify environment)
    incorporated management tasks into daily life with little disruption

Cope with feelings
    Search for meaning
    Attribute causes & outcome
    Make comparisons
    Maintain hope   **parents**
    Use defense mechanisms   **denial: Ethan**

Problem solving/decision making
    group decision making

VI. INDIVIDUAL AND FAMILY DEVELOPMENTAL TASKS

Extent to which accomplishing tasks. Assess each member using appropriate individual tasks.

Individual (Check if problem and explain or describe problem.)

Problem	Individual Developmental Tasks	Explanation
	Establish & maintain healthy growth & nutrition patterns	**no problem**
	Develop & maintain control over body	**yes**
	Understand & relate to the physical world	**appropriate for age**
	Develop & maintain self-awareness & satisfying sense of self	**yes**
	Establish & maintain effective relationships with others	**learning to relate to others but at times will internalize emotions and is uncommunicative**

Family (Check if problem and explain.)

Problem	Family Developmental Tasks	Explanation
	Meet basic physical needs (e.g., food, health care, shelter, money)	**yes**
	Help each member develop individual potential (Appropriate for age, condition)	**baseball & movies as family**
	Meet needs for emotional support	**yes**
X	Communicate effectively	**open, all except Ethan who doesn't share feelings**
	Understanding of needs	**excellent**
	Adapt organization & management (perform roles)	**yes**
	Function in community (organizations belong to)	**synagogue, dance groups**

VII. INDIVIDUAL AND FAMILY SITUATIONAL TASKS

Individual (Check if problem and explain.)

Problem	Individual Situational Tasks	Explanation
	Learn to understand & manage the disease	**excellent understanding**
X	Master feelings associated with the illness	**denial**
?	Contain stress within personally tolerable limits	**not sure**
	Maintain self-esteem	**somewhat**
	Preserve interpersonal relationships	**yes**
	Meet the conditions of the new circumstances	**originally adapted well**
	Master, within limits of the condition, age-appropriate developmental tasks	**yes**
	Preserve sense of control over the situation (make decisions)	**yes**
	Adjust to potential role changes	**yes**
	Maintain control of symptoms of illness (e.g., pain, incapacitation, decreased control of bodily functions)	**basically asymptomatic**
	Prepare for an uncertain future	**not known**

Family (Check if problem and explain.)

Problem	Family Situational Tasks	Explanation
X	Allow individuals to manage illness (appropriate for age, developmental status, & condition)	allow Ethan to assume much (probably too much) responsibility
	Revise impressions of person's physical health	still consider Ethan to be healthy
	Learn how illness affects daily life	yes
	Understand condition, treatment, limitations	excellent understanding
	Learn areas in which person's life and function are not affected by illness and develop plan to assure as much normalcy as possible	encourage normal life
	Meet needs of all family members as well as those of ill person	yes
	Maintain own health	?
	Maintain integrity of each family member	yes
	Adapt family resources	yes
X	Express and share feelings	Ethan needs help, keeps to self

VIII. ABILITIES

Abilities (Check abilities and explain)

Ability	Individual and Family Abilities	Explanation
Tasks of diabetes management	Ability to accomplish tasks	Ethan & parents accomplish
	Use of effective coping strategies	Ethan using denial
	Satisfaction with task accomplishment	all satisfied
	Use family strengths (Identify)	intelligent, supportive, work together

IX. NEEDS

Needs (Check if need exists and explain.)

Need	Individual and Family Needs	Explanation
	Trust	
X	Support	from health care team
X	Guidance and counseling	from health care team
X	Information	on diabetes management
X	Skill training	diabetes tasks
X	Resource identification	needed to be told re diabetes, community resources
	Health	
	Housing	
	Financial assistance	
	Vocational	
	Food	
	Clothing	
	Other	

X. PLAN OF CARE

Date & Priority	Stressor or Need	Client/ Patient	Other	Intervention	Evaluation
4/2–4/28	**Learn to do urine & blood glucose monitoring**	X	parents	instructed by nurses	return demo— good
4/25	**Learn to draw up and give insulin**	X		instructed by nurses	
4/28			mother	instructed by nurses	return demo— good
4/26–4/30	**Learn concepts of diabetes & management, etiology, pathophys, hypo & hyperglycemia (S/S & Tx)— insulin action & regulation**	X	X	instructed by CNS	able to state

Visit #4

Ethan was evaluated. His blood glucose was excellent. Ethan stated "Everything is fine" and mother agrees.

Two weeks later I called mother and told her I would like Ethan to be a "big brother" for a boy with newly diagnosed diabetes. Ethan's mother agreed it was a good idea and said she would discuss it with Ethan. She called me back to tell me that Ethan became furious, his face was bright red, and he screamed, "Absolutely not! I want nothing to do with it!" He refused to discuss it further. His mother was shocked by his reaction, as was I, and we agreed that Ethan obviously had very negative feelings about his diabetes that he never verbalized.

Visit #5

Home blood glucose levels and HbA1 do not match. There is evidence that some are fictitious. This is further evidence of Ethan's denial of his disease. Ethan was taking his insulin and doing blood tests without any parental supervision. Because he assumed diabetes management with such maturity, he had taken over all responsibility for his care. However, he was only 13 at this time, denying his diabetes, taking advantage of this responsibility and clearly needed closer supervision. *Plan:* To work with parents and Ethan regarding feelings and supervision. Possible referral of Ethan for counseling.

Commentary

The utilization of Hymovich's model helps the practicing nurse assess the child and family in an organized manner. The information obtained through this assessment is more comprehensive than data collected without its use. In using this model, it is essential to assess each member of the nuclear family (Lipman, 1989). Hymovich's model provides a systematic, thorough format for family assessment. The information gleaned from a comprehensive assessment will guide the nurse in planning necessary interventions. In addition, it will identify those families at risk for problems with adaptation and disease management at a later time.

Reference

Lipman, T.H. (1989). Assessing family strengths to guide plan of care using Hymovich's framework. *J Pediatr Nurs, 4*(3), 186–196.

Hymovich's Contingency Model of Long-Term Care Clinical Assessment Guidelines

by: Chris Conn, R.N., M.S.

Introduction

DM is a 49-year-old male with a C4-5, C6-7 disc herniation and compression fracture. On November 30, 1990 he dove into a pool, struck his head, and was immediately rendered quadriplegic. Within minutes he was brought to the surface by a friend while his wife called for emergency assistance. DM had been drinking and was intoxicated at the time of the accident. He was diagnosed with a central cord injury and placed in halo traction. After his condition stabilized, DM was admitted to a rehabilitation center on December 12, 1990. Five days after admission to the rehabilitation center, Hymovich's assessment guidelines were utilized with this patient to assess its applicability for use with the adult, physically disabled patient.

DATE: 12/17, 12/19, 12/21 1990
PERSON INTERVIEWED: D.M.
During interviews, DM frequently dozed off and had to be aroused. His answers were very general and vague and provided little insight into his emotional being.

I. IDENTIFYING CHARACTERISTICS

CLIENT
Name: **Donald Mitchell**
Age: **49**
Sex: **Male**
Education (Grade in school or last grade completed): **Two years of community college**
Occupation: **Prior to July 1990 was purchasing manager for Chem-Lawn**
Race: **Caucasian**
Ethnicity: **American**
Religion: **Protestant**

Personality characteristics:
   Introspection: **Poor; unable to recognize contradictions between his actions and verbalizations.**
   Hardiness: **Does not motivate himself or allow others to motivate him in order to achieve independence. So far he has not responded to goal setting or challenges from the staff.**
   Locus of control: **External**
   Dispositional optimism: **"I hope things get better."** Only expresses very general thoughts about his future. Has not thought about options or goals and how to achieve them.
   Temperament: **Passive with all team members regarding his care, schedule, or future goals, however he is very demanding with his wife. Staff state he is verbally abusive toward wife. At other times they act very intimate.**

Developmental level:

Emotional: **Psychologist reports his emotional level is at the adolescent stage.**

Cognitive: **Pt. has been able to function in life as expected for his age and educational level; however, he exhibits very poor problem-solving abilities.**

Social: **Interacts appropriately with other patients and staff. He rarely participates in social activities and when he does, others must initiate the conversation.**

Family Income: **$45,000 per year prior to loss of job in July 1990. No present income from unemployment or disability insurance. DM's wife is not looking for a job at this time. According to DM, she is waiting to see "what type of assistance he will need when discharged." Pt. and wife have been living off savings and investments since July. DM was unable to estimate how long they could live off of savings.**

Family (Other members of household)

Name	Age	Sex	Education	Occupation	Relationship	Roles (e.g., wage earner; student)
C.M.	48	F	1 yr college	Computer programmer	Wife	Homemaker, occ'ly works temp. jobs
A.M.	25	F	H.S.	Customer service rep	Daughter	Married; lives in Illinois
T.M.	23	F	H.S.	Office manager	Daughter	Lives in Illinois

GENOGRAM

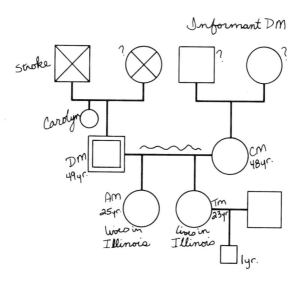

II. TIME AND TIME MANAGEMENT

Past

Relevant past health history & experiences: **"I've always been healthy except for some arthritis that flares up in my right elbow and finger as well as occasional back strain." "Yes, I'm in good health." DM has given different stories regarding vocational, social, and medical background to members of different disciplines.**

Development prior to illness: **Appears normal except for emotional development**

Present

Onset of illness: **On 11/30/90, DM dove into a pool, struck his head and was immediately rendered quadriplegic. Within minutes, he was brought to the surface by a friend while his wife called for emergency assistance. DM was diagnosed with a Central Cord Injury, due to disc herniation and compression fractures at C4–5 and C6–7. He was medically stabilized and placed in halo traction. On 12/12/90, he was admitted to a rehabilitation center. DM failed to mention that he had been drinking alcoholic beverages and was intoxicated at the time of the accident.**

Stage of illness: **Spinal shock is subsiding; demonstrated limited shoulder movement as well as the ability to wiggle his toes bilaterally. Rehabilitation program began 12/12 with an estimated 6-to-8-week stay.**

Future

Goals and plans: **"I focus on getting out of here with motor's intact."° DM takes it day by day. Does not participate in any planning regarding his future, including how he and his wife will deal with his functional changes or their present financial problems.**

TIME MANAGEMENT:

Daily routine (Describe): **Awakened by 7:30; therapies between 8:00 and 3:00. Wife and friends visit in the evening; occasionally he will go out with recreational therapy. Shower and bowel care 3 evenings/week. Asleep by 10pm and often earlier. He is catheterized every 6 hours.**

Treatments:

Schedule: **PT 11am–12n and 1pm–2pm; OT 8am–8:30am and 10am–11am; Biofeedback 2pm–3pm**

How often able to do treatments: **Attends all therapies including Saturday therapies; however, he falls asleep easily during therapies and is rarely concerned if he is late for therapies.**

How interfere with usual schedule: **No resemblance to prior routine. When his level of independence is better established, the rehabilitation team will assist DM develop an adapted routine based on premorbid activities.**

Available help: **All team members (nurse, physician, OT, PT, biofeedback, RT, social worker, psychologist). DM identifies his wife as helpful; however, at this point she has been more of a mother figure. She demonstrates no interest in learning about the physical changes due to DM's**

°[In rehab, we often refer to motor and sensory return; this statement refers to the return of voluntary movement]

injury and leaves the unit when approached by nurses to participate in his care. At this point, she will be his only available help on discharge.

Would client use help: **Readily accepts assistance to meet his physical needs, however withdraws when team members attempt to discuss psychological issues with him. He is beginning to "open up" to the psychologist who has been working with him since his injury. DM did not seek assistance premorbidly to address his financial problems.**

How labor is divided for tasks:
Situational: **DM is dependent for all physical care needs and provides no direction for his care. His day to day routine revolves around his spinal cord injury and efforts to increase independence.**
Developmental: **The developmental delays DM displays, such as problem-solving skills, are addressed primarily by the psychologist with additional emphasis placed on communication and discussion of DM's concerns about his injury and its impact on his spouse and future. Vocational plans have not been addressed.**

PASSAGE OF TIME:
Usually slow or rapid: **"Kind of both."**
When pressured (more slowly or rapidly): **"I'm not sure."**

III. ORIENTATION TO LIFE

Health:
Values placed on health: **"I try to stay healthy, you know eat right. I haven't thought much more about it."**

Beliefs about:
Health: **"I'm healthy now"** (No association with disability and health)
Illness: **"It's when you can't get to work."**
Death: **"I never think about it now. I did when I was first hurt but then I got confused and then was better." Thought he was going to die when in the pool.**

Hospitalization: **First experience as a patient; had no definitive responses.**

Health system beliefs
Satisfaction with past experiences with health system:
Doctors: **"They know what they're doing."**
Nurses: **"They are great."**
Social workers: **Not applicable**
Others: **Not applicable**
Hospitals: **Not applicable**
Has not verbalized any negative comments regarding the effectiveness, efficiency or quality of his care since admission.

Treatment:
Expectations about type of treatment needed: **No exposure to spinal cord injury and rehabilitation prior to injury. Aware of rehabilitation program routine and his role. No thoughts beyond discharge.**

Expectations about outcome: **No future orientation. Has not set goals for himself or family; seems to be just waiting to see what happens.**

Religious beliefs:
    Importance of:
        Religion: **Has never regularly attended church**
        God: **"I don't think much about religion or God."**
        Prayer: **"I don't pray."**
    Amount of reliance on religion when stressed: **None**

Spirituality:
    Source of strength & hope: **Unable to identify any. "Just have to hang in there."**
    If ever asks why this is happening: **"No, it was an accident."**
    If a God or deity functions in daily life: **"No."**

IV. INDIVIDUAL AND FAMILY STRESSORS

Internal Resources

Focal stressor event(s) (Developmental and situational)
1. Onset: **DM lost his job in July 1990.**
    States he did not enjoy the job. States that he and his boss mutually agreed that he should leave. The psychologist reports that DM and his wife were having marital problems and moved to Florida because she wanted to. DM left a job he enjoyed to take his job at Chem-Lawn which he disliked even before taking the job; was fired. The social worker states she was told that he was fired after his company merged with another.
        Manifestations: **Financial difficulties—no income, living off savings, began drinking heavily**
        Duration: **Ongoing financial problems. Experienced questionable period of DTs in acute care. No ETOH since accident.**
        Intensity: **Financial difficulties are DM's primary concern at this time.**

2. Onset: **Spinal Cord Injury 11/30/90**
        Manifestations: **Paralysis from shoulders down; dependent for care**
        Duration: **Ongoing with minimal return of function at this time.**
        Intensity: **Severe**

Health & Energy
    Current health status: **No medical complications**

    Rest & sleep patterns: **Abnormal pattern. Sleeps well during the night; however, it is difficult to keep him awake during the day. No physical basis has been identified for inability to stay awake.**

    Available energy: **Minimal energy; however, patient seems to be more alert when he has visitors.**
    Current difficulties (new, chronic): **This is new since his injury.**

Knowledge & Information
Disease:
    General knowledge about disease: **Can state type of injury and its effects on his body; is aware that the amount of voluntary movement he will recover is unknown at this time. (Although his prognosis is still unknown, there is a good chance that he will get full functional return of his lower extremities. Knowing this may be contributing to his lack of concern.)**

    Name of present illness: **Central Cord Syndrome**

    What caused illness: **Refer to Onset of Illness. DM does not associate his accident with drinking.**

Onset of symptoms: **Immediate onset on November 30**

Initial thoughts about illness: **"I was scared. I couldn't get out of the pool and thought I would drown."**

What illness is doing to self: **No response from patient, he was not sure how to answer.**

Course of disease: **Pt. aware of variability as previously stated.**

Severity: **Still unknown at this time**

Expectations re course (short, long): **DM looks no further than discharge; most of his expectations are based on day to day changes.**

Treatment:
   Purpose: **Per team members: To increase independence and understanding of bodily changes and how to adapt previous life-style and goals to physical changes. DM focuses only on how treatment will assist in the return of voluntary movement.**

   Possible side effects: **None**

   Possible complications: **Variable, depending on future recovery**

   Skills needed: **Ability to perform care or direct another to perform care and prevent complications. Includes urinary catheterization, bowel care, ROM, skin care and others. When asked "Is (e.g., ROM) something you need to learn?", DM is able to identify it; however, he was unable to initiate a list of care needs independently.**

   Unanswered questions about treatment: **None identified**

Resources:
   What is available: **Other than those at the rehabilitation center, patient aware of none.**

   How to use: **Has difficulty expressing needs; most resources are provided based on health care team observations. Prior to SCI, DM did not consult any community resources.**

Feelings
   Self-efficacy or control: **"It's hard not being able to get things I need, but I do what I can. Yes, I can dictate what I need." Observations of behavior show no internal locus of control.**

   Hopefulness: **Minimal to moderate amount**

   Uncertainty: **Great deal of uncertainty exhibited by patient**

FAMILY
   Knowledge of disease and treatment: **Wife did not arrive for an interview as scheduled. Several times I casually met her in the hall and soon after mentioning I would like to speak with her, she disappeared. The nurses and other team members report that she avoids any discussion regarding DM's condition and his future prognosis. She has not shown any interest in learning how to care for him. The team is unsure of the knowledge she has.**

   Relationships (Supportive): **Pt. states wife is primary support, however per observation and psychology report this relationship is based on a very dysfunctional "need" system, and the future is uncertain. Their two daughters live in Illinois. Do not know of other family members. DM and wife have been in Florida since October 1989, and although they have some casual friends here that visit DM, he did not identify them as a support system. After completing the assessment and speaking with other team members, I doubt he would open up to his friends in Florida.**

Changes in responsibilities:

For care of ill person: **At this time, it is difficult to know the amount of care DM will require in the future. Wife has provided no hands on care.**

For other: **Wife will be the only potential wage earner, at least initially. Despite the loss of her husband's income in July, she has not attempted to get a full-time job. DM had no major household duties that the wife has had to take over except for mowing the lawn.**

Role changes & flexibility: **Pt. states no problem foreseen in future. Does not identify wage earner as a role his wife needs to fill.**

Communication (open, closed): **Pt. states it is very open. Nurse and psychologist report openness is variable, with fluctuations among endearments, anger, and verbal abuse with wife. His daughters have not visited since the accident. DM denied any problems with their relationship or disappointment that they had not visited yet. One nurse heard a conversation DM had with one of his daughters on Christmas day and noted that no endearments were exchanged and DM appeared "rude" to his daughter.**

Boundary permeability: **Very closed. They do not seek outside assistance and do not share their feelings with others easily.**

Tolerance for difference: **Not assessed**

Necessity for respite care: **Unable to determine if a need will exist in the future. The team estimates that the long-term physical care wife will need to provide will be minimal.**

External Resources

Informal support

People who provide help when needed: **Mainly nurses at this time. No support identified when DM returns home.**

Feelings about support:

Comfort in asking or accepting it: **Uncomfortable asking for and accepting assistance. Often falls asleep or changes subject.**

Satisfaction with support:

__X__ Yes   _____ No.   Explain

Types of help (Check type or support currently receiving or needed and explain.)

Type of help	Receive	Need	Explanation
Listen	X		Receives from nurses and wife, yet DM rarely discusses his concerns.
Information	X		Receives info re: health care from entire team.
Problem solving		X	Identified by nurse and team members. E.g., unable to identify options to decrease expenses & increase income.
Tangible: food, money		X	No income; living off savings
Child care	N/A		
Household tasks	N/A		
Errands	N/A		
Transportation		X	Possible future need depending on recovery. May need adaptive tools for driving.
Social support outside		X	New to the community, family up North. Greatest needs are financial assistance & family counseling.

Formal support (Check type of support currently receiving or needed and explain.)

Type of help	Receive	Need	Explanation
Educational	X		Re: physical changes, caring for self, increasing independence. Demonstrates little internalization of information or interest in it.
Occupational		X	Depends on progress; vocational assistance.
Financial		X	Will run out of resources without additional income. Pt. unsure how long his resources will last.
Housing		X	Will need if loses home
Child care	N/A		
Respite care	N/A		
Recreational	X		Options are available but he rarely participates.

V. INDIVIDUAL AND FAMILY COPING STRATEGIES

Usual way of coping (Satisfaction with previous coping): **"You just deal with the problem."** Psychologist states DM does not deal with problem; other health care team members concur.

Ability to cope with this event: **Copes mainly by withdrawal, allows others to make his decisions.**

Beliefs about ability to manage: **"We can deal with it."**

Management of illness:
    Seek information: **Rarely**
    Use information: **No**
    Use of skills: **Yes, when asked; will not initiate on his own. At this time skills are limited to participation in feeding with the use of a sling and attempted motor movement.**

    Seek resources: **No**
    Use of resources: **Does not actively utilize resources.**
    Monitor self or other: **No**

    Adhere to regimen: **Allows team members to "treat" him and does not refuse therapies, etc.**

Incorporate illness into life-style: **Not appropriate at this time. DM has not progressed enough emotionally to begin this phase.**

    Manage time: **Does not manage timing of care, therapies, etc.**
    Maintain normalcy: **Unable to do in hospital. Has not begun adapting to prior life-style.**
    Modify roles: **Has not begun yet**
    Modify environment: **Awaiting further recovery before modifying.**

Cope with feelings
    Search for meaning: **States he does not**
    Attribute causes & outcome: **"It was just an accident."**
    Make comparisons: **No**
    Maintain hope: **"I try to think positive."**
    Use defense mechanisms: **Uses sleep as an escape from reality.**

VI. INDIVIDUAL AND FAMILY DEVELOPMENTAL TASKS

Extent to which accomplishing tasks (Assess each member using appropriate individual tasks)

Individual (Check if problem and explain or describe problem.)

Problem	Individual Developmental Tasks	Explanation
	Establish & maintain healthy growth & nutrition patterns	
X	Develop & maintain control over body	**Not internalizing info and utilizing to direct care or monitor own care.**
	Understand & relate to the physical world	
X	Develop & maintain self-awareness & satisfying sense of self	**Unable to identify and/or verbalize feelings of self-worth or personal concerns related to changes brought on by his SCI.**
X	Establish & maintain effective relationships with others	**Does not have many friends; does not initiate social contacts; closed boundaries; questionable relationship with wife**

Family (Check if problem and explain.)

Problem	Family Developmental Tasks	Explanation
X	Meet basic physical needs (e.g., food, health care, shelter, money)	**Eventually all savings will be exhausted and expect increased cost with disability. Needs to learn physical care.**
	Help each member develop individual potential (Appropriate for age, condition)	
X	Meet needs for emotional support	**DM & wife have a dysfunctional relationship; although it previously provided support, unsure if it can now, esp'ly post-discharge.**
X	Communicate effectively	**Same as above. Impaired communication between DM & wife & poor problem-solving skills; ? ability to discuss future.**
X	Understanding of needs	**Not addressing needs beyond the present. Once they are focused on future planning, will reassess this area.**
X	Adapt organization & management (perform roles)	**Family not addressing, once able to discuss they will require assistance with this.**
X	Function in community	**Closed boundaries may inhibit functioning.**

VII. INDIVIDUAL AND FAMILY SITUATIONAL TASKS

Individual (Check if problem and explain.)

Problem	Individual Situational Tasks	Explanation
X	Learn to understand & manage the disease	**Neither wife nor pt. participate actively in physical care**
X	Master feelings associated with the illness	**Pt. not addressing, so assume does not discuss with wife**
	Contain stress within personally tolerable limits	**Sleeping may dec. stress, however, pt. doesn't identify stress as a problem; sleep may not be effective in future**
X	Maintain self-esteem	**Job loss & injury associated with decreased self-esteem; DM does not verbalize this**
X	Preserve interpersonal relationships	**Role change & communication problems**
X	Meet conditions of the new circumstances	**Not addressing**
X	Master, within limits of the condition, age-appropriate developmental tasks	**Demonstrates previous mastery or at least enough for superficial purposes: family, career, etc. Probable regression due to injury. May need assistance with career planning (not happy with previous employment; may be too unable functionally to pursue same level of work)**
X	Preserve sense of control over situation (make decisions)	**Pt. passive, needs to develop control**
X	Adjust to potential role changes	**Pt./wife don't address**
X	Maintain control of symptoms of illness (e.g., pain, incapacitation, decreased control of bodily functions)	**Pt. feels cannot control**
X	Prepare for an uncertain future	**No future orientation**

Family (Check if problem and explain.)

Problem	Family Situational Tasks	Explanation
X	Allow individuals to manage illness (appropriate for age, developmental status, & condition)	**No demonstrated interest in managing care or illness**
X	Revise impressions of person's physical health	**Future physical capabilities still unknown**
X	Learn how illness affects daily life	**Still uncertain**
X	Understand condition, treatment, limitations	**Still uncertain**
X	Learn areas in which person's life & function are not affected by illness & develop plan to assure as much normalcy as possible	**Future abilities still uncertain; problem-solving skills will need to be improved.**
X	Meet needs of all family members as well as those of ill person	**Future role of wife still uncertain**
X	Maintain own health	**Not taking responsibility nor able to direct others at this point**
	Maintain integrity of each family member	
X	Adapt family resources	**Unable to identify resources. Family has problems adapting.**
X	Express & share feelings	**Family may discuss feelings, however do not appear to address sensitive issues**

VIII. ABILITIES (Check ability if present and explain.)

Ability	Individual and Family Abilities	Explanation
	Ability to accomplish tasks	**Unknown at this point**
	Use of effective coping strategies	
	Satisfaction with task accomplishment	
	Use family strengths (Identify)	

IX. NEEDS (Check if need exists and explain.)

Need	Individual and Family Needs	Explanation
	Trust	
X	Support	**Addressed earlier**
X	Guidance and counseling	**Addressed earlier**
X	Information	**About possible career retraining, physical care; how to identify & use community resources**
X	Skill training	**DM & wife need to learn how to meet DM's physical needs**
X	Resource identification	**Especially regarding finances**
	Health	
X	Housing	**Possible need in future**
X	Financial assistance	
X	Vocational	**Possible need in future**
	Food	
	Clothing	
	Other	

X. PLAN OF CARE

Date & Priority	Stressor or Need	Pt/ Client	Other (who)	Intervention	Evaluation
#1	Income	X		1. Consult with social worker re resources	1. Develop source of income.
		X	X	2. Assist family to identify costs & prioritize needs	2. Decrease in monthly costs
		X	X	3. For each cost identify ways to decrease or eliminate; teach how to budget	3. DM & wife able to budget
		X	X	4. Discuss feasibility of wife's obtaining employment	4. Wife to start job
		X	X	5. Assist to identify family resources in Ohio	
		X	X	6. Assist to calculate how long savings will last	
#2	Anticipatory guidance	X		1. Ind'l counseling with psychologist q day	1. Develop future goals & plans to achieve them
		X		2. All therapies to set daily & weekly goals with patient & relate them to anticipated future needs	
		X	X	3. Begin biweekly family counseling sessions	
		X	X	4. Introduce to other couples who have had similar experiences to share experience & problem solving	
		X	X	5. Daily ask pt. & wife if identified any concerns other than financial. List concerns & help them identify interventions.	

X. PLAN OF CARE *Continued*

Date & Priority	Stressor or Need	Pt/ Client	Other (who)	Intervention	Evaluation
#3	Cervical Injury: Manage Disability			1. **Begin VIVA* Instruction daily**	1. **DM able to perform physical care needs and/or instruct a care giver to perform**
		X	X	2. **When providing care, explain action as well as anticipated outcome.**	2. **Wife able to perform all physical needs that DM can not independently perform and/or find a health care worker to perform for them**
		X	X	3. **Encourage participation in care; give rewards for participation**	3. **Both aware of follow-up needs and potential physical complications**
		X		4. **Every shift ask DM if has any concerns about care or education needs**	
		X		5. **Introduce DM to other pts who are proactive; capitalize on their influence**	
#4	**Dysfunctional communication**	X	X	1. **Psychologist to address this issue with follow-up observations by health care team**	1. **Couple to demonstrate communication patterns where both parties can express their feelings**

***VIVA is a computerized program that provides information to spinal cord injured persons about physical changes and care needs due to spinal cord injury. Subjects such as spine anatomy and physiology, respiratory needs, and sexuality are addressed. This is integrated by the nurses into the patient's daily schedule and the information gained by the patients is evaluated and reassessed throughout their stay as well as on outpatient visits.**

These four problems are the highest priority for this family. If no progress is made in these areas, no progress can be made in other identified areas of needs or stress. At that point, plans for discharge would be made. Several scenarios are possible at this point:

1. If DM's wife refuses to learn how to care for him, but will take him home, he will be discharged home despite her lack of knowledge.
2. The wife refuses to learn his care as well as refuses to take him home. At this point other family members would be sought out or nursing home placement. (DM has stated his daughters have no room for him or his wife in their apartments.)
3. The wife leaves her husband prior to discharge.
4. This couple learns to cope with their stressors and DM goes home, with his wife providing the necessary care.

Commentary

It took a total of 3 hours, over three sessions, to complete the assessment using Hymovich and Hagopian's guidelines with DM. In some instances it was difficult to ask short specific questions to elicit the information. Topics particularly difficult were those of beliefs of health, death, religion, and coping. Some of these areas require ongoing observation for complete assessment. Some of the difficulty may have been an attempt to elicit verbal answers when observation was necessary. Also, some patients have little insight into their emotional being and do not have answers readily available. Others may not reveal this information readily, for the topics are sometimes sensitive and emotionally taxing and require more than a simple answer. Some patients may be impaired by age, educational level, language, and illness and have difficulty with some topics. Still others, who may not be able to reply immediately, may think about the questions and want to discuss them at a later date.

It is helpful to prioritize essential information and determine what information is required during the first contact with the patient. Knowing when and how to assess and reassess coping skills is difficult during initial use of the tool. Since it may not be possible to collect all of the information at the initial contact, developing a time frame for gathering certain information may be more realistic. An inservice education program to explain the conceptual framework, the tool, terminology such as "hardiness, locus of control, and situational tasks," and the meaning of terms such as "time management, values placed on health, available energy, and understand and relate to the physical world" is recommended. Also, some nurses may want to prepare a list of questions to elicit certain information.

There may be some duplication or redundancy and some problems may be identified in several areas. For example, concern regarding finances can be identified under "family income," "focal stresses," and/or "role changes." Some people may be bothered by this duplication. On the other hand, this redundancy validates problems, needs and/or strengths, and indicates that many things people deal with are not mutually exclusive and cannot be viewed in isolation but are contingent on and affect many variables in life.

Some specific problems may not be easily identified by the tool. Although alcohol and drug abuse may be identified under ways of coping, specific questions relating to substance abuse may need to be added to the assessment guide.

Hymovich and Hagopian's assessment guidelines, based on the model, are comprehensive and appropriate for use with the adult dealing with physical disability. The intense focus on the family and specific assessment of resources and needs are extremely beneficial to those working in the rehabilitation field. It is recommended that rehabilitation personnel take the time to evaluate the tool for their use and contribute to its development.

CASE EXAMPLE C

Hymovich's Contingency Model of Long-Term Care Clinical Assessment Guide

DATE: 4/21/90
PERSON(S) INTERVIEWED: Ida S.

I. IDENTIFYING CHARACTERISTICS

Name	**Ida S.**
Age	**36 years**
Sex	**F**
Education	**College grad—BS**
Occupation	**grade school teacher until diagnosed 7 years ago**
Race	**W**
Ethnicity	**Italian**
Religion	**Catholic**

Personality characteristics (e.g., introspection, hardiness, locus of control, dispositional optimism, temperament)
even-tempered, outgoing, expressive

Developmental level (Emotional, cognitive, social)
adult

Family (Other members of household)

Name	Age	Sex	Education	Occupation	Roles (e.g., wage earner)
Robert	**42**	**M**	**HS grad**	**construction**	**husband, married 14 yrs wage earner**
Grace	**11**	**F**	**7th grade**	**student**	**daughter**
Bobby	**8**	**M**	**4th grade**	**student**	**son**

Income	**± $45,000/year—no financial difficulty at this time**
Sources	**husband**
Insurance	**BC/BS**
Recreation	**mainly visits with friends**

GENOGRAM

Informant: Ida

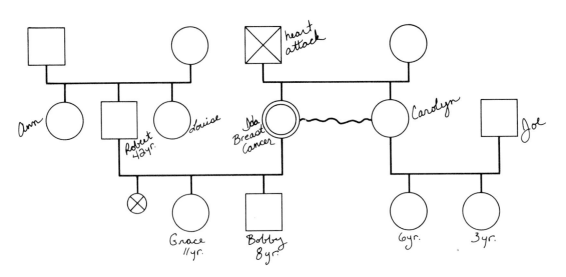

II. TIME AND TIME MANAGEMENT

Past (Relevant past health history and experiences)
Mrs. S. first diagnosed with cancer of breast 7 years ago at age 29. Had a right radical mastectomy (1983). 4 yrs later had mets to ribs & successfully treated with radiation therapy (XRT). Last spring (1989) developed metastases to right humerus & liver. Treated with XRT to humerus & chemotherapy.

Development prior to illness **on time**

Present
Onset of illness **right hip pain developed 2 wks ago. XRT started**
Stage of illness **recurrent disease, pain responding to XRT**
Stage of reaction to illness (shock, anger, denial, despair, guilt, depression) **would not discuss feelings with CNS on this visit; appears to be using a lot of denial re: prognosis**

Future (goals and plans) **for another remission; pain-free life**

TIME MANAGEMENT: Daily routine (Describe)
up at 6:45. Makes breakfast; sends husband to work & children to school; watches TV, sometimes goes back to bed

Treatments (Schedule, how often able to do treatments, how interefere with usual schedule)
goes to XRT daily X 10 days

Available help (Would client use help?)
gets ride with neighbor to XRT at hosp. Mother comes over in pm & cooks supper & helps with housework, shopping, etc.

How labor is divided for situational and developmental tasks
**Everyone pitches in & helps; husband usually does shopping on w/e.
Mrs. S. will go if feels up to it**

PASSAGE OF TIME: (Usually slow or rapid; when pressured more slowly or rapidly) **since XRT time is going more rapidly & she feels there is no time for anything else**

III. ORIENTATION TO LIFE

Health (Values placed on health, beliefs about health, illness, death, hospitalization)
seeks immediate attention for any new symptom & believes good health is a "gift."

Health system (Beliefs about health system)
the system works for her

Satisfaction with past experiences with health system (doctors, nurses, hospitals)
very satisfied with health care system, MDs, RNs, etc.

Treatment (Expectations about type of treatment needed and outcome)
XRT will help; it has helped in past & will help again

Religious beliefs (Importance of religion, God, prayer; amount of reliance on religion when stressed)
Catholic priest visits home once a week. Religion, God & prayer very important. Relies substantially on religion.

Spirituality (Source of strength and hope, if ever asks why this is happening, if a God or deity functions in daily life)
Believes in God. Does not ask "why me?" "It's mine to bear."

IV. INDIVIDUAL AND FAMILY STRESSORS

Internal Resources

Focal stressor event(s) Developmental and situational (Onset, manifestations, duration, intensity) **pain in right hip**

Health & energy (Current health status, rest & sleep patterns, available energy, current difficulties (new, chronic)
fair health; some fatigue; sleeps 8 hours & naps 2 hrs/day; currently has pain in rt hip. XRT should help pain soon; in meantime on Percoset

Knowledge & information

Disease (General knowledge about disease, name of present illness, what caused it, onset of symptoms, initial thoughts, what illness is doing to self, course of disease, severity, expectations re: course [short, long])

well informed about disease & treatment. Knows she has cancer. "Who knows what caused it." "Here we go again" when recurrence was diagnosed.

Treatment (Purpose, possible side effects, complications, skills needed, unanswered questions about treatment)

knows about Rx & side effects

Resources (What is available, how to use)

Was signed up for Wheels but decided to take advantage of neighbor's offer to take her to XRT. May need a walker & wheelchair

Feelings (Self-efficacy or control, hopefulness, uncertainty)

Feels in control; is hopeful about decrease in pain and increase in mobility. "The future is always uncertain."

FAMILY

Health and energy

husband & children in good health

Knowledge of disease and treatment

Husband well informed. Children have been told that their mother has a virus. It is not clear what they really know.

Relationships (Supportive) **Husband very supportive; mother is a strong support; it is questionable how much support children receive.**

How labor is divided **right now husband does most; mother cooks**

Changes in responsibilities (For care of ill person, other)
some modifications

Role changes and flexibility **flexible**

Communication (open, closed) **Open between husband & wife; closed with children (at least re diag.)**

Boundary permeability **Permeable but Mrs. S. not heavily involved in outside activities. Life centers around disease & treatment. Family oriented.**

Tolerance for difference

Necessity for respite care **Mother & neighbors provide some relief for husband.**

External Resources

Informal support

People who provide help when needed
    Mother, 354-6920
    Neighbor, Mrs. G, 543-9876
Feelings about support (Comfort in asking or accepting it)
    Mrs. S does not hesitate to ask for help

Satisfaction with support
  X Yes
  _____ No   Explain

Types of help (Check type or support currently receiving or needed and explain.)

Type of help	Receive	Need	Explanation
Listen	X		
Information	X	X	re talking with children
Problem-solving			no problem
Tangible: food, money			no problem
Child care	X	X	mother helps in pm
Household tasks	X	X	mother
Errands	X		neighbor, mother
Transportation	X		neighbor
Social support outside family			not much, neighbor Mrs. G.

Formal support (Check type of support currently receiving or needed and explain.)

Type of help	Receive	Need	Explanation
Educational	—		
Occupational	—		
Financial	—		
Housing	—		
Child care	X		mother helping
Respite care	X		mother, neighbor
Recreational		?	family doesn't do much together for recreation; everything is focussed on Mrs. S's illness

V. INDIVIDUAL AND FAMILY COPING STRATEGIES

Usual way of coping (Satisfaction with previous coping)
    Talking, getting information; take it in stride; accept & face challenge

Ability to cope with this event   **good**

Beliefs about ability to manage
    believes everyone is managing

Management of illness
Seek information
Use information
Use of skills
Seek resources   **doing well**
Use of resources
Monitor self or other
Adhere to regimen   **very adherent**

Incorporate illness into life style (Manage time, maintain normalcy, modify roles, modify environment)
    coping well

Cope with feelings
    Search for meaning   **doesn't ask**
    Attribute causes & outcome   **"It's mine to bear."**
    Make comparisons   **? not observed**
    Maintain hope   **very hopeful**
    Use defense mechanisms   **not observed**

Problem solving/decision making
    usually husband & wife; children occasionally involved

VI. INDIVIDUAL AND FAMILY DEVELOPMENTAL TASKS

Extent to which accomplishing tasks. Assess each member using appropriate individual tasks.

Individual (Check if problem and explain or describe problem.)

Problem	Individual Developmental Tasks	Explanation
	Establish & maintain healthy growth & nutrition patterns	
?	Develop & maintain control over body	**as much as circumstances allow; does participate in decisions re: health care**
	Understand & relate to the physical world	
	Develop & maintain self-awareness & satisfying sense of self	
	Establish & maintain effective relationships with others	**has limited social network; life revolves around illness; not a problem for Mrs. S.**

Family (Check if problem and explain)

Problem	Family Developmental Tasks	Explanation
	Meet basic physical needs (e.g., food, health care, shelter, money)	
	Help each member develop individual potential (Appropriate for age, condition)	
X	Meet needs for emotional support	**not open communication with children ?? support**
X	Communicate effectively	**?? what do children know; adults communicate with each other but not with children**
X	Understanding of needs	**children not fully informed**
	Adapt organization & management (perform roles)	
	Function in community (organizations belong to)	**not too involved in community except for church**

VII. INDIVIDUAL AND FAMILY SITUATIONAL TASKS

Problem	Individual Situational Tasks	Explanation
—	Learn to understand & manage the disease	
—	Master feelings associated with the illness	**Mrs. S. has lived with cancer for 7 years.**
—	Contain stress within personally tolerable limits	**She seems to be coping well, mobilizing resources, adapting & facing an uncertain future. Sees a psychiatrist prn**
—	Maintain self-esteem	
—	Preserve interpersonal relationships	
—	Meet the conditions of the new circumstances	
—	Master, within limits of the condition, age-appropriate developmental tasks	
—	Preserve sense of control over the situation (make decisions)	
—	Adjust to potential role changes	
X	Maintain control of symptoms of illness (e.g., pain, incapacitation, decreased control of bodily functions)	**this is being managed as well as possible with Rx for pain XRT. Pain decreasing in severity**
	Prepare for an uncertain future	

Problem	Family Situational Tasks	Explanation
	Allow individuals to manage illness (appropriate for age, developmental status, & condition)	**All family members have never been assessed.**
	Revise impressions of person's physical health	**Mr. & Mrs. S. seem to be adapting well. It is not clear how the children are really doing since they have never been told the diagnosis: each new recurrence is still referred to as a virus.**
	Learn how illness affects daily life	
	Understand condition, treatment, limitations	
	Learn areas in which person's life & function are not affected by illness & develop plan to assure as much normalcy as possible	
	Meet needs of all family members as well as those of ill person	
	Maintain own health	
	Maintain integrity of each family member	
	Adapt family resources	
	Express & share feelings	

VIII. ABILITIES

Abilities (Check abilities and explain)

Ability	Individual and Family Abilities	Explanation
X	Ability to accomplish tasks	
X	Use of effective coping strategies	
X	Satisfaction with task accomplishment	
X	Use family strengths (Identify)	**Adaptability & flexibility. Strong religious faith.**

IX. NEEDS

Needs (Check if need exists and explain)

Need	Individual and Family Needs	Explanation
	Trust	
	Support	
X	Guidance and counseling	
X	Information	re: communicating with children
X	Skill training	
	Resource identification	
	Health	
	Housing	
	Financial assistance	
	Vocational	
	Food	
	Clothing	
X	Other **physical**	**pain relief; increased mobility; transportation prn**

X. PLAN OF CARE

Date & Priority	Stressor or Need		Client/ Patient	Other	Intervention	Evaluation
4/30/90		open, honest communication with children	X	X children husband	Discuss parental feelings & later reasons for open & honest communication with children. Offer assistance in telling children; assess children	
4/30/90		pain relief	X		Continue XRT & pain medication	
4/30/90		mobility			Assist to get wheel chair &/or walker if pain continues	
4/30/90	XRT	information			Reevaluate knowledge of XRT, skin care; teach new information as necessary	
4/30/90	Transportation (potential need)				Neighbor now providing rides; may not continue; look into alternatives	Assess each visit

Hymovich's Contingency Model of Long-Term Care Guidelines for Assessment Interview

DATE:_____

PERSON(S) INTERVIEWED:_____

I. IDENTIFYING CHARACTERISTICS

CLIENT
Name
Age
Sex
Education (Grade in school or last grade completed)
Occupation
Race
Ethnicity
Religion

Personality characteristics
   Introspection
   Hardiness
   Locus of control
   Dispositional optimism
   Temperament
Developmental level
   Emotional
   Cognitive
   Social

Family income
Insurance
Recreation

Family (Other members of household)

Name	Age	Sex	Education	Occupation	Relationship	Roles (e.g., wage earner)

GENOGRAM

II. TIME AND TIME MANAGEMENT

Past
Relevant past health history & experiences

Development prior to illness

Present
Onset of illness

Stage of illness

State of reaction to illness (eg., shock, anger, denial, despair, guilt, depression)

Future
Goals and plans

TIME MANAGEMENT:
Daily routine (Describe)

Treatments
Schedule
How often able to do treatments
How they interfere with usual schedule

Available help
Would client use help?

How labor is divided for tasks
Situational
Developmental

PASSAGE OF TIME:
Usually slow or rapid
When pressured (more slowly or rapidly)

III. ORIENTATION TO LIFE

Health
Values placed on health

Beliefs about
Health
Illness
Death
Hospitalization

Health system beliefs

Satisfaction with past experiences with health system
  Doctors
  Nurses
  Social workers
  Others
  Hospitals

Treatment
  Expectations about type of treatment needed
  Expectations about outcome

Religious beliefs
  Importance of
    Religion
    God
    Prayer
  Amount of reliance on religion when stressed

Spirituality
  Source of strength & hope
  If ever asks why this is happening
  If a God or deity functions in daily life

IV. INDIVIDUAL AND FAMILY STRESSORS

INTERNAL RESOURCE STRESSORS

INDIVIDUAL

Focal stressor event(s) (Developmental and situational)
  Onset
  Manifestations
  Duration
  Intensity

Health & Energy
  Current health status
  Rest & sleep patterns
  Available energy
  Current difficulties (new, chronic)

Knowledge & Information
  Disease
    General knowledge about disease
    Name of present illness
    What caused illness
    Onset of symptoms
    Initial thoughts about illness
    What illness is doing to self
    Course of disease
    Severity
    Expectations regarding course (short, long)

  Treatment
    Purpose
    Possible side effects
    Possible complications
    Skills needed
    Unanswered questions about treatment

  Resources
    What is available
    How to use

Feelings
  Self-efficacy or control
  Hopefulness
  Uncertainty

FAMILY

  Health & Energy
  Knowledge of disease and treatment

  Relationships (supportive)
  How labor is divided
  Changes in responsibilities
    For care of ill person
    For other

  Role changes & flexibility

  Communication (open, closed)   ·

  Boundary permeability

  Tolerance for difference

  Necessity for respite care

EXTERNAL RESOURCES

Informal support
People who provide help when needed

Feelings about support
   Comfort in asking for or accepting it

Satisfaction with support
____Yes
____No. Explain

Types of help (Check type or support currently received or needed and explain)

Type of help	Receive	Need	Explanation
Listen			
Information			
Problem solving			
Tangible: food, money			
Child care			
Household tasks			
Errands			
Transportation			
Social support outside family			
Other			

Formal support (Check type of support currently receiving or needed and explain)

Type of help	Receive	Need	Explanation
Educational			
Occupational			
Financial			
Housing			
Child care			
Respite care			
Recreational			
Other			

V. INDIVIDUAL AND FAMILY COPING STRATEGIES

Usual way of coping (Satisfaction with previous coping)

Ability to cope with this event

Beliefs about ability to manage

Management of illness

Seek information
Use information
Use of skills
Seek resources
Use of resources
Monitor self or other
Adhere to regimen

Incorporate illness into life-style
      Manage time
      Maintain normalcy
      Modify roles
      Modify environment

Cope with feelings
      Search for meaning
      Attribute causes & outcome
      Make comparisons
      Maintain hope
      Use defense mechanisms

Problem solving/Decision making

VI. INDIVIDUAL AND FAMILY DEVELOPMENTAL TASKS

Extent to which accomplishing tasks (Assess each member using appropriate individual tasks.)

Individual (Check if problem and explain or describe problem.)

Problem	Individual Developmental Tasks	Explanation
	Establish & maintain healthy growth & nutrition patterns	
	Develop & maintain control over body	
	Understand & relate to the physical world	
	Develop & maintain self-awareness & satisfying sense of self	
	Establish & maintain effective relationships with others	

Family (Check if problem and explain)

Problem	Family Developmental Tasks	Explanation
	Meet basic physical needs (e.g., food, health care, shelter, money)	
	Assist each member develop individual potential (appropriate for age, condition)	
	Meet needs for emotional support	
	Communicate effectively	
	Understanding of needs	
	Adapt organization & management (perform roles)	
	Function in community (organizations belong to)	

VII. INDIVIDUAL AND FAMILY SITUATIONAL TASKS

Individual (Check if problem and explain.)

Problem	Individual Situational Tasks	Explanation
	Learn to understand & manage the disease	
	Master feelings associated with the illness	
	Contain stress within personally tolerable limits	
	Maintain self-esteem	
	Preserve interpersonal relationships	
	Meet conditions of the new circumstances	
	Master, within limits of the condition, age-appropriate developmental tasks	
	Preserve sense of control over situation (make decisions)	
	Adjust to potential role changes	
	Maintain control of symptoms of illness (e.g., pain, incapacitation, decreased control of bodily functions)	
	Prepare for an uncertain future	

Family (Check if problem and explain.)

Problem	Family Situational Tasks	Explanation
	Allow individuals to manage illness (appropriate for age, developmental status, & condition)	
	Revise impressions of person's physical health	
	Learn how illness affects daily life	
	Understand condition, treatment, limitations	
	Learn areas in which person's life and function are not affected by illness, and develop plan to assure as much normalcy as possible	
	Meet needs of all family members as well as those of ill person	
	Maintain own health	
	Maintain integrity of each family member	
	Adapt family resources	
	Express and share feelings	

VIII. ABILITIES

Abilities (Check ability if present and explain.)

Ability	Individual and Family Abilities	Explanation
	Ability to accomplish tasks	
	Use of effective coping strategies	
	Satisfaction with task accomplisment	
	Use family strengths (identify)	
	Other	

IX. NEEDS

Needs (Check if need exists and explain.)

Need	Individual and Family Needs	Explanation
	Trust	
	Support	
	Guidance and counseling	
	Information	
	Skill training	
	Resource identification	
	Health	
	Housing	
	Financial assistance	
	Vocational	
	Food	
	Clothing	
	Other	

X. PLAN OF CARE

Date & Priority	Stressor or Need		Client/ Patient	Other	Intervention	Evaluation

Glossary

A

abuse An intentional act of commission.

accommodation Cognitive process of modifying existing schemata or formation of new ones for stimuli that do not fit existing schemata.

adaptation The extent to which the individual or family system is accomplishing its developmental and situational tasks.

ambiguity Incongruence between elements that fall outside the specified range of normal variations and for which there is no typical alternative to account for the variation.

assets System strengths, abilities, or capabilities.

assimilation The cognitive process of integrating new stimuli into already schemata.

attitudes Hypothetical constructs of existing predispositions to social objects that guide and direct behavior.

attribution The use of causal thinking following an important life event in order to make sense of and control life.

B

beliefs Personally formed notions and meanings an individual has about the environment.

body image A part of a person's self-concept that consists of one's idea about the person's size, shape, and functioning of the body and its parts.

C

capabilities The system's strengths, abilities, or assets.

chaotic family An impermeable family with rigid boundaries and few interactions with the outside world.

chronic condition A long-term health problem leading to actual or potential interference with a system's level of functioning. Is synonymous with the terms chronic illness, chronic health problem, long-term condition.

chronic health problem A long-term illness or condition leading to actual or potential interference with a system's level of functioning. Synonyms: chronic illness, chronic condition, long-term condition.

chronic illness A long-term health problem or condition leading to actual or potential interference with a system's level of functioning. Synonyms: chronic condition, chronic health problem, long-term condition.

chronic sorrow A prolonged sadness that persists throughout life.

client A person of any age with a chronic illness who is receiving or needs assistance from health care providers; is synonymous with the terms individual, person, and patient.

closed systems Tight boundaries which are self-contained, and do not interact with the environment but exchange information only within themselves (Hymovich & Chamberlin, 1980; Pasquali et al, 1985; von Bertalannfy, 1986).

cognitive appraisals Continuous evaluative processes of categorizing the facts and significance of the event to oneself.

cognitive reappraisals Strategies that change the meaning of the situation without changing it objectively. Also known as cognitive restructuring or cognitive therapy.

cognitive therapy "A structured short-term treatment for depression and anxiety based on helping the client to identify and change distorted thought patterns that trigger and perpetuate one's distress" (Childress & Burns, 1981, p. 1024). Also called cognitive reappraisal or cognitive restructuring.

commitment One's dedication to a belief in such a way as to influence behavior.

community A system composed of the family's neighborhood, health, recreational, educational, social, and political institutions that affect its functioning.

contingency variables Mediators that influence the impact a chronic condition has on system functioning. These variables are the system orientation to life, stressors, coping strategies, strengths, and needs.

contract A mutually arrived at agreement between a client and the health provider about goals to be achieved.

control "The **real** or **perceived** ability to determine outcomes of an event" (Gatchel & Baum, 1983, p. 80). Self-efficacy.

coping A cognitive, affective, and behavioral process to manage perceived stressors or potential stressors in the environment or internal to the system that tax or exceed the system's current resources for responding.

coping function The purpose a coping strategy serves for the system.

coping outcome The effect a coping strategy has in relieving the stressor.

coping pattern Coping disposition, trait, or style.

coping resource Capability available to help the system tolerate, master, or reduce the nature of the stressor.

coping strategy System members' cognitive, affective, or behavioral means of minimizing or relieving their perceived stressors.

coping style The relatively stable and consistent manner in which a person generally responds to stressors.

coping trait The relatively stable and consistent manner in which a person generally responds to stressors.

courtesy stigma The spread of the disability to those who are affiliated with the stigmatized person and are regarded by others as having a spoiled identity.

crisis A state precipitated by a focal stressor event for which the system's current coping strategies are ineffective.

crisis intervention A process of short-term therapy focusing on rapid mobilization of one's emotional resources to resolve the immediate psychological crisis and to restore persons to their premorbid state.

D

developmental disability A substantial chronic disability likely to continue indefinitely that results from a physical and/or a mental impairment manifested in a person before 22 years of age.

developmental stressors Stressful events that occur during the normal course of one's growth and development and can strain or surpass the system's ability to cope.

developmental tasks Growth responsibilities that arise at a particular stage in the person's or family's life cycle that must be accomplished in order to perform tasks that follow.

disability The consequences of an impairment in terms of the person's functional performance and activities.

disease Describes the pathological process representing a basic underlying disturbance at the cellular level. Synonyms are defect, disorder, and condition.

disengaged family A family with rigid boundaries, whose members function separately and autonomously rather than interdependently.

dispositional optimism A tendency to judge expectations in an optimistic rather than pessimistic way.

downward comparison A person's attempt to cope with a threatening experience and enhance subjective well-being by comparing himself or herself to those who are less fortunate.

E

ecomap An assessment tool to diagram relationships between a family and its supra systems.

enmeshed family A family with somewhat permeable and diffuse boundaries with little differentiation between the members.

emotion-focused coping Attempts to reduce or eliminate the emotional distress associated with the stressful event, that is, to make the system feel better.

energy The capacity to do work needed to meet the demands of the chronic condition and other family and individual demands.

entropy The energy available within a system.

explanatory models (EMS) Beliefs and perceptions about a specific disease that are held by the individual.

extended family Refers to those family members who do not share a household with the parents and children comprising the immediate family. It also includes the grandparents, uncles, and aunts of the immediate family members who may be living in the same household with the client.

F

family A system of interdependent interacting individuals who are related to one another by marriage, birth, adoption, or mutual consent.

focal stressor or focal stressor event An actual or potential developmental or situational circumstance or event that causes the individual or family system to evaluate its situation and determine the presence of a need.

G

generalized resistance resources (GRRs) Any factor within the individual that helps to organize tension.

genogram A graphic representation of a family tree, over at least three generations, that contains information about family structure, critical events, and relationships.

H

habilitation Establishing fundamental capabilities, knowledge, experiences, and attitudes needed for as near normal living as possible.

handicap The social disadvantages a person experiences as the result of an impairment or disability.

hardiness A set of attitudes toward challenge, commitment, and control that mediate one's response to stress.

hassles Repeated or chronic strains of everyday life.

health The ability to function physically, psychologically, and socially in a manner that is deemed satisfying to the individual.

health belief model A theoretical decision-making model that explains behaviors directed at prevention, decisions to seek health care, and compliance with medical regimes.

health locus of control An individual or family system's belief that health is a function of one's own control or of external control.

health status The person's or health professional's appraisal of physical and mental well-being. The relationship between stressors, coping, and tasks.

helplessness A noncontingent relationship between response and behavior, that is, the chances that something may happen are independent of what the person does.

high touch Refers to seeing the person as a human being, separate from the machines and pathology.

hope A feeling or belief that something desired will occur.

hopelessness A state in which a person believes that nothing can be done to change a situation, does not feel worthy of help, and has feelings of giving up.

I

identifying characteristics A complex set of variables that help to define a system.

identity spread Related to the assumptions that the ill person cannot work, act, or be like others.

illness The secondary personal and social responses to disease.

immediate family Spouses or parents and children living within a single household and the unmarried children who are away at school or college.

impairment "Any loss or abnormality of physiological or anatomical structure or function" (WHO, 1980, p. 46).

individual A person of any age with a chronic condition who is receiving or needs assistance from health care providers. Is synonymous with the terms *person, patient,* and *client.*

individual system The person's biological, emotional, social, cognitive, and spiritual subsystems.

instruction The process whereby one individual intentionally influences the learning of another by structuring the environment in such a way that the latter will learn some desired behavior.

L

labeling Designation of a term or title for a particular condition.

learning A relatively permanent change in behavior due to practice or experience.

level of functioning The system's current performance as determined by the extent to which it is accomplishing its developmental and situational tasks.

life review "A naturally occurring, universal mental process characterized by the return to the consciousness of past experiences, and particularly the resurgence of unresolved conflicts" (Butler, 1963, p. 65). It provides an opportunity to reminisce and finish any unfinished business of life.

locus of control A psychologic construct that refers to the extent to which a person believes his or her own actions influence events in the world.

long-term condition Any chronic or permanent health problem that interferes with the person's ordinary physical, psychologic, or social functioning. Synonymous with chronic condition, chronic health problem, chronic illness.

long-term care "A range of services that address the health, social, and personal care needs of persons who are unable to care for themselves because of a physical or mental impairment caused by a chronic condition" (Reif & Estes, 1982, p. 151).

N

need Motivating force that initiates behavior with the purpose of maintaining internal consistency and harmony with the external environment. A condition identified by the individual, family, or health team as requiring resources or relief.

negentropy Negative entropy. The utilization of energy within a system.

neglect An act of omission of needed care.

normalization The response of the family to negate illness or abnormal behavior in order to maintain valued social roles for people. The process of maintaining normalcy.

nursing care The deliberate activities of a nurse to help the individual and family systems meet their needs.

O

objective time Time measured by a clock or calendar.

open system Those systems with permeable boundaries that interact with the outside environment.

orientation to life The way a system views the world in terms of its values, attitudes, and beliefs.

P

patient A person of any age with a chronic illness who is receiving or needs assistance from health care providers. Is synonymous with the terms *individual, person,* and *client.*

person A person of any age with a chronic illness who is receiving or needs assistance from health care providers. Is synonymous with the terms *individual, client,* and *patient.*

potential stressors Events or conditions known to be stressors, that for some individuals under certain circumstances have the probability of becoming stressors.

powerlessness A feeling that ones' actions will not affect an outcome.

problem-focused coping Actions taken to remove or alleviate the source of stress.

R

reciprocity The perception of bidirectional exchange of valued resources (Tilden & Gaylen, 1987).

rehabilitation "An approach, a philosophy, an attitude, and a process" to facilitate a person's movement toward health (Dittmar, 1989, p. 2).

religion "A unified system of beliefs, and practices relative to sacred things [that] unite into one single moral community called a church by all those who adhere to them" (Giddens, 1978, p. 92).

resources System strengths, assets, and capabilities.

role "A set of activities that are expected of a person by virtue of his or her occupancy of a particular position in social space" (Kahn & Antonucci, 1980, p. 261).

S

self-care The practice of activities that people initiate and perform on their own behalf.

self-concept "The beliefs and feelings that one holds about oneself at a given time" (Andrews & Roy, 1985, p. 124).

self-efficacy An expectation that one can achieve personal mastery and determine the outcome of an event. Control.

self-esteem An evaluation of one's worth in relationship to one's ideal and to the performance of others. A major component of self-concept.

situational stressors Stressful events that arise as the result of a stressful event and can strain or surpass the system's ability to cope. They are superimposed on developmental stressors and tasks. They are circumstances or events that family members indicate are problematic or potentially problematic for themselves or other family members.

situational tasks Functional requirements that arise as a result of a stressor and are superimposed on the developmental tasks.

society The large political, economic, and social system under which each of the other systems (individual, family, community) function.

spiritual distress "Distress of the human spirit . . . a disruption in the life principle which pervades a person's entire being and which integrates and transcends one's biological and psychosocial nature" (Kim, McFarland & McLane, 1987, p. 314).

spiritual well-being Satisfaction in a relationship with God, perception of life as having meaning, and a satisfaction with one's life.

spiritualism A belief that the dead survive as spirits and can cause harm to the living.

spirituality "The core of one's being; a sense of personhood; what one is and is becoming" (Stoll, 1989, p. 6).

spread The extension of a perception of one attribute about a person to other attributes of that person.

stigma The incongruence between the ideal social identity and the real social identity.

strengths System assets, abilities, and resources.

stress A transaction between a person and the environment that is cognitively appraised by the person as exceeding personal resources to cope with it.

stress inoculation training A cognitive-behavioral approach to prepare patients for upcoming stressful events by providing them with a set of skills to be used in a stressful situation.

stressors Any stimuli, or the absence of stimuli, in the environment or internal to the system, that can tax or exceed system resources for adapting and accomplishing tasks and that elicit a response from the system.

subjective time That which is measured by "a set of mental schemata and concepts that individuals and cultures have developed for various purposes" (Gorman & Weissman, 1977, p. 217).

subsystem A system in the hierarchy beneath the point of reference (e.g., if the family system were the point of reference, the individual would be a subsystem).

support The help available that has the potential to enhance a person's coping with stressors.

suprasystem A system in the hierarchy above the point of reference (e.g., if the family system were the point of reference, the community would be the suprasystem).

system A complex of elements or components that interact with each other in a more or less stable way within any particular period of time.

T

tasks Duties that a given system is expected to accomplish in order to continue its growth and functioning.

teaching The process of passing facts, ideas, and part of oneself to others.

time "An indefinite, unlimited duration in which things are considered as happening in the past, present, or future" (Guralnik, 1984, p. 1489).

trajectory The way disease progression is perceived over time by those involved. It includes the ideas of direction, movement, shape, and predictability.

trust "The expectancy held by an individual that the communication behaviors of another individual or other individuals can be relied upon" (Northouse, 1979, p. 366.)

U

uncertainty The experience of lack of information or knowledge that results from an unpredictable situation.

V

values Standards or principles of worth that influence and shape a system's behavior.

References

Andrews, H., & Roy, C. (1985). *Essentials of the Roy adaptation model.* Norwalk: CT: Appleton-Century-Crofts.

Butler, R.N. (1963). The life review. *Psychiatry, 26,* 65–76.

Childress, A.R., & Burns, D.D. (1981). The basics of cognitive therapy. *Psychosomatics, 22*(12), 1017–1027.

Dittmar, S.S. (1989). Scope of rehabilitation. In S.S. Dittmar (Ed.), *Rehabilitation nursing: Process and application* (pp. 2–15). St. Louis: Mosby.

Gatchel, R.J., & Baum, A. (1983). *An introduction to health psychology.* Reading, MA: Addison Wesley.

Giddens, A. (1978). *Emile Durkheim.* New York: Penguin.

Gorman, B.S., & Wessman, A.E. (1977). Images, values, and concepts of time in psychological research. In B.S. Gorman, & A.E. Wessman (Eds.), *The personal experience of time* (pp. 217–263). New York: Plenum.

Guralnik, D.B. (Ed.). (1984). *Webster's new world dictionary of the American language* (2nd ed). New York: Simon & Schuster.

Kahn, R.L., & Antonucci, T.C. (1980). Convoys over the life course: Attachment, roles and social support. In P.B. Baltes & O.G. Brim (Eds.), *Life-span development and behavior* (pp. 253–286). New York: Academic.

Kim, M.J., McFarland, G.K., & McLane, A.M. (1987). *Pocket guide to nursing diagnosis.* 2nd ed. St. Louis: C.V. Mosby.

Northouse, P.G. (1979). Interpersonal trust and empathy in nurse-nurse relationships. *Nurs Res, 28*(6), 365–368.

Reif, L., & Estes, C.L. (1982). Long-term care: New opportunities for professional nursing. In L.H. Aiken (Ed.), *Nursing in the 1980s: Crises, opportunities, challenges* (pp. 147–181). Philadelphia: Lippincott.

Stoll, R. (1989). The essence of spirituality. In V.B. Carson *Spiritual dimensions of nursing practice.* Philadelphia: W.B. Saunders.

Tilden, V.P., & Gaylen, R.D. (1987). Cost and conflict: The darker side of social support. *West J Nurs Res, 9*(1), 13–18.

Index